Microbiology Nuts & Bolts

Key Concepts of Microbiology & Infection

3rd Edition

Dr David Garner
BM MSc MRCPCH FRCPath

About the Author

The author has been described as a gifted teacher and educator, who has an exceptional level of microbiology and infectious diseases knowledge, with an even greater ability to translate that knowledge so that others can also understand this often complicated subject. His award-winning teaching is the highlight of many medical students' clinical attachments and as a result of his dedication to the subject, many junior colleagues have been motivated and inspired to enter a career in Microbiology.

He qualified from Southampton University Medical School in 1997 and has worked in diverse areas of medicine, general surgery, emergency medicine and paediatrics. Now, as a Consultant Clinical Microbiologist in a United Kingdom NHS hospital, he spends his days diagnosing, treating and managing infections as well as teaching others how to do this safely and effectively.

Microbiology textbooks often considered by students to be dull and contain long lists of boring bacterial names; they appear to have little relevance to clinical medicine. The author recognised there was a need for a clinically-orientated no-nonsense microbiology book, so he decided to get on and write one. The feedback has been amazing, with both the first and second editions of Nuts & Bolts regularly making the list of top 3 microbiology textbooks on Amazon.co.uk. The website and accompanying Bug Blog are read worldwide by thousands of interested people every week and it is clear that many of you out there really value "Nuts & Bolts".

The author is ever grateful for your continuing support.

www.microbiologynutsandbolts.co.uk

Introduction

Microbiology Nuts & Bolts helps doctors and healthcare staff to confidently identify the microorganisms causing an infection and understand how to treat them. The book is set out by condition rather than microorganism allowing for quick reference in a clinical setting. Readers regularly comment just how amazing it is that so much information has been packed into such a small book. It is not an all-encompassing reference text and is deliberately not referenced extensively in order to keep its presentation simple. It is concise enough to be of use on a daily basis, be it on a ward or in a clinic, yet detailed enough to promote a thorough understanding of microorganisms, their management and the treatment of patients. It has received fantastic feedback in reviews by the Royal College of Physicians, the Royal College of Pathologists, the Royal Pharmaceutical Society, the Hospital Infection Society, the British Society for Antimicrobial Chemotherapy, the Institute of Biomedical Science and the Society for Applied Microbiology.

The book is divided into six parts: Basic Concepts, Microbiology, Infection Control, Clinical Scenarios, Antibiotics and Emergencies. It is best to read Basic Concepts and Microbiology first, as this gives the building blocks to understanding infection. After that, the Clinical Scenarios and Antibiotics sections aid diagnosis and management of specific infections.

Emergencies have been separated into their own section to ensure they can be found quickly. Flowcharts help guide initial emergency treatment, which often needs to be implemented immediately in order to save lives, although they are not a replacement for experienced senior support. Infection Control does not go into depth regarding policies and politics but gives practical advice about preventing the spread of infections and what to do when you have too many patients for the side rooms available.

The previous editions were well received by doctors and healthcare staff and as always their valuable feedback has been instrumental in shaping this, the latest edition. Existing sections have been fully updated and new sections have been added for acute bronchitis, necrotising pancreatitis and Lyme disease as well as new antibiotics and updates for the management of sexually transmitted infections and infection control precautions for viral haemorrhagic fevers. The Emergencies section has undergone extensive revision to take into account changes in UK national guidelines for the management of sepsis, meningitis, encephalitis and malaria. The size has also changed to accommodate larger text but we hope it still remains small enough to be your go to pocket book.

We have been asked many times why is there no App for Microbiology Nuts & Bolts? The short answer is that Apps are great at giving answers but less able to "teach", leading to healthcare staff blindly following algorithms and proformas instead of understanding the fundamental principles of medicine...so no, there is no App!

The ultimate aim of the book is to empower doctors and healthcare staff to manage patients with infections better; if it achieves this then it is a success.

P.S. Don't forget to write a review on Amazon and like us on FaceBook where you'll find the latest edition of the Bug Blog.

Hard work, artwork and front cover: J Garner
Editor Chief in Charge: J Garner

A clinically focused, no-nonsense pocket book to the key elements
of microbiology and infection. A must-have guide to stop common
and often unnecessary mistakes that occur in everyday medicine
and antibiotic prescribing.

Dedication
To Jenny and the cat club who are still helping and hindering in equal measure
and using inappropriate terms in an untimely manner such as "that should be
straight-forward" and "it will be simple"!

If you like this book, recommend it to someone else. If you don't,
then tell us why at...

www.microbiologynutsandbolts.co.uk

Table of Contents

Abbreviations

A&E	Accident and Emergency Department also known as ED or Emergency Department
ABW	Adjusted Body Weight
ACE	Angiotensin Converting Enzyme
AICU	Adult Intensive Care Unit
AIDS	Acquired Immune Deficiency Syndrome
ALT	Alanine Transaminase
ANA	Anti-nuclear Antibody
ANCA	Anti-neutrophil Cytoplasmic Antibody
APTT	Activated Partial Thromboplastin Time
ASOT	Anti-Streptolysin O Titre
AST	Aspartate Transaminase
BAL	Bronchoalveolar Lavage
BBV	Blood-borne Virus
BD	Bis in die (Latin), twice daily
BDG	(1,3)-Beta-d-glucan
BE	Base Excess
BHIVA	British HIV Association
BNF	British National Formulary (cBNF is the Children's BNF)
BP	Blood Pressure
bpm	Beats or breaths per minute
BSAC	British Society for Antimicrobial Chemotherapy
BSE	Bovine Spongiform Encephalopathy
CAP	Community Acquired Pneumonia
CCDC	Consultant in Communicable Disease Control
CDAD	*Clostridium difficile* Associated Disease
CFT	Complement Fixation Test
CJD	Creutzfeldt-Jakob Disease
CLL	Chronic Lymphocytic Leukaemia
CMV	*Cytomegalovirus*
CNS	Central Nervous System
COPD	Chronic Obstructive Pulmonary Disease
CrCl	Creatinine Clearance
CRP	C-Reactive Protein
CSF	Cerebrospinal Fluid
CT	Computerised Tomography
CTA	Cardiac CT Angiography
CTX-M	Cefotaxime-Munich (an ESBL)
CVA	Cerebrovascular Accident
CVC	Central Venous Catheter
CVID	Common Variable Immune Deficiency

CVP	Central Venous Pressure
DAA	Direct Acting Antivirals
D&V	Diarrhoea and Vomiting
DNA	Deoxyribonucleic Acid
DRESS	Drug Reaction with Eosinophilia and Systemic Symptoms
EBNA	Epstein-Barr Nuclear Antigen
EBV	*Epstein Barr Virus*
ECG	Electrocardiogram
EDTA	Ethylenediaminetetraacetic Acid
eGFR	Estimated Glomerular Filtration Rate
ELISA	Enzyme Linked Immunosorbent Assay
EMU	Early Morning Urine
ERCP	Endoscopic Retrograde Cholangio-Pancreatography
ESBL	Extended-Spectrum Beta-Lactamase
ESR	Erythrocyte Sedimentation Rate
ETT	Endotracheal Tube
EUCAST	European Committee on Antimicrobial Susceptibility Testing
EVD	External Ventricular Drain
FBC	Full Blood Count
FFP	Fresh Frozen Plasma
G6PD	Glucose-6-Phosphate Dehydrogenase
GCS	Glasgow Coma Scale
GFR	Glomerular Filtration Rate
GI	Gastrointestinal
GISA	Glycopeptide Intermediate *Staphylococcus aureus*
GMC	General Medical Council
GP	General Practitioner or Primary Care Physician
GRE	Glycopeptide Resistant *Enterococcus*
GRSA	Glycopeptide Resistant *Staphylococcus aureus*
GU	Genitourinary
GUM	Genitourinary Medicine
HACEK	Oral Gram-negative bacilli causing infective endocarditis, each letter represents a different bacterial species
HAP	Hospital Acquired Pneumonia
HBIG	Hepatitis B Immunoglobulin
HBV	*Hepatitis B Virus*
HCV	*Hepatitis C Virus*
HDU	High Dependency Unit
HDV	*Hepatitis D Virus*
HEV	*Hepatitis E Virus*
HHV	*Human Herpes Virus*

Hib	*Haemophilus influenzae* Type b
HIV	*Human Immunodeficiency Virus*
HLIU	High Level Isolation Unit
HSV	*Herpes Simplex Virus*
HUS	Haemolytic Uraemic Syndrome
IBW	Ideal Body Weight
ICD	Infection Control Doctor
ICP	Intracranial Pressure
ICT	Infection Control Team
ICU	Intensive Care Unit
ID	Infectious Diseases
IGRA	Interferon Gamma Release Assay
IMP	Imipenem carbapenemase
INR	International Normalised Ratio
IUCD	Intra-uterine Contraceptive Device
IV	Intravenous
IVDU	Intravenous Drug User
KPC	*Klebsiella pneumoniae* Carbapenemase
LFTs	Liver Function Tests
LP	Lumbar Puncture
MABP	Mean Arterial Blood Pressure
MAOI	Monoamine Oxidase Inhibitor
MBC	Minimum Bactericidal Concentration
MC&S	Microscopy, Culture and Sensitivities
MDCTA	Electrocardiogram-gated Multidetector CT Angiography
MDR	Multidrug Resistant
MERS-CoV	Middle-Eastern Respiratory Syndrome Coronavirus
MIC	Minimum Inhibitory Concentration
MRI	Magnetic Resonance Imaging
mRNA	Messenger Ribonucleic Acid (RNA)
MRSA	Meticillin Resistant *Staphylococcus aureus*
MSM	Men who have sex with men
MSSA	Meticillin Sensitive *Staphylococcus aureus*
MSU	Midstream Urine
MTB	*Mycobacterium tuberculosis*
NDM	New Delhi Metallo-Beta-Lactamase
NEWS	National Early Warning Score
NICE	National Institute for Health and Care Excellence
NPA	Nasopharyngeal Aspirate
NPV	Negative Predictive Value

NSAID	Non-Steroidal Anti-inflammatory Drug
OCP	Ova, Cysts and Parasites
OD	Omne in die (Latin), once daily
OXA	Oxacillinase
PABA	Para-aminobenzoic Acid
PBP	Penicillin Binding Protein
PCP	Pneumocystis Pneumonia
PCR	Polymerase Chain Reaction
PegIFN	Pegylated Interferon
PEP	Post-Exposure Prophylaxis
PEPSE	Post-Exposure Prophylaxis following Sexual Exposure
PET CT	18F-fluorodeoxyglucose Positron Emission Tomography CT
PEWS	Paediatric Early Warning Score
PHE	Public Health England (prev. Health Protection Agency)
PHEC	Public Health England Centre (prev. Health Protection Unit)
PICC	Peripherally Inserted Central Catheter
PICU	Paediatric Intensive Care Unit
PID	Pelvic Inflammatory Disease
PML	Progressive Multifocal Leukoencephalopathy
PO	Per os (Latin), orally or by mouth
PPE	Personal Protective Equipment
PPI	Proton Pump Inhibitor
PPV	Positive Predictive Value
PR	Per Rectum
PrEP	Pre-Exposure Prophylaxis
PUO	Pyrexia of Unknown Origin
PVL	Panton-Valentine Leukocidin
QDS	Quater die sumendus (Latin), four times per day
qSOFA	Quick Sepsis-Related Organ Failure Assessment
RBC	Red Blood Cell
RCA	Root Cause Analysis
RNA	Ribonucleic Acid
RPR	Rapid Plasma Reagin
RSV	*Respiratory Syncytial Virus*
SARS	Severe Acute Respiratory Syndrome
SAT	Stool Antigen Test
SC	Subcutaneous
SCBU	Special Care Baby Unit
SCID	Severe Combined Immunodeficiency
SHV	Sulfhydryl variable (an ESBL)

SLE	Systemic Lupus Erythematosus
SOFA	Sepsis-Related Organ Failure Assessment
sp./spp.	Species (singular/plural)
SPA	Suprapubic Aspirate
STD	Sexually Transmitted Disease
SVR	Sustained Virological Response
TB	Tuberculosis
TDM	Therapeutic Drug Monitoring
TDS	Ter die sumendum (Latin), three times per day
TEM	Named after Temoniera (an ESBL)
TOE	Transoesophageal Echocardiography
TOP	Topical application
TPPA	*Treponema pallidum* Particle Agglutination
tRNA	Transfer Ribonucleic Acid (RNA)
TSS	Toxic Shock Syndrome
TTE	Transthoracic Echocardiography
U&Es	Urea and Electrolytes
UBT	Urease Breath Test
UKAS	United Kingdom Accreditation Service
URT	Upper Respiratory Tract
URTI	Upper Respiratory Tract Infection
UTI	Urinary Tract Infection
VAP	Ventilator Associated Pneumonia
VCA	Viral Capsid Antigen
VDRL	Venereal Disease Research Laboratory test
VHF	Viral Haemorrhagic Fever
VIM	Verona Integron-encoded Metallo-beta-lactamase
VRE	Vancomycin Resistant *Enterococcus*
VZV	*Varicella Zoster Virus*
WBC	White Blood Cell
XDR	Extensively Drug Resistant
ZN	Ziehl-Neelsen

Basic Concepts

<u>**What is Infection? Infection vs. Colonisation vs. Contamination**</u>

Infection is the presence of microorganisms causing damage to body tissues, usually in the presence of acute inflammation (pain, swelling, redness, heat and loss of function). For example *Staphylococcus aureus* on intact skin does not cause a problem; it is the normal flora for skin. However, if you cut your skin, *Staphylococcus aureus* can cause infection in the cut with associated inflammation and tissue damage.

Microorganisms can also cause damage in the absence of inflammation but it is unusual, e.g. in neutropaenic patients with angio-invasive fungal infections causing tissue infarction.

Colonisation describes when bacteria grow on body sites exposed to the environment, without causing infection. This is a normal process. These bacteria may form part of the normal flora of the individual; however colonisation is not necessarily normal flora. Occasionally, bacteria which are not normally regarded as part of the normal flora can also colonise body areas e.g. *Pseudomonas* spp. in a wound is not normal flora of the skin or a wound but it is not actually causing tissue damage or infection; it is just growing in the warm wet conditions of the wound. *Pseudomonas* spp. are the normal flora of warm wet places. Likewise, some prosthetic devices can also become colonised with bacteria without causing infection e.g. urinary catheters.

Colonisation does not normally harm the patient and does not usually need treating with antibiotics e.g. *Neisseria meningitidis* can be found in up to 30% of the healthy population in their oropharynx. However, infection can result in harm and often needs treatment with antibiotics e.g. if *Neisseria meningitidis* enters the bloodstream from the oropharynx to cause septicaemia, then it needs urgent treatment.

Examples of colonisation

Body Site or Prosthetic Device	Bacterial Colonisation
Pressure sores	• Skin flora e.g. *Staphylococcus* spp. • Enteric flora e.g. *Enterococcus* spp., *Escherichia coli*, *Pseudomonas* spp.
Breaks in the skin e.g. wounds	• Skin flora e.g. *Staphylococcus* spp. • Enteric flora e.g. *Enterococcus* spp., *Escherichia coli*, *Pseudomonas* spp.
Upper respiratory tract	• Mixed enteric flora in patients given antibiotics or who have been in healthcare settings for more than 4 days e.g. *Enterococcus* spp., *Escherichia coli*, *Pseudomonas* spp.
Urinary catheter	• Enteric flora e.g. *Enterococcus* spp., *Escherichia coli*, *Pseudomonas* spp.
Endotracheal tube **OR** Tracheostomy tube in a ventilated patient	• Mixed enteric flora in patients given antibiotics or who have been in healthcare settings for more than 4 days e.g. *Enterococcus* spp., *Escherichia coli*, *Pseudomonas* spp.

Warning

In the absence of good clinical information on request forms (see section – Microbiology, Why Bother Completing Request Forms?) microbiology laboratories are unable to distinguish between colonisation and infection and so will just report the presence of bacteria. It is then up to the clinician to decide if these bacteria are causing infection.

Better filled in request forms lead to better clinical advice from microbiology services.

Contamination is the presence of a microorganism that has been introduced into a microbiology sample from an external source e.g. poor technique when taking the sample, a swab touching a surface before being used, sneezing over a patient whilst they provide a sputum sample. Contamination can also occur when a sample is not collected correctly and the patients "normal flora" (microorganisms growing in their normal environment) gets into the sample e.g. urine taken incorrectly can contact perineal skin and pick up the "normal microorganisms" which then grow in the laboratory (the presence of epithelial cells in the urine sample indicates definite contact with skin and therefore a risk of contamination).

<u>**Source of Infection: Endogenous vs. Exogenous**</u>

It is important to understand how infections arise in patients in order to manage them appropriately.

Endogenous infections are caused when the patient's own bacterial flora gets into a site it should not be in. This is responsible for about 85% of all infections. Knowledge of the patient's normal flora aids the management of these types of infections. For example, pneumonia tends to be caused by bacteria from the URT; knowing what the normal flora of the URT is allows prediction of the antibiotics necessary to treat pneumonia.

Exogenous infections are much less frequent than endogenous and occur when the patient acquires a microorganism that directly invades and causes disease. Knowledge of methods of transmission aids the management of outbreaks of these types of infections. For example, knowing that *Norovirus* is transmitted by the faecal-oral route allows the precautions of hand hygiene, individual toilets, isolation of infected patients and environmental cleaning to be implemented to prevent transmission and control outbreaks.

<u>**Bacteraemia vs. Septicaemia**</u>

Many healthcare professionals use the terms bacteraemia and septicaemia to mean the same thing, however they are different. **Bacteraemia** is the presence of bacteria in blood. **Septicaemia** is the presence of bacteria in blood **PLUS** clinical features of sepsis e.g. temperature >38.3°C or <36°C, heart rate >90bpm, respiratory rate >20 bpm, WBC <4x10^9/L or >12x10^9/L, blood glucose >7.7mmol/L or altered mental state (see section – Emergencies, Sepsis). **WARNING:** patients can be septic without being septicaemic if they have the clinical features of sepsis but do not have bacteria in their blood.

A patient can be bacteraemic without being septicaemic **BUT** cannot be septicaemic without being bacteraemic.

Bacteraemia may be:
- **Significant** causing the patients infection or indicating where the infection is occurring e.g. *E. coli* in pyelonephritis, *Staphylococcus aureus* in cellulitis or Alpha-haemolytic *Streptococcus* spp. in infective endocarditis
- **Non-significant** a contaminant in the specimen (e.g. coagulase-negative *Staphylococcus* spp. from skin) or temporarily in the blood from another site, known as "translocation" e.g. bacteria can be pushed into blood by simply brushing your teeth (Alpha-haemolytic *Streptococcus* spp.), grazing your leg (coryneform bacteria) or squeezing a big spot (*Staphylococcus aureus*). None of these are a "problem" as the body "deals" with them and "clears" the blood

BUT the examples use the same bacteria! How do you know if they are significant or not? Answer: do they have the clinical features of the infection? E.g. *Staphylococcus aureus* in cellulitis presents with a hot, red, swollen leg whereas non-significant bacteraemia has no symptoms or signs, the test was just done at an opportune moment to "catch" the presence of, or be contaminated by, the bacteria.

Types of Infectious Microorganisms

Bacteria

Bacteria are free-living single cell microorganisms with no cell nucleus. Their genes are found on chromosomes, free within the cell cytoplasm. They reproduce by cell division to create identical daughter cells (clonal expansion). Bacteria are widely spread throughout the environment with only a small number causing human disease. There are approximately 15,000 times more bacteria on 1 human, than humans on the earth. You can see them with a light microscope in a laboratory. Examples: *Staphylococcus aureus*, *Escherichia coli*, *Listeria monocytogenes*.

Viruses

Viruses are small microorganisms consisting of genetic elements surrounded by a protein coat. They cannot self-replicate. Viruses invade other cells and use their host's reproductive mechanism to replicate. They are too small to be seen with a light microscope and can only be seen with an electron microscope. Examples: *Varicella Zoster Virus* (VZV), *Influenza Virus*, *Rhinovirus*.

Parasites

Parasites are organisms that grow on, feed off and are sheltered by another living organism but which contribute nothing to the survival of that organism. They are often multi-cellular and relatively large compared to bacteria and viruses. All are visible with a light microscope but some are large enough to see with the naked eye. A female *Ascaris* roundworm can be up to 30cm long. They usually reproduce by sexual reproduction. Examples: *Plasmodium falciparum* (malaria), *Giardia lamblia*, *Ascaris lumbricoides*.

Fungi

Fungi are multi-cellular organisms with eukaryotic DNA and a chitinous cell wall. They feed on organic matter and produce spores which can survive for long periods of time in the environment. These spores aid the spread of the fungi. Fungi are usually bigger than bacteria and are visible with a light microscope and occasionally with the naked eye. They usually reproduce by sexual reproduction. Examples: *Candida albicans*, *Aspergillus* spp., *Mucor* spp. (Zygomycetes).

Prions

Prions are infectious proteins folded in an abnormal way. When they enter another cell they cause all the similar proteins to refold in the abnormal fashion resulting in disease. They are very rare and not considered further in this book. Examples: Creutzfeldt Jakob Disease (CJD), Kuru, Bovine Spongiform Encephalopathy (BSE).

The Anatomy of a Bacterium

Bacteria are the most common microorganisms treated with specific antibiotics. Antibiotics have different mechanisms of action related to which part of the bacterium they act upon; therefore it is helpful to know the basic anatomy of a bacterium.

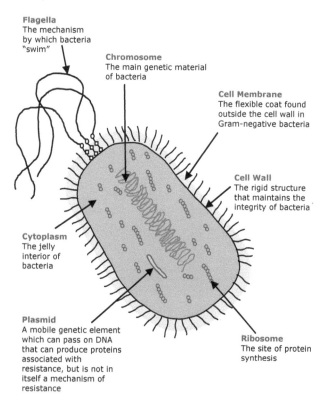

Flagella
The mechanism by which bacteria "swim"

Chromosome
The main genetic material of bacteria

Cell Membrane
The flexible coat found outside the cell wall in Gram-negative bacteria

Cell Wall
The rigid structure that maintains the integrity of bacteria

Cytoplasm
The jelly interior of bacteria

Plasmid
A mobile genetic element which can pass on DNA that can produce proteins associated with resistance, but is not in itself a mechanism of resistance

Ribosome
The site of protein synthesis

<u>What is Normal Flora and why is it Important?</u>

Normal flora is the community of microorganisms that live on another living organism (human or animal) or inanimate object without causing disease. The human body is not sterile; we become colonised with bacteria from the moment we are born. We are covered with, and contain within our intestines, approximately one hundred trillion (10^{14}) bacteria that form the normal flora of our bodies. This normal flora helps prevent us being colonised with dangerous bacteria, which might lead to infection.

Microbiome is the term for a community of normal microorganisms.
Dysbiosis is the term for the disruption of the microbiome, removing normal microorganisms or the growth of abnormal microorganisms.

Many circumstances can change normal flora. For example, the normal flora of the human body begins to change after admission to a hospital or long-term care facility. The process usually begins around day 4 of admission; this is why after 4 days of admission the antibiotics for hospital acquired infections change. It is not because the severity of the illness is different.

Knowledge of the normal flora of the human body allows:
- Prediction of the pathogens causing infection as bacteria tend to grow in specific body sites e.g. *Streptococcus pneumoniae* from the upper respiratory tract causing pneumonia or *Staphylococcus aureus* from the skin causing intravenous cannula infections
- Investigation for underlying abnormalities in specific areas of the body when bacteria are isolated from normally sterile sites e.g. *Escherichia coli* isolation from blood cultures indicates probable intra-abdominal pathology as *E. coli* is part of the normal gastrointestinal flora, or growth of an Alpha-haemolytic *Streptococcus* sp. in blood cultures may indicate infective endocarditis as a result of poor dentition as Alpha-haemolytic *Streptococcus* spp. are part of the normal mouth flora

Nothing is 100% accurate but knowing where bacteria normally live can help work out when they are in the wrong place. This allows predictions of the likely causes of disease and hence the choice of suitable antibiotics for empirical therapy. Knowing which factors affect normal flora allows predictions to be made as to what the flora will become under the influence of those factors, e.g. exposure to antibiotics removes sensitive bacteria, so if a patient with a cut hand, and a sensitive *Staphylococcus aureus* (MSSA) in their normal flora, is given Flucloxacillin for the cut, a void will be left behind which could be filled by a Flucloxacillin resistant bacterium such as Meticillin resistant *Staphylococcus aureus* (MRSA).

Myth
Bacteria have no place in our environment. **FALSE** - Bacteria are part of the normal environment. Almost everything has its own normal flora. Hospitals, the community, soil, animals, air conditioning units and swimming pools all have their own "normal flora". However, certain things like surgical instruments and synovial fluid should be sterile. If something contains its normal flora it is normal; if it grows something else's normal flora e.g. synovial fluid grows skin flora, it is abnormal. Knowing where normal flora comes from allows you to identify the likely cause of infection or know where to investigate.

Circumstances Affecting Normal Flora

Certain circumstances allow microorganisms the opportunity to become part of a person's normal flora. It is usually a combination of factors: right person, in the right place at the right time... (or wrong place at the wrong time if you are the person).

Right Person
The right personal circumstances to allow colonisation.
- Patients are more easily colonised because their diseases, treatments or medical procedures often remove or bypass the normal mechanisms for preventing colonisation e.g. cannulae breach the skin barrier, antacid drugs reduce gastric acid production, steroids prevent white blood cells from functioning properly and cystic fibrosis patients do not clear mucus from their lungs effectively due to changes in the mucociliary escalator
- Contact with companion animals. Companion animals often share normal flora with their owners. The normal flora of a cat owner will often contain *Pasteurella multocida*; part of a cat's normal URT flora
- Lifestyle choices (smoking, alcohol misuse, drug abuse or obesity) can alter normal flora damaging tissue, breaching barriers, acting as an immunosuppressant, or creating microorganism-loving environments

Right Place
The right environmental circumstances to allow colonisation.
- Hospitals admit patients with infections caused by microorganisms that can be readily transferred to other people, e.g. each gram of stool from a patient with *Norovirus* contains 1 billion infectious particles
- Antibiotic resistant bacteria are more common in hospitals as antibiotics are frequently used to treat patients with infections. This creates a selective pressure, removing sensitive bacteria and leaving resistant bacteria behind to settle in the environment e.g. Flucloxacillin given for skin infections may select out MRSA
- The hospital environment can become seeded with bacteria which remain in the environment after a patient has been discharged, e.g. *Clostridium difficile* produces spores which are difficult to kill and can survive for up to 6 months in an environment without proper cleaning

Right Time
The right moment to colonise.
- Exposure to antibiotics removes sensitive bacteria from normal flora; leaving a void other bacteria will fill. Coming into contact with a microorganism whilst on, or having recently taken, an antibiotic allows the opportunity for the new microorganism to establish itself as part of the normal flora
- Bacteria in the food chain can become part of a person's normal flora after eating contaminated food e.g. GRE in chickens and ESBL-positive *Escherichia coli* in "pre-washed" salads. These microorganisms do not necessarily make the person ill at the time of acquisition but can later cause infection if they get into the wrong body site, e.g. ESBL-positive *Escherichia coli* causing a UTI

MSSA = O   MRSA = ▲

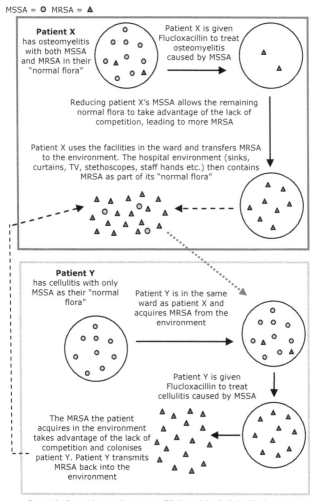

Patient X
has osteomyelitis with both MSSA and MRSA in their "normal flora"

Patient X is given Flucloxacillin to treat osteomyelitis caused by MSSA

Reducing patient X's MSSA allows the remaining normal flora to take advantage of the lack of competition, leading to more MRSA

Patient X uses the facilities in the ward and transfers MRSA to the environment. The hospital environment (sinks, curtains, TV, stethoscopes, staff hands etc.) then contains MRSA as part of its "normal flora"

Patient Y
has cellulitis with only MSSA as their "normal flora"

Patient Y is in the same ward as patient X and acquires MRSA from the environment

Patient Y is given Flucloxacillin to treat cellulitis caused by MSSA

The MRSA the patient acquires in the environment takes advantage of the lack of competition and colonises patient Y. Patient Y transmits MRSA back into the environment

Bacteria from the environment fill the niche left behind when antibiotics remove normal flora.

23

Bacterial Flora in a Normal Person in the Community

Below are body sites and their common normal flora; isolating these microorganisms from their normal body site is normal and does not indicate infection. Knowing where microorganisms are normally found helps identify a cause if they migrate from their normal body site into another body site. The microorganisms listed below are also most likely to cause disease if they migrate to another body site. For example, *Escherichia coli* from the gastrointestinal tract gets into the urogenital tract causing a UTI.

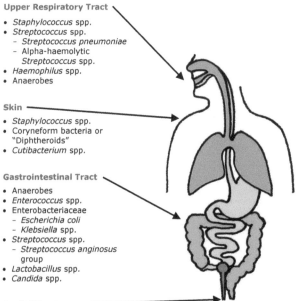

Upper Respiratory Tract

- *Staphylococcus* spp.
- *Streptococcus* spp.
  - *Streptococcus pneumoniae*
  - Alpha-haemolytic *Streptococcus* spp.
- *Haemophilus* spp.
- Anaerobes

Skin

- *Staphylococcus* spp.
- Coryneform bacteria or "Diphtheroids"
- *Cutibacterium* spp.

Gastrointestinal Tract

- Anaerobes
- *Enterococcus* spp.
- Enterobacteriaceae
  - *Escherichia coli*
  - *Klebsiella* spp.
- *Streptococcus* spp.
  - *Streptococcus anginosus* group
- *Lactobacillus* spp.
- *Candida* spp.

Genital Tract

- *Lactobacillus* spp.
- *Streptococcus* spp.
  - *Streptococcus agalactiae*

In the community, normal flora is generally sensitive to antibiotics.

Bacterial Flora in a Normal Person in a Hospital or Long-term Care Facility

Below are body sites and their common normal flora for a hospital patient or a person in a long-term care facility. They are different to community normal flora because of exposure to different microorganisms, physiological changes, immunosuppressants and selective pressures. Isolating these microorganisms from their normal body site in hospitals or long-term care facilities is normal and does not indicate infection.

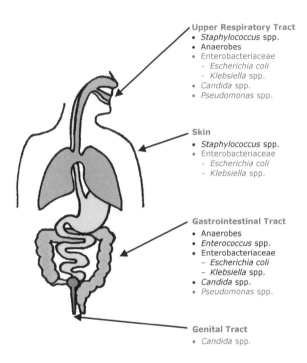

Upper Respiratory Tract
- *Staphylococcus* spp.
- Anaerobes
- Enterobacteriaceae
  - *Escherichia coli*
  - *Klebsiella* spp.
- *Candida* spp.
- *Pseudomonas* spp.

Skin
- *Staphylococcus* spp.
- Enterobacteriaceae
  - *Escherichia coli*
  - *Klebsiella* spp.

Gastrointestinal Tract
- Anaerobes
- *Enterococcus* spp.
- Enterobacteriaceae
  - *Escherichia coli*
  - *Klebsiella* spp.
- *Candida* spp.
- *Pseudomonas* spp.

Genital Tract
- *Candida* spp.

In hospital environments most of the normal flora remains sensitive to antibiotics but added to these are normal flora that are resistant to antibiotics and environmental factors, such as drying, alcohol hand scrubs or detergents (these more resistant microorganisms are shown in red)

25

Significance of Bacteria in the Bloodstream (Bacteraemia)

Organism in Blood	Site of Normal Flora
Staphylococcus aureus	Skin Nose
Coagulase negative *Staphylococcus*	Skin
Streptococcus pyogenes	Not normal flora
Streptococcus agalactiae	GI tract
Group C Beta-haemolytic *Streptococcus*	Not usually normal flora
Group G Beta-haemolytic *Streptococcus*	GI tract
Enterococcus spp.	GI tract
Streptococcus anginosus	GI tract
Streptococcus gallolyticus	GI tract
Streptococcus pneumoniae	URT
Alpha-haemolytic *Streptococcus* spp.	URT
Diphtheroids	Skin
Cutibacterium spp.	Skin
Haemophilus influenzae	URT
Enterobacteriaceae e.g. *Escherichia coli, Klebsiella* spp., *Enterobacter* spp.	GI tract
Pseudomonas spp.	GI tract
Anaerobes e.g. *Clostridium* spp., *Bacteroides* spp.	GI tract

Common Causes of Bacteraemia	Uncommon Causes of Bacteraemia
• Cellulitis • Septic arthritis • Osteomyelitis • CVC infection	• Infective endocarditis
• Common contaminant • CVC infection	• Infective endocarditis
• Tonsillitis • Cellulitis • Septic arthritis • Osteomyelitis	• Necrotising fasciitis
• Septic arthritis • Osteomyelitis • Cellulitis in diabetes	• Infective endocarditis • GI malignancy
• Tonsillitis • Cellulitis • Septic arthritis • Osteomyelitis	
• Tonsillitis • Cellulitis • Septic arthritis • Osteomyelitis	• Infective endocarditis • GI malignancy
• Peritonitis • Cholecystitis • Cholangitis	• Infective endocarditis • GI malignancy
• Abscess • Peritonitis • Cholecystitis • Cholangitis	
• Infective endocarditis	• GI malignancy
• CAP/HAP	• Meningitis • Septic arthritis
• Infective endocarditis	
• Common contaminant	• Infective endocarditis
• Common contaminant	
• CAP/HAP	• Meningitis • Septic arthritis
• UTI • Peritonitis • Cholecystitis • Cholangitis	• VAP
• Catheter-associated UTI • Soft tissue in diabetes	• CAP/HAP/VAP • Burns • Skin grafts
• Peritonitis • Cholecystitis • Cholangitis	• GI malignancy • Necrotising fasciitis

Diagnosing Infection: History

It may sound obvious but in order to manage a patient with an infection safely and effectively you first have to work out what is wrong with them. This is done through the dynamic process of formulating a **differential diagnosis**. The process begins the moment the patient is referred (e.g. you are told the patient has a cough; you narrow questioning to the respiratory system and a differential diagnosis that includes diseases like pneumonia, lung cancer, COPD etc.). By taking a **history**, **examination** and requesting targeted **investigations** you narrow down the differential diagnosis until you get to a single diagnosis.

A **differential diagnosis** is a list of potential diseases or infections that a patient might have. The simplest and most effective method of formulating a differential diagnosis is:
- **Immediately life-threatening** conditions e.g. meningitis, encephalitis, necrotising fasciitis
- **Common** conditions e.g. UTI, pneumonia, cellulitis, heart failure
- **Uncommon** conditions e.g. infective endocarditis

In the **history**, the key infection-related aspects to concentrate on are:

History	Examples of Significance
The patient's specific symptoms	• Cough indicating chest or upper respiratory tract • Right upper quadrant pain indicating possible cholangitis
A chronological timeline of when and how symptoms developed	• Chicken Pox followed by haemorrhagic skin lesions pointing towards invasive Group A Beta-haemolytic *Streptococcus* and necrotising fasciitis
Contact with people with infections or symptoms	• Tuberculosis contact
A list of recent travel (countries and regions)	• Malaria endemic regions
The patient's vaccination history	• Primary childhood courses as well as travel-related vaccines
The patient's current and former occupations	• Healthcare staff and blood-borne viruses • Plumber and exposure to *Legionella pneumophila*
The patient's pastimes and hobbies	• Water sports and exposure to rats in leptospirosis
Any pets or contact with animals	• Zoonotic infections e.g. *Pasteurella multocida* and cat bites, *Chlamydophila psittaci* and parrots
A sexual history	• Sexually transmitted diseases and blood-borne viruses
The patient's ethnic origin	• Exposure to relatives with tropical infections
The patient's country of birth	• Chronic tropical infections • Exposure to relatives with tropical infections

The key infection-related aspects to examination are:

Examination	Examples of Significance
General observations	• Inhalers, bedside medications, finger clubbing, splinter haemorrhages • Presence of new onset confusion
Presence and pattern of fever	• Hyperthermia (>38°C) **OR** hypothermia (<36°C) • Vivax and Ovale malaria fever every 48 hours, Malariae malaria fever every 72 hours, Falciparum malaria fever more frequent than 24 hours
Heart rate	• Tachycardia >90 bpm in sepsis • **BEWARE** Beta-blockers falsely decrease heart rate **OR** arrhythmias can falsely increase heart rate
Blood pressure	• Systolic pressure <90mmHg **OR** decreased >40mmHg from baseline • **BEWARE** "normotensive" patients may actually be "hypotensive" if they are normally "hypertensive"
Skin lesions	• Blanching and non-blanching rashes can occur in meningococcal sepsis • Erythema marginatum occurs in rheumatic fever • **BEWARE** if symptoms are more severe than clinical features **THEN** consider necrotising fasciitis
Upper respiratory tract	• Tonsillar pus and presence of quinsy • Swelling and erythema of the tympanic membrane in otitis media
Chest	• Decreased expansion, dullness to percussion, bronchial breathing and increased vocal resonance (tactile vocal fremitus) in consolidation
Heart	• New murmurs in infective endocarditis • **BEWARE** if severe valve damage, there may be no murmurs as no turbulence of blood flow
Abdomen	• Right upper quadrant pain in cholangitis • Loin pain in pyelonephritis
Central nervous system	• Acute confusion in the elderly (also part of CURB-65 score in CAP) • Neck stiffness and meningism in meningitis

Radiology

Test	Interpretation
Chest X-ray	• British Thoracic Society states consolidation on a chest X-ray is required for a diagnosis of pneumonia in hospital (**BEWARE** neutropaenic patients may not be able to produce consolidation on a chest X-ray)

Haematology

Test	Result	Interpretation
Full Blood Count	Total White Blood Cell (WBC) Count	• High (>12x10^9/L) **OR** low (<4x10^9/L) both indicators of potential sepsis
	Differential WBC Count	In general: • Neutrophils increase or decrease in bacterial and fungal infection • Lymphocytes increase or decrease in viral infection • Eosinophils increase in parasitic infection
	Platelets	• Acute phase reactant, may rise in infection
Clotting	International Normalised Ratio (INR)	• Increases in sepsis and invasive Group A Beta-haemolytic *Streptococcus* infection (streptokinase)
Erythrocyte Sedimentation Rate	ESR	• Acute phase reactant, may rise in infection, in particular bone and joint infections

Biochemistry

Test	Result	Interpretation
Urea, Creatinine and Electrolytes	Urea	• Raised (>7mmol/L) in severe CAP (CURB-65 score)
	Creatinine	• Rising in *Clostridium difficile* is a sign of increased severity • Renal function is required in order to dose antibiotics safely
C-Reactive Protein	CRP	• Rises in bacterial infection, usually over 200mg/L • **BEWARE** patients in liver failure may not be able to produce CRP (check INR and albumin to assess synthetic liver function)

Procalcitonin	Procalcitonin	Rises in bacterial infection, (normal <0.1ng/ml):
		• Pneumonia:
		  – unlikely (<0.25ng/ml)
		  – possible (0.25 - <0.5ng/ml)
		  – likely (≥0.5ng/ml)
		• Sepsis:
		  – unlikely (<0.5ng/ml)
		  – possible (0.5 - <2 ng/ml)
		  – likely (≥2ng/ml)
		  – severe sepsis (≥10ng/ml)

Paul-Bunnell or Monospot test	Glandular fever or infectious mononucleosis screen	Detect EBV induced (heterophile) antibodies: • PPV = >96% • NPV = 1st week 75%, 3rd week 95%

Immunodeficiency States

An immunodeficiency state is any condition which makes a person more at risk of frequent or severe infections. Immunodeficiency states can also leave patients at risk of opportunistic infections e.g. fungal infections like candidiasis or normally non-infectious bacteria like skin microorganisms during IV cannulation.

Primary Immunodeficiency

Antibody deficiency	X-linked agammaglobulinaemia
	Common Variable Immunodeficiency (CVID)
	Immunoglobulin class deficiencies
T cell deficiency	Di George syndrome
	Severe Combined Immunodeficiency (SCID)

Secondary Immunodeficiency

Viral	HIV
Drugs	Anti-cancer chemotherapy
	Steroids
	Anti-transplant rejection e.g. Ciclosporin, Mycophenalate, Tacrolimus, Sirolimus
	Steroid-sparing agents e.g. Methotrexate, Azathioprine
	Biologics and biosimilars e.g. Adalimumab, Rituximab, Infliximab, Abatacept, Tocilizumab
Haematological malignancy	Leukaemia
	Myeloma
Metabolic	Trauma
	Renal failure
	Liver failure
	Vitamin deficiency
Immunoglobulin loss	Nephrotic syndrome
	Protein-losing enteropathy
Other	Pregnancy
	Splenectomy
	Intravenous devices e.g. cannulas, central venous catheters
	Urinary catheters
	Endotracheal tube
	Tracheostomy
	External Ventricular Device (EVD)
	Peritoneal dialysis catheter
	Chest or abdominal drain

Microbiology

How to Take Microbiology Specimens

Aseptic Technique
Aseptic technique is a procedure that is designed to minimise contamination. Microbiology samples should be taken aseptically to prevent contamination with bacteria e.g. if you take blood cultures without aseptic technique it is likely that the result will be a skin contaminant rather than the cause of the infection.

Examples of techniques to minimise the risk of contamination:
- Blood cultures and CSF - clean the skin with 2% Chlorhexidine and wear gloves
- Midstream urine specimen (MSU) - part the labia or retract the foreskin, void the first part of the urine stream (10-20mls at least) and then collect the next portion (approx. 10-20mls)
- Wound swabs - remove slough (which is dead and detached tissue and is not a sign of infection), debride the wound to reveal the fresh tissue beneath, swab the fresh tissue
- Sputum - ask patients to cough sputum immediately into the specimen container rather than holding it in the mouth whilst looking for a container

Sample Before Treatment
If safe to do so, take microbiology samples before starting antibiotics otherwise those antibiotics may inhibit the growth of bacteria, causing negative cultures.

Blood Cultures First
Always take blood cultures before any other blood samples because other blood sample collection bottles are not necessarily sterile and can therefore contaminate the blood culture collection kit. This will lead to contaminated blood cultures, known as pseudobacteraemia.

Aerobic Bottle First
Take the aerobic bottle before the anaerobic bottle in case there is not enough blood for both bottles e.g. if the needle comes out of the patient's arm. You are more likely to diagnose infection from the aerobic blood culture bottle because more pathogenic bacteria grow in this type of bottle than the anaerobic bottle.

Cerebrospinal Fluid
Do not forget to take a sample for peripheral blood glucose, at the same time as CSF protein and CSF glucose. The glucose levels need to be compared and therefore done at the same time. As glucose levels vary, if peripheral blood glucose is forgotten you will not be able to take the sample later as the comparison will not be valid. The comparison allows a distinction to be made between bacterial meningitis and other causes of meningitis (see section – Emergencies, Meningitis).

Avoid a Quick Swab
If possible send pus or tissue rather than swabs because pus and tissue can be Gram stained allowing recognition of bacteria or fungi that are present but which have failed to grow on culture.

What's the difference between cultures and Gram stains? **Microscopy** includes any investigation using a microscope, including the Gram stain. **Culture** is whatever grows after incubation e.g. on the agar plate. They are not necessarily the same; antibiotics can inhibit growth in culture, microorganisms may not grow fast enough or may have specific growth requirements that prevent them being cultured even though they can be seen on microscopy. Therefore microscopy may give a more complete view whereas culture may not. Culture, however, will give the microorganisms names and provide antibiotic **sensitivities**. Microscopy, Culture and Sensitivities are often abbreviated to MC&S.

For example: At the time of appendicectomy the patient is on Cefuroxime and Metronidazole. The intra-abdominal pus sample is sent to the laboratory, the result later shows:

Result

Specimen	Pus
Appearance	–
Microscopy	Gram-positive cocci in chains Gram-negative bacilli Yeasts
Culture	Enterococcus faecium - Amoxicillin resistant - Vancomycin sensitive

The microscopy shows a mixture of bowel flora, but the *Enterococcus faecium* is the only bacterium that grows on culture because it is inherently resistant to Cefuroxime and Metronidazole. The yeast may not have had sufficient time to grow on culture. It would be a mistake to only treat the *Enterococcus faecium* as the microscopy clearly shows the presence of other bowel flora.

Why Bother Completing Request Forms?

Clinical details are essential, so complete request forms fully and accurately. You'll get a better microbiology service if you do.

This is why...
- The sample will not be "rejected" due to inadequate information. Many laboratories are now refusing to process samples with inadequately completed request forms...it is embarrassing to explain to your patient that you need to do the sample again as you didn't fill out the form correctly
- Clinical details aid the laboratory in selecting the correct tests for the condition/sample. If clinical details are incomplete, the laboratory cannot do the tests you should have asked for, even if you forgot to ask for them
- State any antibiotic therapy the patient is on or which you intend to start. The laboratory can then ensure that appropriate antibiotic sensitivities are released, related to that therapy
- Clinical details are essential to the Microbiologists when they give advice along with the result. Consider: swab from a superficial laceration of a knee or intra-operative swab from the synovial surface; both can be labelled "knee swab" but the treatment can be no antibiotics or 6 weeks of antibiotics...the clinical details are required to give the correct advice
- If the patient may have an easily transmissible infection e.g. typhoid, meningitis, *Escherichia coli* O157, ensure staff in the laboratory are not put at risk by labelling the sample "High-Risk". Laboratory acquired infections in technical staff do occur and are usually due to inadequate labelling of specimens

> **Warning**
> Your sample will be rejected if inadequate information is given due to:
> - Not knowing what the specimen is
> - Unclear who the patient is, ward they are on or doctor requesting
> - Unclear which tests to perform
> - Unable to interpret the results
> - Unknown risk to the laboratory staff

What is Relevant Information for a Request Form?

- Patient identifying information: name, date of birth, hospital number, NHS number
- Where the result is to go back to: ward/location, Consultant/GP details, person requesting, contact number
- Presenting complaint and provisional diagnosis
- Other clinical conditions: pregnancy, cystic fibrosis, diabetes and other co-morbidities
- Kidney function
- Current, recent or planned treatment

Considerations When Contacting a Microbiologist for Advice

- Ask your own seniors first. They know the patient better than the Microbiologist, and they have direct responsibility for the patient
- Call your cover Consultant oncall before a Microbiologist oncall. They have probably dealt with the issue before and can advise you
- If you call the Microbiologist...Know your patient
  - History and examination - you'll be asked for these details (see section – Basic Concepts, Diagnosing Infections)
  - Have the notes, observations, drug chart and investigation results available before you contact the Microbiologist
- If the call is **NOT URGENT** restrict routine calls to normal working hours
  - Microbiology departments are small and do not have many doctors. Calls out-of-hours can make it very difficult for microbiology departments to provide a full service within hours
  - **REMEMBER** the oncall Microbiologist out-of-hours is at home and therefore may not be able to access any results

Hints and Tips

Remember, the Microbiologist does not have the patient in front of them, and is unable to make clinical judgements based upon their own observations. They have no notes, blood results or X-rays. They are entirely reliant upon what they are told by the referring doctor. Unless they are provided with accurate and detailed information they may give the wrong advice.

Consider the patient who had a pyrexia of unknown origin in whom the fact that they had a prosthetic heart valve was left out of the story. The Microbiologist did not consider infective endocarditis as a potential diagnosis and as a result the patient went into heart block and required a pacemaker. Their heart valve then failed and needed replacing and they suffered an ischaemic stroke during the surgery. This is a serious clinical incident because all of this could have been avoided if the information about the prosthetic heart valve had been given to the Microbiologist during the initial referral.

This is why the Microbiologist will ask a series of questions in order to try and get a detailed history including information that has otherwise been omitted from the story presented by the referring doctor.

Information is based upon a District General Hospital laboratory service.

Microorganism or Condition	Test	Sample	Container
Adenovirus	PCR	NPA Sputum BAL Stool	See Tests by Specimen Type Table
Aspergillus spp.	Galacto-mannan	Serum	Red or yellow vacutainer
	(1,3)-Beta-d-glucan	Serum	Red or yellow vacutainer
Bartonella spp.	IgM IgG	Serum	Red or yellow vacutainer
Bordetella pertussis (Whooping cough)	IgG	Serum	Red or yellow vacutainer
	Culture	Pernasal swab	Pernasal swab
	PCR	NPA	Sterile universal
Borrelia burgdorferi (Lyme disease)	PCR	CSF	Sterile universal
	ELISA	Serum	Red or yellow vacutainer
Brucella spp.	IgM IgG	Serum	Red or yellow vacutainer
Candida spp.	(1,3)-Beta-d-glucan	Serum	Red or yellow vacutainer
Clostridium difficile toxin	Toxin	Stool	Blue stool container
Chlamydia spp.	PCR	Swab	Red/Orange Chlamydia swab
Coxiella burnetii (Q fever)	IgM IgG	Serum	Red or yellow vacutainer

Laboratories may vary slightly, if in doubt check with your local service.

Minimum Volume Required	Turnaround Time from Lab Receipt
See Tests by Specimen Type Table	10 days
1 tube	7 days
1 tube	7 days
1 tube	14 days
1 tube	10 days
1 swab	Up to 7 days
2-5mls	7 days **Note:** all +ves are phoned out
0.5-1ml	2-5 days **Note:** all +ves are phoned out
1 tube	3 days (+ve samples sent to Ref Lab for confirmation)
1 tube	10 days
1 tube	7 days
5ml	1 day
Eyes - 2 swabs (1 per eye) Genital - 1 swab	3 days
1 tube	21 days

Microorganism or Condition	Test	Sample	Container
Cryptococcus neoformans	Cryptococcal antigen	Serum	Red or yellow vacutainer
	Microscopy and culture	CSF	Sterile universal
Culture Negative Pneumonia	Mycoplasma pneumoniae, Chlamydophila pneumoniae and Viruses	Serum Complement Fixation Test (CFT)	Red or yellow vacutainer
	PCR	Sputum	Sterile sputum container
Cytomegalovirus (CMV)	IgM IgG	Serum	Red or yellow vacutainer
	PCR	Whole blood	Purple EDTA vacutainer
Dengue Virus	IgM IgG	Serum	Red or yellow vacutainer
	PCR	Whole blood	Purple EDTA vacutainer
Epstein Barr Virus (EBV)	IgM IgG	Serum	Red or yellow vacutainer
	PCR	Whole blood	Purple EDTA vacutainer
Enterovirus	PCR	Throat swab Stool CSF	See Tests by Specimen Type Table
Fungal Skin and Nail Infection	Microscopy and culture	Skin scrapings or nail clippings	Folded black paper square
Gonorrhoea (Neisseria gonorrhoeae)	Culture	Swab	Charcoal swab
	PCR	Swab	Red/Orange genital swab

Minimum Volume Required	Turnaround Time from Lab Receipt
1 tube	10 days
0.5-1ml	Microscopy 1 day Culture 2 days
1 tube	7 days
2-5ml	7 days
1 tube	3 days
1 tube	10 days
1 tube	14 days
1 tube	7 days
1 tube	5 days
1 tube	7 days
See Tests by Specimen Type Table	2 days
N/A	Microscopy 1 day Culture 7 days
1 swab	2-4 days
1 swab	3 days

Microorganism or Condition	Test	Sample	Container
Group A Beta-haemolytic *Streptococcus*	Anti-Streptolysin O Titre (ASOT)	Serum	Red or yellow vacutainer
Helicobacter pylori	IgG	Serum	Red or yellow vacutainer
	Antigen	Stool	Blue stool container
	Culture	Duodenal biopsy	Dent's media (special request from laboratory)
Hepatitis A Virus	IgM IgG	Serum	Red or yellow vacutainer
Hepatitis B Virus	HBsAg Anti-HBs Anti-HBc	Serum	Red or yellow vacutainer
	Viral Load	Whole blood	Purple EDTA vacutainer
Hepatitis C Virus	IgG	Serum	Red or yellow vacutainer
Herpes Simplex Virus (HSV)	PCR	Swab	Green viral swab
		CSF	As per CSF
Human Immunodeficiency Virus (HIV)	Antibody Antigen	Serum	Red or yellow vacutainer
	Viral load	Whole blood	Purple EDTA vacutainer
Influenza Virus	PCR	Nose and Throat Swab	Green viral swab

Minimum Volume Required	Turnaround Time from Lab Receipt
1 tube	5 days
1 tube	3-4 days
5mls	7 days
1 biopsy sample	Up to 14 days
1 tube	3-4 days
1 tube	Routine 4 days or 1 day, if needlestick injury
1 tube	7 days
1 tube	3-4 days
1 swab	5 days
As per CSF	
1 tube	1 day **Note:** all +ves are phoned out
1 tube	10 days
1 swab each site	Routine 3 days or 1 day, if Outbreak

Microorganism or Condition	Test	Sample	Container
Leptospirosis	IgM IgG	Serum	Red or yellow vacutainer
	PCR	Whole blood	Purple EDTA vacutainer
Measles Virus	IgG	Serum	Red or yellow vacutainer
	PCR	Buccal swab	Swab direct from PHEC
MRSA	Culture	Swab	Charcoal swab
Mumps Virus	IgG	Serum	Red or yellow vacutainer
Mycobacteria spp.	Microscopy and culture	Sputum BAL	Sterile universal
Neisseria meningitidis (Meningococcal PCR)	PCR	Whole blood	Purple EDTA vacutainer
		CSF	Sterile universal
Norovirus	Antigen	Stool	Blue stool container
	PCR		
Parvovirus	IgM IgG	Serum	Red or yellow vacutainer
Pneumocystis jirovecii	(1,3)-Beta-d-glucan	Serum	Red or yellow vacutainer
	PCR	Whole blood	Purple EDTA vacutainer
		BAL	Sterile universal

Minimum Volume Required	Turnaround Time from Lab Receipt
1 tube	7 days
1 tube	7 days
1 tube	3 days
1 swab	2-3 days

1 swab each from:
  – Nose
  – Groin
  – Wounds
	2 days

1 tube	3 days
2-5mls	Microscopy 1 day Culture up to 42 days
1 tube	2-5 days
0.5-1ml	2-5 days
5mls	1 day
5mls	2 days
1 tube	7 days
1 tube	7 days
1 tube	7 days
2-5mls	7 days

Microorganism or Condition	Test	Sample	Container
Psittacosis (*Chlamydophila psittaci*)	Antibody	Serum Complement Fixation Test (CFT)	Red or yellow vacutainer
	PCR	Sputum	Sterile sputum container
Respiratory Syncytial Virus (RSV)	Antigen	NPA Fluid	Sterile universal
	PCR	NPA Fluid	Sterile universal
		Throat swab	Green viral swab
Rotavirus	Antigen	Stool	Blue stool container
	PCR		
Rubella Virus	IgG	Serum	Red or yellow vacutainer
Streptococcus pneumoniae (Pneumococcal PCR)	PCR	Whole blood	Purple EDTA vacutainer
		CSF	Sterile universal
Syphilis (*Treponema pallidum*)	ELISA RPR TPPA IgM	Serum	Red or yellow vacutainer
Toxoplasma gondii	IgM IgG	Serum	Red or yellow vacutainer
Trichomonas vaginalis	Microscopy	Swab	Charcoal swab
Tropical Infectious Diseases	IgM IgG	Serum	Red or yellow vacutainer
	PCR	-	-

Minimum Volume Required	Turnaround Time from Lab Receipt
1 tube	7 days
2-5ml	7 days
2-5mls	1 day during season
2-5mls	2 days
1 swab	2 days
5mls	1 day
5mls	2 days
1 tube	10 days
1 tube	2-5 days
0.5-1ml	2-5 days
1 tube	10 days
1 tube	5 days
1 swab	1-2 days
Discuss with microbiology laboratory before taking samples	

Microorganism or Condition	Test	Sample	Container
Tuberculosis	IGRA (Quantiferon)	Blood	Specific vacutainer tubes from laboratory
	IGRA (T Spot)	Blood	Green lithium heparin or blue citrate vacutainer
	Microscopy and culture	Early morning urine (EMU)	250ml container
		Sputum BAL	Sterile universal
	PCR	Sputum BAL CSF	Sterile universal
Varicella Zoster Virus (VZV) (Chicken Pox)	IgG	Serum	Red or yellow vacutainer
	PCR	Viral swab	Green viral swab
		CSF	Sterile universal
West Nile Virus	IgM IgG	Serum	Red or yellow vacutainer
		CSF	Sterile universal
	PCR	Urine	Sterile universal
		CSF	Sterile universal
Zika Virus	IgG IgM	Serum	Red or yellow vacutainer
	PCR	Serum	Red or yellow vacutainer
		Urine	Sterile universal
16sRNA (all bacteria)	PCR	-	-

Minimum Volume Required	Turnaround Time from Lab Receipt
Fill all tubes to line	7 days
1 tube	1-2 days (samples sent to Ref Lab, service not available at weekends)
Full first urine of the day (for 3 consecutive days)	Microscopy 1 day Culture up to 42 days
2-5mls 2-5mls	2-5 days
2-5mls 2-5mls 0.5-1ml	2-5 days
1 tube	Routine 3 days or 1 day, if Chicken Pox contact
1 swab	5 days
As per CSF	-
1 tube	7 days
As per CSF	7 days
1 tube	7 days
As per CSF	7 days
1 tube	5 days
1 tube	5 days
20-25mls	5 days
Discuss with microbiology laboratory before taking samples	

Specimen Type	Test	Sample	Container
Antimicrobial Assay	Peak and Trough levels (see section – Antibiotics, TDM)	Serum	Red or yellow vacutainer
Ascitic Fluid	Microscopy and culture	Fluid	Sterile universal **PLUS** paediatric blood culture bottle
Bacterial Eye Swab	Culture	Swab	Charcoal swab
Bronchoalveolar Lavage (BAL)	Microscopy and culture	Fluid	Sterile universal
Blood Culture (Adults)	Culture	Whole blood	Aerobic and Anaerobic bottles
Blood Culture (Children)	Culture	Whole blood	Paediatric bottle
Cerebrospinal Fluid (CSF)	Microscopy and culture	Fluid	Sterile universal **PLUS** Grey fluoride oxalate vacutainer
Ear Swab	Culture	Swab	Charcoal swab
Endocervical Swab	Culture	Swab	Charcoal swab
High Vaginal Swab (HVS)	Culture	Swab	Charcoal swab
Intra-uterine Contraceptive Device (IUCD)	Culture	IUCD	Sterile universal
Nasopharyngeal Aspirate (NPA)	Culture	Fluid	Sterile universal
	PCR	Fluid	Sterile universal

Minimum Volume Required	Turnaround Time from Lab Receipt
1 tube	Up to 2 days depending on antimicrobial tested
2ml each container	Microscopy 2 hours if urgent Culture 2-4 days
2 swabs (1 per eye)	2-5 days
1ml in 3 containers for bacteria, mycobacteria and viruses as required	Microscopy 1 day Culture 2-4 days Viral 10 days Mycobacteria up to 42 days
5-10ml each bottle	Up to 5 days **Note:** all +ves are phoned out
1-5ml (higher bacterial load than adults)	Up to 5 days **Note:** all +ves are phoned out
4 universals with 0.5-1ml in each **PLUS** 40 drops for glucose in the fluoride oxalate vacutainer	Microscopy and biochemistry 2 hours Culture 2 days
1 swab	2-4 days
1 swab	2-4 days
1 swab	2-4 days
-	2-4 days Actinomycosis 10 days
2-5mls	2-4 days
2-5mls	5-7 days

Specimen Type	Test	Sample	Container
Pleural Fluid	Microscopy and culture	Fluid	Sterile universal **PLUS** paediatric blood culture bottle
Pus	Microscopy and culture	Fluid	Sterile universal
Semen	Culture	Fluid	Sterile universal
Sputum	Culture	Fluid	Sterile sputum container
Stool	Ova, cysts & parasites	Stool	Blue stool container
	Culture		
	PCR		
Synovial Fluid	Microscopy and culture	Fluid	Sterile universal **PLUS** paediatric blood culture bottle
	White Blood Cell (WBC) count		Purple EDTA vacutainer
Throat swab	Culture (Bacterial)	Swab	Charcoal swab
	PCR (Viral)		Green viral swab
Tissue	Microscopy and culture	Tissue	Sterile universal
Urine	Microscopy and culture	– Midstream urine (MSU) – Suprapubic aspirate (SPA) – Clean catch urine	Sterile universal with boric acid (if <8mls **DO NOT** use boric acid)
Wound Swab	Culture	Swab	Charcoal swab

Minimum Volume Required	Turnaround Time from Lab Receipt
2-5mls in each container	Microscopy 1 day Culture 2-5 days
2-5mls	Microscopy 1 day Culture 2-5 days
1-2ml	2-4 days
2-5ml	2-4 days
5ml	5 days
5ml	5 days
5ml	2 days
1-2mls in each container	Microscopy 2 hours Culture 2-5 days
2-5mls	2 days
1 swab	2-4 days
-	Microscopy 1 day Culture 2-5 days
20-25mls (if not using a sterile universal then fill to the containers fill line)	Microscopy 1 day Culture 2-3 days
1 swab each wound	2-4 days

Specimen Type	Appearance	Microscopy
Sputum or BAL	• Salivary – not sputum, URT contamination likely • Mucoid – no evidence of inflammation, may not be sputum, URT contamination possible • Purulent – inflammation but not necessarily infection e.g. asthma • Bloodstained – consistent with infection but not specific	• Gram stain • Ziehl-Neelsen (ZN) stain for acid fast bacilli such as *Mycobacteria* spp.

Urine (MSU, SPA & Clean Catch)	Not Applicable	• White blood cell count
		  – >100x10^6/L definitely significant
		  – >10x10^6/L significant if MSU or Clean Catch
		• Any white blood cells significant if SPA
		• Epithelial cells indicate contact with perineal skin and therefore probable contamination with perineal flora

Stool	• Formed – not diarrhoea • Semi-formed • Liquid	• Ova, cysts and parasites (OCP) e.g. *Giardia lamblia*, *Cryptosporidium*, intestinal worms
CSF	• Clear • Colourless • Turbid – high WBC count or lots of bacteria • Yellow – Xanthochromia or drug-related e.g. Rifampicin	• White blood cell count • Red blood cell count • Normal white blood cell to red blood cell ratio 1:600 • Gram stain • Protein and Glucose
Synovial Fluid	• Clear • Turbid – white blood cells or crystals • Purulent – inflammation, not necessarily infection	• Crystals • Gram stain
Pus, Bone or Tissue	Not Applicable	• Gram stain
Blood Cultures	Not Applicable	• When positive on automated incubator: Gram stain

Culture and Sensitivity	Other Tests Available

Is it consistent with diagnosis?
  – Bacteria
  – Fungi
  – Mycobacteria
	• Viral PCR
	• PCP PCR
	• *Mycoplasma pneumoniae* and *Chlamydophila pneumoniae* PCR

Is it consistent with diagnosis?
  – Bacteria
  – Candida
	• Early morning urine for TB culture
	• Legionella and pneumococcal antigens in CAP

Is it consistent with diagnosis?
  – *Campylobacter* spp.
  – *Shigella* spp.
  – *Salmonella* spp.
  – *Escherichia coli* O157
	• Foreign travel - *Vibrio* spp.
	• *Clostridium difficile* toxin
	  – All inpatients >2 years old, all outpatients >65 years old and where requested if <65 years
	• Antigen for *Norovirus* or *Rotavirus*
	• Viral, bacterial and parasite PCR

Is it consistent with diagnosis? – Bacteria	• Viral PCRs if consistent clinical details • *Neisseria meningitidis*, *Streptococcus pneumoniae* and *Listeria monocytogenes* PCR
Is it consistent with diagnosis? – Bacteria	• White blood cell count
Is it consistent with diagnosis?	-
Is it consistent with diagnosis?	-

How to Interpret Microbiology Results – Bacteriology

There are methods to systematically read chest X-rays (see Appendix 1), and a similar approach should be taken to laboratory results. They are multipart results and reading the parts in isolation means you will misinterpret the significance of the result. In order to correctly interpret a bacteriology report all three parts (if given) need to be considered in this order:

Appearance
- A description of the appearance of the sample e.g. purulent, bloodstained, turbid, clear
- Is there evidence of inflammation or disease e.g. purulent sputum, pus or liquid stool
- Is there evidence of contact with a non-sterile site or absence of disease e.g. salivary sputum, formed stool

Microscopy
- A list of the different appearances of microorganism present e.g. the report states a Gram-positive coccus in chains seen on the Gram film
- Is there evidence of contact with a non-sterile site or absence of disease e.g. epithelial cells in urine
- Is it consistent with the diagnosis e.g. the patient has symptoms of cough, SOB and fever; a possible diagnosis is pneumonia and pneumonia can be caused by a Gram-positive coccus in chains

> **Warning**
> **BEWARE** neutropaenic patients may be unable to mount a white blood cell response. They can grow bacteria and have significant infections in the absence of inflammation.

Culture and sensitivity
- A list of the microorganisms which have grown
- Is it consistent with the diagnosis e.g. *Streptococcus pneumoniae* is cultured from a patient with pneumonia
- A list of antibiotics used to treat the bacteria that were cultured; it is not usually necessary to give every sensitive antibiotic listed.
  - The list of antibiotics allows choices based around potential allergies to antibiotics
  - You may have to use combinations of antibiotics to treat mixed infections e.g. *Escherichia coli* and *Bacteroides* spp. with Cefuroxime and Metronidazole

> **Common Mistake**
> Some doctors assume that if bacteria are grown from a patient's specimen then antibiotics should be given. **This is a mistake.** Growth of bacteria in the absence of inflammation (i.e. normal microscopy or no white blood cells), or growth of bacteria in the presence of other factors (e.g. epithelial cells in urine) is an indication of probable contamination or colonisation, not infection. Do not over interpret the significance of these results.
> **REMEMBER** Bacteria are normal in certain places as colonisers or normal flora.

Occasionally other tests are performed and reported separately as they do not fit the usual sequence of Appearance, Microscopy and Culture. They are performed when the clinical details alert the laboratory to the need for further or specific testing.

- **Antigen detection**
    - Clinical details state CAP e.g. the laboratory conducts the tests for urine Pneumococcal and Legionella antigens
    - Clinical details state an outbreak of diarrhoea and vomiting e.g. the laboratory conducts the tests for *Norovirus* and *Rotavirus* in stool
- **Molecular detection of nucleic acid or Polymerase Chain Reaction (PCR)**
    - Clinical details state meningitis e.g. the laboratory conducts the tests for *Neisseria meningitidis* and *Streptococcus pneumoniae* PCR on EDTA blood or CSF
- **Toxin detection**
    - Clinical details state diarrhoea after starting Ciprofloxacin e.g. the laboratory conducts the tests for *Clostridium difficile* toxin in stool

Examples of Bacteriology Requests, Results and Interpretations

Clinical Details on the request form:
Right upper quadrant pain, fever and jaundice
Result

Specimen	Blood culture
Appearance	-
Microscopy	Gram-negative bacilli
Culture	Escherichia coli - Amoxicillin sensitive - Gentamicin sensitive

How is this Interpreted?
The Gram-negative bacillus identifies as *E. coli*. *E. coli* is normal flora for the gut; finding it in a blood culture indicates a significant infection below the diaphragm, probably involving either the urinary tract or a gastrointestinal tract related structure. In the clinical details (above) the patient has Charcot's triad (fever, RUQ pain and jaundice) indicating a probable diagnosis of cholangitis (infection of the biliary tract). Appropriate antibiotics have been provided for treatment.

Clinical Details on the request form:
Cough and shortness of breath
Result

Specimen	Sputum
Appearance	Salivary
Microscopy	Gram-negative bacilli
Culture	Escherichia coli

How is this Interpreted?
The salivary appearance of the sample indicates that it has been held in the mouth and is likely to be contaminated with upper respiratory tract bacteria. The Gram-negative bacillus *E. coli* is not a common cause of LRTI, but is a common URT bacterium in hospitalised patients. This result therefore indicates URT contamination, not infection, and the *E. coli* does not need treating. No antibiotics have been released to discourage unnecessary prescribing.

Clinical Details on the request form:
Acutely hot, painful, swollen knee
Result

Specimen	Synovial fluid
Appearance	Turbid
Microscopy	Gram-positive cocci in clumps
Culture	Staphylococcus aureus - Flucloxacillin sensitive - Fusidic Acid sensitive

How is this Interpreted?
The presence of Gram-positive cocci in clumps on microscopy is significant as synovial fluid should be sterile. The identification of *Staphylococcus aureus* confirms the diagnosis of septic arthritis. The patient should normally be treated with IV Flucloxacillin and PO Fusidic Acid.

Clinical Details on the request form:
Acute confusion in an elderly patient

Result

Specimen	Urine
Appearance	–
Microscopy	WBCs <10x10^6/L Epithelial cells ++
Culture	Pseudomonas aeruginosa

How is this Interpreted?
The culture result cannot be interpreted without first assessing whether a UTI is likely from the microscopy. The absence of white blood cells (<10x10^6/L) shows there is no evidence of inflammation in the urinary tract. However, there is evidence that the urine has been in contact with the skin of the perineum (presence of epithelial cells). *Pseudomonas aeruginosa* represents contamination from the perineum and not infection. In addition, *Pseudomonas* spp. are not common causes of UTI except in the presence of a urinary catheter. Seek another reason for the confusion.

Clinical Details on the request form:
Left iliac fossa pain, diverticular abscess found at laparotomy

Result

Specimen	Pus
Appearance	–
Microscopy	Gram-negative bacilli Gram-positive cocci in chains
Culture	Klebsiella pneumoniae - Amoxicillin resistant - Co-amoxiclav sensitive Enterococcus faecalis - Amoxicillin sensitive

How is this Interpreted?
The bacteria seen on microscopy are consistent with what has grown on culture, mixed bowel flora, and in keeping with the diagnosis of a diverticular abscess. There will be anaerobes present in a diverticular abscess because they make up most of the bowel flora, however they have not grown as they do not survive in air (anaerobes) and therefore are difficult to transport alive to the laboratory. This patient will need treatment with an antibiotic active against anaerobes, as well as the bacteria cultured.

Clinical Details on the request form:
Returned traveller, diarrhoea 2 weeks

Result

Specimen	Stool
Appearance	Liquid
Microscopy	Giardia lamblia oocysts seen
Culture	Salmonella, Shigella, Campylobacter and E. coli O157 not isolated

How is this Interpreted?
No bacterial cause for the diarrhoea has been found. However, the history of travel has prompted the laboratory to look for parasites which has diagnosed giardiasis. There are no antibiotics given under culture as the microorganism has been seen not grown (you cannot grow a parasite). The treatment of giardiasis is PO Metronidazole. If the travel history had not been mentioned, the diagnosis would not have been made.

The reason you can't do every test is because no test is 100% accurate. When interpreting results you are not concerned about whether a positive result is a true positive or a negative is a true negative because you expect all positive results to only occur in patients who have the disease (**true positive**, TP) and all negative results to occur in those without disease (**true negative**, TN). Unfortunately life isn't so simple; results are not always that clear cut or reliable! Some positive results occur in patients without disease (**false positive**, FP) and some negative results occur in patients with the disease (**false negative**, FN).

When performing laboratory tests it is important to know how likely the test is to be positive or negative to give an indication of the risk of a false positive or false negative result. The likelihood of a false result is based upon the probability of a true positive or true negative and is shown by the Positive or Negative Predictive Value (PPV or NPV).

- **PPV** is the percentage of genuine positive tests for an infection e.g. PPV of 60% means that 60% of people with a positive test have the infection, however it also means 40% of patients with a positive test actually do not have the infection (false positives)
- **NPV** is the percentage of genuine negative tests for an infection e.g. NPV of 97% means that 97% of people with a negative test do not have the infection, however it also means 3% of patients with a negative test actually do have the infection (false negatives)

PPV and NPV are dependent upon how common the infection is in the population being studied, so a test for a common infection will have a higher PPV and a lower NPV whereas a test for a rare infection will have a lower PPV and a higher NPV.

> **Common Mistake**
> Some doctors routinely request laboratory tests for conditions that are extremely unlikely, if not impossible. **This is a mistake.** If an infection is extremely unlikely then any positive test is almost certainly a false positive and any negative test is a true negative. The PPV is virtually 0%; the NPV is probably 100%, so it isn't necessary to do the test in the first place. For example, acute poliomyelitis (polio) can cause flaccid paralysis but if a patient has never left the UK the chance of them having polio is almost 0% because they won't have come into contact with someone with polio. Therefore don't test them for polio as the inherent inaccuracy of the test might just produce a positive result, but as polio has been eradicated in Europe the result is clearly wrong. Laboratory testing is not 100% accurate.

The next step in trusting a result is the **likelihood ratios** which represent how likely it is that a patient will have a particular infection if they have a positive or negative test. Likelihood ratios are calculated using a standard statistical equation (see below) from the **sensitivity** and **specificity** of the test in that specific patient population compared to a known/confirmed result. This "validates" the test against the known result. For example, if you want to calculate the sensitivity and specificity of a urine dipstick in women you first need to test how effective a urine dipstick is in diagnosing a UTI in this population group. If you take 200 women (100 with confirmed UTI and 100 without a UTI) and test their urine with a urine dipstick, the results would look like this:

	UTI	No UTI	
+ve dipstick	**77** (true positive)	**30** (false positive)	107
-ve dipstick	**23** (false negative)	**70** (true negative)	93
	100	100	200

Sensitivity = $\dfrac{TP}{(TP+FN)}$ = $\dfrac{\mathbf{77}}{(\mathbf{77 + 23})}$ = **0.77** or 77%

Specificity = $\dfrac{TN}{(FP+TN)}$ = $\dfrac{\mathbf{70}}{(\mathbf{30+70})}$ = **0.70** or 70%

These figures can now be used to calculate the two likelihood ratios; one is called the +ve likelihood ratio, the other is called the −ve likelihood ratio. The +ve likelihood ratio indicates the possibility that a positive test result is a genuine positive; the −ve likelihood ratio indicates the possibility that a negative result is actually incorrect.

+ve Likelihood Ratio = $\dfrac{\text{Sensitivity}}{(1\text{-Specificty})}$ = $\dfrac{\mathbf{0.77}}{(1\text{-}\mathbf{0.70})}$ = 2.57 ratio

-ve Likelihood Ratio = $\dfrac{(1\text{-Sensivity})}{\text{Specificity}}$ = $\dfrac{(1\text{-}\mathbf{0.77})}{\mathbf{0.70}}$ = 0.33 ratio

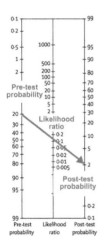

Fagan nomogram

REMEMBER likelihood ratios represent how likely it is that a patient will have a particular infection if they have a positive or negative test.

The likelihood ratios are combined with the **pre-test probability** of the infection (the prevalence of a specific infection within the population, expressed as a percentage) to give **post-test probabilities** of the infection. This uses the Fagan nomogram.

Starting with the pre-test probability value on the left axis (e.g. 20%), draw a straight line through the likelihood ratio value on the middle axis (e.g. 0.1), and end the line on the post-test probability value on the right axis (e.g. 2%). The post-test probability is the probability of the patient having the infection when the test result is known e.g. only 2%, or 2 in 100 people.

The test would be poor at diagnosing the disease if you were using the +ve likelihood ratio as only 2% of patients with a positive result would have the disease. However, it would be a good test for excluding a diagnosis if you were using the −ve likelihood ratio as only 2% of patients with a negative result would actually have the disease.

Both need to be plotted on a chart giving 2 post-test probability results to work out how likely a positive test result indicates the patient does have an infection, and how likely a negative result indicates that the patient doesn't have an infection.

Examples of Pre and Post-test Probability Results and Interpretations

In the clinical examples below the red line uses the +ve likelihood ratio and the blue line uses the −ve likelihood ratio.

Clinical Details:
Older woman with fever. Urine dipstick (sensitivity 77%, specificity 70%)

Result

Pre-Test Probability	10%
+ve Likelihood Ratio	2.57
−ve Likelihood Ratio	0.33
Post-Test Probability of +ve being genuine	25% Poor
Post-Test Probability of −ve being incorrect	3% Low

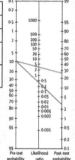

How is this Interpreted?
Post-test probability of a positive result being genuinely positive is 25% which is the same as 75% of positive results being falsely positive. Post-test probability of a negative result actually being a positive result is 3%, which means 3 out of 100 patients with a negative test would actually have a UTI. This is a poor test for diagnosing a UTI but a reasonable test for excluding a UTI in elderly women with a fever.

Clinical Details:
Child with fever, rash and low blood pressure. Blood meningococcal PCR (sensitivity 99.7%, specificity 90%)

Result

Pre-Test Probability	75%
+ve Likelihood Ratio	997
−ve Likelihood Ratio	0.003
Post-Test Probability of +ve being genuine	>99% Good
Post-Test Probability of −ve being incorrect	0.2% Very Low

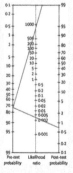

How is this Interpreted?
Post-test probability of a positive result being genuinely positive is >99% which is the same as <1% of positive results being falsely positive. Post-test probability of a negative result actually being a positive result is 0.2%, which means 2 out of 1000 patients with a negative test would actually have meningococcal sepsis. This is a good test for both diagnosing and excluding meningococcal sepsis in children with a fever, rash and low blood pressure.

Clinical Details:

Adult with fever and consolidation on a chest x-ray. Urinary *Streptococcus pneumoniae* antigen (sensitivity 86%, specificity 94%)

Result

Pre-Test Probability	40%
+ve Likelihood Ratio	14.3
-ve Likelihood Ratio	0.14
Post-Test Probability of +ve being genuine	90% Mediocre
Post-Test Probability of -ve being incorrect	8% Poor

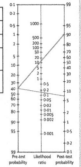

How is this Interpreted?

Post-test probability of a positive result being genuinely positive is 90% which is the same as 10% of positive results being falsely positive. Post-test probability of a negative result actually being a positive result is 8%, which means 8 out of 100 patients with a negative test would actually have *S. pneumoniae* pneumonia. This is at best a mediocre test for diagnosing, but a poor test for excluding, *S. pneumoniae* in adults with fever and consolidation on a chest x-ray. In total 18 out of 100 patients would have an incorrect result with this test.

Hints and Tips

Still confused? Let's look at this in a non-medical analogy. The chances of me getting a Husky dog, with its strong prey drive to eat my cats, means there is a very low **"pre-test probability"** that I will have a Husky. Whereas a Field Spaniel, which is unlikely to attack my cats, means there is a higher **"pre-test probability"** that I will have a Field Spaniel.

However the **"+ve likelihood ratio"** that my wife would allow me to have any dog is very low as she doesn't really like dogs. With these factors combined the **"post-test probability"** that we will ever get a Husky is extremely low i.e. it will never happen, whereas having a Field Spaniel, whilst still unlikely, is more likely than having a Husky.

Alternatively the **"pre-test probability"** and the **"likelihood ratio"** of us having more cats are both very high; therefore it is almost inevitable we will get a sixth cat!

How to Use Pre-test Probability, Likelihood Ratios and Post-test Probabilities in the Clinical Setting

There are two ways of using pre-test probability, likelihood ratios and post-test probabilities in clinical practise:
- Find the pre-test probability in the population, then find the sensitivity and specificity for the test required (from the manufacturer), calculate the likelihood ratios and then use the Fagan nomogram to determine the exact post-test probabilities.

OR
- Make a rough assessment using an approximate pre-test probability (common, uncommon and rare) and an approximate assessment of how good the test is (good, okay or poor) and then use the box below:

		Disease		
		Common	**Uncommon**	**Rare**
Test	**Good**	Believe the result	Probably correct	Probably not correct if another explanation
	Okay	Probably correct	Probably not correct if another explanation	Probably not correct
	Poor	Probably not correct if another explanation	Probably not correct	Don't even do the test!

Now apply this to these examples:
- A patient with pneumonia has a positive urinary *Streptococcus pneumoniae* antigen test. This is an "okay test" for a "common condition" therefore the positive result is "probably correct". But if you had a negative result then this is in fact a "poor test" for a "common condition", the result is then "probably not correct if another explanation" e.g. you have other reasons to support the diagnosis; there is *Streptococcus pneumoniae* in the blood culture which is a "good test" for a "common condition", and therefore "trumps" the urine *Streptococcus pneumoniae* antigen test.
- A patient with a sore throat has a rapid antigen test which is negative and a throat swab culture which is positive for Group A Beta-haemolytic *Streptococcus*. The rapid antigen test is considered "probably not correct" because it is a "poor test" for a "common condition" and there is an alternative "explanation"; the positive culture from the throat swab is a "good test" for a "common condition", and therefore "trumps" the rapid antigen test.

> **Hints and Tips**
> If all the tests for the common causes of a disease are negative, rather than doing the tests for the very rare causes it would be more appropriate to repeat the tests for the common causes because it is more likely that a test has a false negative result for a common cause than a true positive result for a very rare cause. If the repeat tests for the common causes are negative **THEN** consider moving onto the tests for the very rare causes.

Basic Bacterial Identification by Microscopy

There are too many microorganisms to remember easily so they need to be separated into groups with similar features. Microbiologists use a number of terms to describe the different appearances of bacteria; Gram-positive or Gram-negative, coccus or bacillus etc. For example, the Microbiologist might telephone with a result, saying "the cause is a Gram-negative bacillus growing both aerobically and anaerobically". This may appear to be pointless jargon but using a simple system of firstly identifying the staining method, then the shape of the microorganism and finally the microorganism's growth requirements, a doctor can begin to eliminate microorganisms, like in a game of Cluedo®, in order to identify the most likely cause of the infection.

If a microorganism is Gram-negative, it cannot be any of the Gram-positives or acid-fast bacilli and therefore these can be discounted. If the microorganism is bacillus-shaped then all of the cocci can be discounted. If the microorganism is then described as growing anaerobically, the aerobes can be discounted; and if it is also described as growing aerobically as well as anaerobically the anaerobes can also be discounted. This identifies the microorganism as a Gram-negative bacillus growing as a facultative anaerobe e.g. an Enterobacteriaceae, *Haemophilus* spp., *Eikenella* spp., *Pasteurella* spp. or *Capnocytophaga* spp. The clinical history can then narrow the list further because if the patient has CAP it is probably a *Haemophilus* spp., if they have a cat bite it is probably *Pasteurella* spp., and if they have pyelonephritis it will be one of the Enterobacteriaceae.

Identifying the staining method

Ziehl-Neelsen Stain	Acid-fast	Stains red using the ZN method, bacteria have mycolic acid in their cell wall
Gram Stain	Gram-positive	Stains purple with Gram's method, bacteria have a thick cell wall and no cell membrane
	Gram-negative	Stains red with Gram's method, bacteria have a cell membrane outside a thin cell wall

Identifying the shape

Coccus	Shaped like a sphere
Bacillus	Shaped like a rod

Identifying the growth requirements

Aerobic	Grows in the presence of oxygen
Anaerobic	Grows in the absence of oxygen
Facultative Anaerobe	Able to grow in the presence or absence of oxygen
Microaerophilic	Grows in the presence of oxygen at lower concentrations than in air

Knowledge of bacterial identification from the Gram film appearance helps predict the cause of an infection from the microscopy result up to 48 hours before the culture result is available. By using both the Basic Bacterial Identification diagrams and the Table of Bacterial Causes of Infection (following pages) you can identify the likely bacteria from the Gram film appearance on the microscopy result. For example:

- The patient clinically has meningitis; the Gram film of the CSF shows Gram-positive cocci in chains. Meningitis is caused by *Streptococcus pneumoniae*, *Listeria monocytogenes*, *Neisseria meningitidis*, *Haemophilus influenzae* and *Mycobacterium tuberculosis*. We know it is Gram-positive therefore ruling out *Neisseria meningitidis* and *Haemophilus influenzae*, which are Gram-negative, and *Mycobacterium tuberculosis*, which is an acid-fast bacillus. The microscopy also states coccus, which rules out *Listeria monocytogenes* as this is a bacillus. This leaves *Streptococcus pneumoniae*, a chain-forming Gram-positive coccus

- The patient clinically has septic arthritis; the Gram film of the synovial fluid shows Gram-positive cocci in clumps. Septic arthritis is caused by *Staphylococcus aureus*, Beta-haemolytic *Streptococcus* (Groups A, B, C, G), *Escherichia coli* and other Enterobacteriaceae. As it is Gram-positive this rules out *Escherichia coli* and other Enterobacteriaceae, which are Gram-negative. The microscopy also states clumps, which rules out *Streptococcus* spp. as these form chains. This leaves *Staphylococcus aureus*, a clump-forming Gram-positive coccus

- The patient clinically has peritonitis; the Gram film of the peritoneal fluid shows Gram-positive cocci in chains, Gram-positive bacilli and Gram-negative bacilli. Peritonitis is caused by bowel flora including: *Enterococcus* spp., *Clostridium* spp., *Bacteroides* spp., *Escherichia coli* and other Enterobacteriaceae. The mixed Gram film appearance shows the presence of the entire bowel flora. This indicates the patient has probably perforated their bowel rather than developed spontaneous bacterial peritonitis. Even this result is helpful as it indicates there is a hole in the bowel. The patient needs surgery not just antibiotics, as no antibiotic tablet is large enough to plug the hole! Antibiotics will only help if the hole is surgically repaired

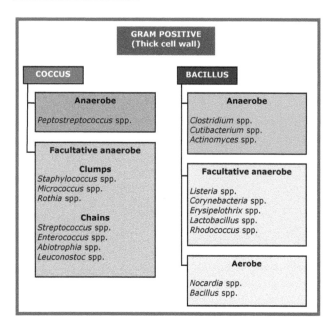

GRAM NEGATIVE
(Thin cell wall and cell membrane)

COCCUS

Facultative Anaerobe

Neisseria spp.
Moraxella spp.
Kingella spp.

Aerobe

Pseudomonas spp.
Stenotrophomonas spp.
Acinetobacter spp.
Legionella spp.
Bordetella spp.
Aeromonas spp.
Vibrio spp.

Microaerophilic

Campylobacter spp.
Helicobacter spp.

BACILLUS

Facultative anaerobe

Enterobacteriaceae
- *Escherichia coli*
- *Klebsiella* spp.
- *Enterobacter* spp.
- *Citrobacter* spp.
- *Proteus* spp.
- *Serratia marcescens*
- *Salmonella* spp.
- *Shigella* spp.
Haemophilus spp.
Eikenella spp.
Pasteurella spp.
Capnocytophaga spp.

Anaerobe

Bacteroides spp.
Fusobacterium spp.

ACID FAST BACILLI
(Mycolic acid in cell wall)

Mycobacterium spp.

NON-CULTURABLE
(No cell wall)

Mycoplasma spp.
Ureaplasma spp.
Chlamydia spp.

Table of Bacterial Causes of Infection

✓ = Common Cause   – = Not a Common cause

Clinical Scenarios	Gram-positive Bacteria								Anaero-	
	Staphylococcus aureus (MSSA)	Staphylococcus aureus (MRSA)	Coagulase Negative Staphylococcus	Beta-haemolytic Streptococcus (A, B, C, G)	Enterococcus faecalis	Enterococcus faecium	Streptococcus pneumoniae	Listeria monocytogenes	Clostridium perfringens	Clostridium difficile
Respiratory Infections										
Community Acquired Pneumonia (CAP)	✓1	–	–	–	–	–	✓	–	–	–
Hospital Acquired Pneumonia (HAP)	✓	✓	–	–	–	–	✓	–	–	–
Ventilator Associated Pneumonia (VAP)	✓	✓	–	–	–	–	✓	–	–	–
Aspiration Pneumonia	✓	–	–	–	–	–	✓	–	–	–
Exacerbation of COPD	✓	–	–	–	–	–	✓	–	–	–
Acute Bronchitis	–	–	–	–	–	–	–	–	–	–
Head and Neck Infections										
Otitis Media	–	–	–	–	–	–	✓	–	–	–
Otitis Externa	✓	–	–	✓	–	–	–	–	–	–
Orbital Cellulitis	✓	–	–	✓	–	–	✓	–	–	–
Sinusitis	✓	–	–	✓	–	–	–	–	–	–
Urogenital Infections										
Urinary Tract Infection (UTI)	–	–	–	–	–	–	–	–	–	–
Prostatitis	–	–	–	–	–	–	–	–	–	–
STDs	–	–	–	–	–	–	–	–	–	–
Skin, Soft Tissue, Bone and Joint Infections										
Cellulitis	✓	✓	–	✓	–	–	–	–	–	–
Cellulitis in Diabetes & Vascular Insufficiency	✓	✓	–	✓	–	–	–	–	✓	–
Bites	✓	–	–	✓	–	–	–	–	✓	–
Burns, Skin Grafts, Post-Operative	✓	✓	–	✓	–	–	–	–	✓	–
Intravenous Device Associated Infection	✓	✓	–	–	–	–	–	–	–	–
Osteomyelitis	✓	✓	–	✓	–	–	–	–	–	–
Septic Arthritis	✓	✓	–	✓	–	–	–	–	–	–

Gram-negative Bacteria									Non-Culturable		
bes											
Bacteroides fragilis	Neisseria meningitidis	Neisseria gonorrhoeae	Haemophilus influenzae	Escherichia coli	ESBL-positive Escherichia coli	Enterobacteriaceae	Pseudomonas aeruginosa	Moraxella catarrhalis	Legionella pneumophila	Mycoplasma pneumoniae	Chlamydia spp.
–	–	–	✓	–	–	–	–	–	✓	✔	✓
–	–	–	✓	?2	?2	✓	✓	–	–	–	–
–	–	–	✓	✓	✓	✓	✓	–	–	–	–
✓	–	–	✓	✓	✓	✓	–	–	–	–	–
–	–	–	✓	–	–	–	–	✓	–	–	–
–	–	–	–	–	–	–	–	–	–	–	–
–	–	–	✓	–	–	–	–	–	–	–	–
–	–	–	–	–	–	–	–	–	–	–	–
–	–	–	–	–	–	–	–	–	–	–	–
✓	–	–	✓	–	–	–	–	–	–	–	–
–	–	–	–	✓	✓	✓	?3	–	–	–	–
–	–	–	–	✓	✓	✓	?3	–	–	–	–
–	–	✓	–	–	–	–	–	–	–	–	✓
–	–	–	–	–	–	–	–	–	–	–	–
✓	–	–	–	✓	–	✓	✓	–	–	–	–
✓	–	–	✓	–	–	–	–	–	–	–	–
✓	–	–	–	✓	–	✓	✓	–	–	–	–
–	–	–	–	–	–	?4	?4	–	–	–	–
–	–	–	–	?5	–	?5	–	–	–	–	–
–	–	–	–	?5	–	?5	–	–	–	–	–

✓ = Common Cause   − = Not a Common cause

Clinical Scenarios	Gram-positive Bacteria								Anaero-	
	Staphylococcus aureus (MSSA)	Staphylococcus aureus (MRSA)	Coagulase Negative Staphylococcus	Beta-haemolytic Streptococcus A, B, C, G)	Enterococcus faecalis	Enterococcus faecium	Streptococcus pneumoniae	Listeria monocytogenes	Clostridium perfringens	Clostridium difficile
Gastrointestinal Infections										
Peritonitis	−	−	−	−	✓	✓	−	−	✓	−
Cholecystitis & Cholangitis	−	−	−	−	✓	✓	−	−	✓	−
Necrotising Pancreatitis	−	−	−	−	✓	✓	−	−	✓	−
Other Infections										
Infective Endocarditis	✓	−	✓	−	✓	✓	−	−	−	−
Emergencies										
Sepsis	✓	✓	−	✓	−	−	✓	✓	−	−
Neonatal Sepsis	−	−	−	✓7	−	−	−	−	−	−
Neutropaenic Sepsis	✓	✓	−	−	−	−	−	−	−	−
Meningitis	−	−	−	−	−	−	✓	−	−	−
Neonatal Meningitis	−	−	−	✓7	−	−	−	✓	−	−
Epiglottitis	−	−	−	✓	−	−	−	−	−	−
Epidural Abscess	✓	−	−	−	−	−	−	−	−	−
Necrotising Fasciitis	−	−	−	✓	−	−	−	−	✓	−
Toxic Shock Syndrome	✓	−	−	✓	−	−	−	−	−	−

1. *Staphylococcus aureus* is an uncommon cause of CAP except after Influenza or out-of-hospital cardiac arrest
2. *Escherichia coli* occasionally causes HAP in particularly debilitated patients
3. *Pseudomonas aeruginosa* can cause UTIs and prostatitis in patients with anatomically abnormal urinary tracts or catheters
4. Enterobacteriaceae and *Pseudomonas aeruginosa* can cause central venous catheter infections, particularly in the immunodeficient

? = Uncommon Cause OR only under specific circumstances (see notes)

	Gram-negative Bacteria									Non-Culturable		
Bacteroides fragilis	Neisseria meningitidis	Neisseria gonorrhoeae	Haemophilus influenzae	Escherichia coli	ESBL-positive Escherichia coli	Enterobacteriaceae	Pseudomonas aeruginosa	Moraxella catarrhalis	Legionella pneumophila	Mycoplasma pneumoniae	Chlamydia spp.
✓	–	–	–	✓	?6	✓	?6	–	–	–	–
✓	–	–	–	✓	?6	✓	?6	–	–	–	–
✓	–	–	–	✓	?6	✓	?6	–	–	–	–
–	–	–	–	–	–	–	–	–	–	–	–
–	✓	–	–	✓	–	✓	✓	–	–	–	–
–	–	–	–	✓	–	?8	–	–	–	–	–
–	–	–	–	✓	–	✓	✓	–	–	–	–
–	✓	–	✓	–	–	–	–	–	–	–	–
–	–	–	–	✓	–	?8	–	–	–	–	–
–	–	–	✓	–	–	–	–	–	–	–	–
–	–	–	–	✓	–	✓	–	–	–	–	–
–	–	–	–	–	–	✓	–	–	–	–	–
–	–	–	–	–	–	–	–	–	–	–	–

5. *Escherichia coli* and Enterobacteriaceae can cause osteomyelitis and septic arthritis in the elderly, particularly following haematogenous seeding from UTIs
6. ESBL-positive *Escherichia coli* and *Pseudomonas aeruginosa* are more common in intra-abdominal infections following surgery
7. Group B Beta-haemolytic *Streptococcus* is the most common cause of neonatal sepsis and meningitis
8. Enterobacteriaceae such as *Klebsiella* spp., *Salmonella* spp. and *Serratia marcescens* are unusual but severe causes of neonatal sepsis and meningitis

Serology is the investigation of a component of blood i.e. serum, to look for evidence of infection, past infection, immunity to infection or susceptibility to infection. Bacteriology looks for living microorganism whereas serology is not reliant on the microorganism being alive. Antigen and antibody tests are performed on serum, removed after the blood has clotted, whereas PCR requires the whole blood sample.

Reasons to send samples to a serology or molecular laboratory are:
- The organism cannot be cultured e.g. a virus or the non-culturable bacteria e.g. *Mycoplasma* spp., *Chlamydia* spp. or *Treponema pallidum*
- The patient may be on an antibiotic that prevents the microorganism from being cultured e.g. patient with meningitis is correctly given Benzylpenicillin by the GP before admission into hospital, which will stop *N. meningitidis* from growing but PCR will still detect bacteria
- To assess the risk of a patient acquiring an infection after exposure to the infectious microorganism e.g. testing for *Varicella Zoster Virus* antibody in a pregnant woman exposed to Chicken Pox
- To assess whether a patient has had an infection in the past or been immunised against that infection e.g. a patient exposed to blood contaminated with *Hepatitis B Virus* has evidence of antibodies against the virus and so cannot acquire it from this needlestick injury
- To detect a microorganism that might be too small to see on microscopy e.g. viruses

In general, there are three types of serology report:
- **Antigen detection**
    - Either molecules from infected cells or fragments of infecting microorganisms
    - Detects acute infection
    - Cheap, usually a rapid result on the same day as sample received
- **Antibody detection**
    - Indicating the individual's response to infection
    - IgM indicates acute or recent infection
    - IgG indicates past infection or immunity
    - Cheap, usually a rapid result on the same day as sample received
- **Molecular detection of nucleic acid or Polymerase Chain Reaction (PCR)**
    - Detects microorganism genes by multiplying undetectable amounts of DNA or RNA to a level that can be detected
    - Detects acute infection e.g. *Enterovirus* PCR in CSF, but can also detect reactivated past infections e.g. CMV in HIV-positive patients
    - Can be affected by contamination as small amounts of microorganism genes can give positive results if they get into the sample after it has been taken
    - Expensive and requires specialist laboratory staff

Combination antibody results e.g. *Epstein Barr Virus* serology
Some infections are diagnosed using combinations of antibody tests e.g. EBV. Viral capsid antigen (VCA) IgM and IgG are present at the onset of symptoms; IgM starts to disappear after 3 months whilst IgG persists for life. Epstein-Barr nuclear antigen (EBNA) IgG starts to appear 6-12 weeks after onset of symptoms when the virus begins to become latent.

The results can be interpreted as follows:

Antibody response	Interpretation	Antibody response	Interpretation
VCA IgM -ve VCA IgG -ve EBNA IgG -ve	Susceptible to infection	VCA IgM -ve VCA IgG +ve EBNA IgG -ve	Evidence of possible recent EBV infection (repeat in 1-2 weeks to look for EBNA IgG)
VCA IgM +ve VCA IgG +ve EBNA IgG -ve	Evidence of acute EBV infection	VCA IgM -ve VCA IgG +ve EBNA IgG +ve	Evidence of past EBV infection

Examples of Serology / Virology Requests, Results and Interpretations

Clinical Details on the request form:
3 month old with bronchiolitis
Result

Specimen	Nasopharyngeal Aspirate (NPA)
Result	Respiratory Syncytial Virus (RSV) antigen detected

How is this Interpreted?
The child is shown to have the most common cause of bronchiolitis: RSV. An antigen test has been used as it is cheap and quick, giving the paediatricians a rapid answer for why the child is unwell. Treatment is usually supportive only, although in certain patients Ribavirin is used under the guidance of a Consultant Paediatrician.

Clinical Details on the request form:
Healthcare staff member post-immunisation against *Hepatitis B Virus*
Result

Specimen	Blood
Result	Anti-HBs antibody positive >100mIU/ml

How is this Interpreted?
The healthcare staff member has responded well to the vaccination course. An antibody test has been used because evidence of immunity is being sought not evidence of infection (as in antigen tests). The healthcare staff member is now immune to *Hepatitis B Virus* and protected from this virus should they sustain a needlestick injury.

Clinical Details on the request form:
Acute confusion, fever and seizures
Result

Specimen	Cerebrospinal Fluid (CSF)
Result	Herpes Simplex Virus DNA detected by PCR

How is this Interpreted?
The patient has clinical features of possible encephalitis and the detection of HSV by PCR confirms HSV encephalitis. A molecular test has been used as it detects the presence of a virus and therefore infection. PCR is an expensive test but there is no antigen test available to detect viruses in CSF. HSV encephalitis requires treatment with at least 2 weeks of IV Aciclovir. It is a serious and potentially life-threatening infection.

Notifiable Infectious Diseases in the UK

Notifiable Infectious Diseases either represent a significant threat to public health or a failure of public health strategy e.g. vaccination programs. Doctors and laboratories in the UK have a legal responsibility to notify specific infectious diseases under the Health Protection (Notification) Regulations 2010.

The following are infections notifiable to the local Public Health England Centre (PHEC) by the doctors responsible for the patient, either by telephone, letter or secure fax using the PHEC reporting form available on the PHE website.

- Acute encephalitis
- Acute infectious hepatitis
- Acute meningitis
- Acute poliomyelitis
- Anthrax
- Botulism
- Brucellosis
- Cholera
- Diphtheria
- Enteric fever (typhoid or paratyphoid fever)
- Food poisoning
- Haemolytic Uraemic Syndrome (HUS)
- Infectious bloody diarrhoea
- Invasive Group A Streptococcal disease
- Legionnaires' Disease
- Leprosy
- Malaria
- Measles
- Meningococcal septicaemia
- Mumps
- Plague
- Rabies
- Rubella
- Scarlet fever
- Severe Acute Respiratory Syndrome (SARS)
- Smallpox
- Tetanus
- Tuberculosis
- Typhus
- Viral Haemorrhagic Fever (VHF)
- Whooping cough
- Yellow fever

The notification of infectious diseases allows public health doctors to manage outbreaks of diseases in order to protect the public. They also help inform future healthcare policy and vaccination strategies.

Infection Control

What is Infection Control?

Infection control is implemented to prevent the spread of infections within hospitals and other healthcare settings. Infection control policies centre on preventing transfer of infections from patient-to-patient, patients-to-staff and staff-to-patients. The infection control toolkit includes hand hygiene, Personal Protective Equipment (PPE), isolation of patients, environmental cleaning and decontamination, staff vaccination, antimicrobial stewardship, surveillance and Root Cause Analysis (RCA).

Root Cause Analysis (RCA)

Root Cause Analysis (RCA) is the process by which an untoward event can be evaluated in order to identify learning points, which can prevent that event happening again. All healthcare staff should be prepared to contribute to the RCA process as their action or inaction may have inadvertently been the root cause e.g.

- The cleaner who fails to wash all the surfaces in a side room
- The nursing staff who fail to inform another department of a patient with an infection control risk
- The physiotherapist who washes a tracheostomy tube in a sink
- The doctor who prescribes the wrong antibiotic
- The maintenance staff who fail to repair the hand wash sinks
- The theatre staff who fail to check the air flow ventilation routinely

The **root cause** is the earliest point at which something went wrong leading to the untoward event. RCA is a bit like a young child continuing to ask "Why?" They keep asking "Why?" until there are no more answers to give. In the case of RCA this point is usually the root cause.

RCA is commonly used to investigate cases of MRSA bacteraemia and *Clostridium difficile* Associated Disease (CDAD) in the NHS.

Common Root Causes

- Inappropriate choice of antibiotic e.g. Clindamycin is a common predisposing antibiotic for CDAD and so should only be used when there is no alternative
- Transmission of microorganisms between patients due to poor infection control practice e.g. poor hand hygiene or environmental cleaning
- Unnecessarily prolonged courses of antibiotics e.g. 7 days of Co-amoxiclav for a simple UTI (rather than the correct duration of 3 days) predisposing to MRSA colonisation
- Multiple courses of antibiotics e.g. recurrent treatments selecting out antibiotic resistant Gram-negative bacteria
- Failure to isolate patients in a timely manner e.g. patients with *Norovirus* infecting other patients on wards because they did not get put in a side room

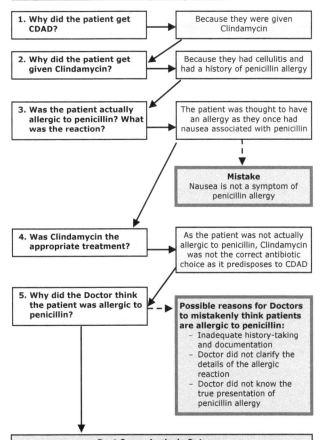

1. Why did the patient get CDAD?

Because they were given Clindamycin

2. Why did the patient get given Clindamycin?

Because they had cellulitis and had a history of penicillin allergy

3. Was the patient actually allergic to penicillin? What was the reaction?

The patient was thought to have an allergy as they once had nausea associated with penicillin

Mistake
Nausea is not a symptom of penicillin allergy

4. Was Clindamycin the appropriate treatment?

As the patient was not actually allergic to penicillin, Clindamycin was not the correct antibiotic choice as it predisposes to CDAD

5. Why did the Doctor think the patient was allergic to penicillin?

Possible reasons for Doctors to mistakenly think patients are allergic to penicillin:
- Inadequate history-taking and documentation
- Doctor did not clarify the details of the allergic reaction
- Doctor did not know the true presentation of penicillin allergy

Root Cause Analysis Outcome
Inadequate knowledge of doctor regarding allergy history and significance

Recommendation:
- Educate doctors to recognise symptoms of true penicillin allergy
- Ensure a full allergy history is explored when symptoms are vague or ambiguous
- Improve allergy documentation in the medical notes

Isolation of Patients

There are 2 main types of patient isolation:
- **Source isolation** protects staff and other patients from acquiring infections
- **Protective isolation** prevents vulnerable patients from catching infections

A patient cannot be forced to stay in their side room; a hospital cannot deny a patient their liberty. However, if the patient should leave their room they should leave the clinical area e.g. visit the canteen or hospital shop. They should be encouraged to wash their hands on leaving the room. Patient's rooms should be clearly labelled with the type of precautions in place. Every healthcare staff member has a responsibility to follow their hospital's guidelines for these types of precautions.

Source Isolation

Patients with transmissible infectious diseases should be nursed in single occupancy rooms (side rooms) with en-suite toilet and separate hand hygiene facilities. The door should remain closed at all times. Some patients need to be nursed in negative pressured rooms, which draw air into the room thereby preventing airborne microorganisms exiting to other clinical areas.

Protective Isolation

Patients who are immunodeficient should be nursed in single occupancy rooms (side rooms) with en-suite toilet and separate hand hygiene facilities. The door should remain closed at all times. Some patients will need to be nursed in positive pressured rooms, which push air out of the room thereby preventing airborne microorganisms entering the room and exposing the patient.

Hand Hygiene

Hands are the most common source of contamination leading to patient-to-patient transmission of infectious microorganisms. Effective hand hygiene is therefore the single most important step healthcare staff can take in order to prevent transmission of infections between patients.

The World Health Organisation's 5 Key Moments of Hand Hygiene:
1. Before patient contact
2. Before an aseptic task
3. After body fluid exposure risk
4. After patient contact
5. After contact with the patient's surroundings

When to use Soap and Water or Alcohol Hand Gel:

Soap and Water	When hands are visibly soiled After caring for patients with diarrhoea
Alcohol Hand Gel	When hands appear clean but require antisepsis Between patient contacts Before and during aseptic techniques

Personal Protective Equipment (PPE)

Personal protective equipment is used to prevent members of staff acquiring infections as well as preventing their clothing from becoming contaminated with infectious microorganisms. PPE includes gloves, plastic aprons, goggles, visors and face masks.

Gloves (contact)
- Should be worn when handling blood and other body fluids, drainage material, invasive devices such as catheters and equipment that has been in contact with infective patients
- Should **NOT** be worn continuously but should be removed when the task has been completed and definitely between patients

Plastic Aprons (splashes)
- Should be worn when there is a risk of splashing with body fluids
- Should **NOT** be worn continuously but should be removed when the task has been completed and definitely between patients

Goggles or Medical Visors (splashes)
- Should be worn when there is a risk of splashing of body fluids into the eyes or mouth e.g. intubation, nasopharyngeal aspiration, tracheostomy care, chest physiotherapy, bronchoscopy, cardiopulmonary resuscitation, open suctioning of the airway
- Should **NOT** be worn continuously but should be removed when the task has been completed and definitely between patients

Face Masks (airborne)
- Should only be worn when there is a risk of airborne spread of infection such as during aerosol-generating procedures (as per procedures under Goggles or Medical Visors above)
- Should **NOT** be worn continuously but should be removed when the task has been completed and definitely between patients

PPE Usage and Side rooms
It is necessary for staff to put on PPE every time they enter a side room. Exceptions to PPE usage for staff, patients and visitors include:
- Where there will be no contact with the patient or their immediate environment e.g. members of the MDT on a ward round who are observing
- In an emergency situation e.g. patient about to remove CVC or ETT or fall. Attend to the emergency and then decontaminate. Encourage Emergency Medical Team (Crash Team) to use PPE if situation allows
- Porters moving patients around the hospital who are only dealing with the patient's environment. Deliver the patient and then decontaminate self and equipment e.g. hands/trolley/wheelchair
- Visitors of a patient should be encouraged to wash their hands on exit. They may choose to wear PPE if assisting in care-giving but as they do not risk transferring microorganisms to another patient they are not obliged to wear PPE
- Patients who are in a side room can leave without PPE but they should be encouraged to wash their hands on exit. For MDR TB the patient must wear a FFP3 mask when moving around the hospital. For precautions regarding MDR TB (see section - Infection Control, Multidrug Resistant TB)

Summary of Isolation Priority and Infection Control Precautions

"Help! I have 3 patients and only 2 side rooms" is a common problem for an oncall Microbiologist. Below is the priority for use of side rooms for the most common scenarios.

Microorganism	Priority	Isolation
Viral Haemorrhagic Fever	1	See section – Infection Control, Viral Haemorrhagic Fever: Control Measures
Influenza	2	Up to 7 days after onset, 14 days if immunodeficient
Open Pulmonary Tuberculosis	3	Until 2 weeks of completed antibiotic treatment **OR** until discharge
Measles	4	Until 5 days after onset of rash
Varicella Zoster Virus (VZV) Chicken Pox and Shingles	5	Until vesicles dry and crusted over
Meningitis	6	Bacterial meningitis only Until 24 hours after antibiotics started
Clostridium difficile Associated Disease (CDAD)	7	Until diarrhoea resolved for 48 hours
Diarrhoea and Vomiting	8	Until diarrhoea and vomiting resolved for 48 hours
Antibiotic Resistant Gram-negative Bacteria	9	Until discharge unless higher priority case requires isolation
MRSA	10	Until discharge unless higher priority case requires isolation
Glycopeptide resistant *Enterococcus* (GRE)	11	Until discharge unless higher priority case requires isolation
Group A Beta-haemolytic *Streptococcus*	12	Until 24 hours after antibiotics started
Cellulitis	13	Until 24 hours after antibiotics started

If there are more patients than side rooms discuss the situation with the hospital Bed Manager, rather than a Microbiologist, as they will be able to help with up-to-date bed allocation and prioritisation.

PPE	Additional Information
See section – Infection Control, Viral Haemorrhagic Fever: Control Measures	Viral haemorrhagic fever takes priority over everything!
Universal precautions	Surgical face mask, gloves and apron required if within 1 metre of patient **OR** when patient receiving nebulised medication. Gloves, gowns and FFP3 face protection for aerosol-generating procedures
Universal precautions FFP2 face mask for aerosol-generating procedures	FFP3 face mask if caring for patient with open pulmonary MDR-TB in negative pressure room
Universal precautions	Staff caring for patient must be immune
Universal precautions	Staff caring for patient must be immune
Universal precautions Face mask required for aerosol-generating procedures	
Universal precautions	Separate toilet facilities Hand hygiene with soap and water
Universal precautions	Separate toilet facilities Hand hygiene with soap and water
Universal precautions	
Universal precautions	
Universal precautions	
Universal precautions	
Universal precautions	

Influenza

There are 3 types of *Influenza Virus*, which commonly affect patients: A, B and C. Although influenza B and C can spread easily, from an infection control perspective, influenza A is of greater significance as it can cause pandemics. Influenza A spreads readily in healthcare settings with a high mortality in at-risk groups (see section – Clinical Scenarios, Influenza).

Influenza A Virus can undergo antigenic drift and antigenic shift:
- **Drift** is due to small changes in the genetics of the virus, meaning people become infected but as they have experienced a similar virus their bodies can recognise a large element of the new virus. Relatively few people are infected and have milder symptoms. This is seasonal flu, which genetically changes slightly but continuously
- **Shift** occurs when the virus acquires new genes from a different *Influenza Virus*. This creates a new virus people have not been exposed to yet, capable of causing a pandemic. Pandemic "Swine Flu" and "Bird Flu" are examples of antigenic shift in an animal, e.g. the pig had both human and avian flu and genes swapped between them to create a new *Influenza Virus*. These pandemic viruses tend to become the "next" seasonal virus after the population has been exposed

Mode of Transmission
- Transmission usually occurs via droplets and aerosols.

Incubation Period
- 1-4 days, although most infections occur within 2 days of exposure.

Period of Communicability
- Potential cross-infection can occur any time the patient continues to shed virus from the upper respiratory tract. This is usually 3-5 days, although children and the immunodeficient can shed the virus for 10-14 days.

Best Practice Control Measures

Careful antibiotic prescribing	Oseltamivir or Zanamivir should be started as early as possible, ideally within 48 hours of the onset of symptoms
Hand hygiene	With soap and water or alcohol hand gel
PPE	Surgical face mask, gloves and apron required if within 1 metre of patient or when patient receiving nebulised medication. Gloves, gowns and FFP3 face protection for aerosol-generating procedures. Remove **ALL** PPE before leaving room
Isolation	Side room with own toilet facility for 7 days or 14 days if immunodeficient Door to be kept closed
Environmental decontamination	Deep cleaning of the clinical area daily and after patient is discharged
Patient care	If patients require investigations in other departments, inform those departments of patient's condition in advance Patient should be last on a list and deep cleaning commence after patient's departure

Tuberculosis (TB)

Tuberculosis refers to infections caused by bacteria of the *Mycobacterium tuberculosis* (MTB) complex, which includes *M. tuberculosis*. The infection control concern regarding TB is its ability to spread by aerosols and droplets between patients and members of staff. It is difficult to treat and increasing antibiotic resistance is leading to increased mortality again.

Mode of Transmission
- Aerosol
- Very rarely, MTB complex bacteria can be acquired through ingestion

Incubation Period
- 2-10 weeks

Period of Communicability
- Patients are infectious whilst viable bacteria are present in sputum. In practical terms this includes patients with cough and/or smear positive for acid fast bacilli in sputum samples
- Only admit to hospital if clinically required
- Patients in whom TB is suspected should be isolated until 3 sputum samples on 3 separate days are negative on staining for acid fast bacilli
- If a TB patient remains in hospital, they should be kept isolated until:
  - They have received at least 2 weeks of antibiotic therapy
  - Their cough has reduced
  - They have been afebrile for 1 week and have clinically improved
  - There are no immunocompromised patients in the area they are being moved to
  - They do not have extensive pulmonary involvement e.g. cavitation
  - They do not have laryngeal TB

Best Practice Control Measures

Antibiotic treatment	Treatment should be guided by an experienced Respiratory or Infectious Diseases Physician
Hand hygiene	With soap and water or alcohol gel
PPE	See section – Infection Control, Personal Protective Equipment Remove **ALL** PPE before leaving room FFP2 face mask for aerosol-generating procedures
Isolation	Negative pressure side room with own toilet facility if available otherwise normal side room with own toilet facility Door to be kept closed Relatives must be symptom free before visiting
Environmental decontamination	Deep cleaning of the clinical area daily and after patient is discharged
Patient care	If patients require investigations in other departments, inform those departments of patient's condition in advance Patient should be last on a list and deep cleaning commence after patient's departure

Multidrug Resistant Tuberculosis (MDR TB)

Multidrug resistant TB (MDR TB) is resistant to antibiotics commonly used to treat tuberculosis. All patients suspected of having TB should be assessed for the risk of MDR TB. Approximately 4% of new TB in the UK is MDR TB.

Definition of Resistant TB
MDR TB - Resistant to Isoniazid and Rifampicin
XDR TB - Resistant to Isoniazid, Rifampicin, fluoroquinolones and aminoglycosides

Risk Factors for MDR or XDR TB
- Previous TB treatment
- Current TB treatment failure
- Contact with patient with known MDR TB
- HIV co-infection
- London residence
- Male aged 25-44
- Travel to or from a country with ≥5% rate of MDR TB
  - At time of writing principally Eastern Europe, the former Soviet States and Russia although rates are increasing across all continents
  - Check World Health Organisation website for up-to-date information

MDR TB - Control Measures

Antibiotic treatment	Treatment should be guided by an experienced Respiratory or Infectious Diseases Physician using a 6 drug treatment regimen
Hand hygiene	With soap and water or alcohol gel
PPE	See section – Infection Control, Personal Protective Equipment Remove **ALL** PPE before leaving room FFP3 face mask when entering patients room
Isolation	Negative pressure side room with own toilet facility if available otherwise normal side room with own toilet facility until able to transfer to unit with negative pressure side room Door to be kept closed Relatives must be symptom free before visiting
Environmental decontamination	Deep cleaning of the clinical area daily and after patient is discharged
Patient care	If patients require investigations in other departments, inform those departments of patient's condition in advance Patient should be last on a list and deep cleaning commence after patient's departure The patient should wear an FFP3 mask when moving around the hospital On discharge from hospital inform the local Health Protection England Centre

Respiratory Spread Viral and Bacterial Infections

There are a number of microorganisms spread by droplets from the respiratory tract of infected patients, but which do not present with respiratory symptoms. As a result, healthcare staff can forget that these infections require specific infection control measures and other patients can be put at risk of cross-transmission.

These microorganisms include:
- *Measles Virus*
- *Varicella Zoster Virus* (Chicken Pox and Shingles)
- *Neisseria meningitidis*
- Group A Beta-haemolytic *Streptococcus*

Mode of Transmission
- Transmission usually occurs via droplets, but can also occur from direct contact with lesions.

Incubation Period
- *Measles Virus* – 7-18 days
- *Varicella Zoster Virus* (Chicken Pox) – 10-21 days
- *Neisseria meningitidis* - 2-10 days, average 4 days
- Group A Beta-haemolytic *Streptococcus* - 1-3 days

Period of Communicability
- *Measles Virus* – 4 days before to 4 days after rash
- *Varicella Zoster Virus* (Chicken Pox and Shingles) – 2 days before vesicles appear until all vesicles are dry and crusted over
- *Neisseria meningitidis* - until 24 hours after starting antibiotics
- Group A Beta-haemolytic *Streptococcus* - until 24 hours after starting antibiotics

Best Practice Control Measures

Hand hygiene	With soap and water or alcohol gel
PPE	See section – Infection Control, Personal Protective Equipment Remove **ALL** PPE before leaving room
Isolation	Side room with own toilet facility Door to be kept closed
Staffing	Patients with *Measles Virus* or *Varicella Zoster Virus* should only be cared for by staff who are known to be immune to these infections
Environmental decontamination	Deep cleaning of the clinical area daily and after patient is discharged
Patient care	If patients require investigations in other departments, inform those departments of patient's condition in advance Patient should be last on a list and deep cleaning commence after patient's departure

Clostridium difficile Associated Disease (CDAD)

The bacterium *Clostridium difficile* was reclassified in 2016 to *Clostridioides difficile* but as this has not yet become mainstream this book will continue to use the old name. It is the most common cause of antibiotic associated diarrhoea. It spreads very readily in the hospital environment unless infection control measures are put in place. Clinical features of *Clostridium difficile* Associated Disease (CDAD) range from asymptomatic carriage through to diarrhoea, toxic megacolon and death.

Mode of Transmission
- Faecal-oral spread
- *Clostridium difficile* can survive for long periods of time in the environment as spores which, if not removed, can then infect new patients

Incubation Period
- Unknown
- Symptoms can occur at any time after prescribing antibiotics, however usually 5-10 days

Period of Communicability
- Patients should remain in isolation until 48 hours after symptoms resolve

Best Practice Control Measures

Careful antibiotic prescribing	Where possible avoid the use of antibiotics which are regarded as particularly predisposing to CDAD – the "**4Cs**" • **C**ephalosporins • **C**iprofloxacin and other quinolones • **C**lindamycin • **C**o-amoxiclav Reduced Ciprofloxacin usage was the main driver for decreasing CDAD in the UK
Hand hygiene	With soap and water, alcohol gel is **NOT** effective
PPE	See section – Infection Control, Personal Protective Equipment Remove **ALL** PPE before leaving room
Isolation	Side room preferably with own toilet facility
Environmental decontamination	Deep cleaning of the clinical area daily and after patient is discharged
Patient care	Accurate recording of symptoms Stool sample for *Clostridium difficile* toxin testing Do not prescribe anti-motility agents If patients require investigations in other departments, inform those departments of patient's condition in advance Patient should be last on a list and deep cleaning commence after patient's departure

Antibiotics cause CDAD. **FALSE** - Antibiotics do not cause CDAD they only predispose to CDAD. If a patient does not come into contact with *Clostridium difficile* bacteria the patient will not get CDAD even if they have many predisposing factors (e.g. over 65 years old, cancer, bowel surgery, previous antibiotics, nasojejunal tubes, Proton Pump Inhibitors, hospitalisation or living in a long-term care facility). Eradicating *Clostridium difficile* from the environment by good cleaning practices is of fundamental importance in the control of CDAD.

The attitude that certain antibiotics should be avoided at all cost so as to avoid CDAD **is potentially dangerous**. The correct antibiotic for the infection should be given whilst being aware of the risk of predisposing to CDAD. For example, an elderly patient with urosepsis who is allergic to Penicillin, the doctors don't want to use Ciprofloxacin as it predisposes to CDAD and don't like using Gentamicin because it can cause renal failure. As a result they choose a seemingly random antibiotic such as Teicoplanin...Why? This is like putting diesel in a petrol car...it is simply wrong. The antibiotic needs to be active against the causative microorganism and able to penetrate the infected site.

Teicoplanin is probably the worst possible choice because it has no activity against the common causes of urosepsis and therefore the patient may die as a result of avoiding the use of Ciprofloxacin for fear of causing CDAD infection. Interestingly, doctors don't worry about prescribing Ceftriaxone for meningitis even though this antibiotic also predisposes to CDAD.

Don't select the wrong antibiotic for the infection the patient currently has because you are worried they may acquire another infection in the future.

In order to try and reduce the incidence of CDAD, hospitals are restricting the use of high risk predisposing antibiotics. As a result there is an increasing reliance on a small pool of antibiotics to treat a broad range of infections. The heavy use of these antibiotics is leading to increasing bacterial resistance. For example, an empirical guideline that uses a lot of Beta-lactam-Beta-lactamase inhibitor combinations (Co-amoxiclav and Piptazobactam) leads to increased numbers of infections with AmpC and ESBL-positive bacteria.

The increased rates of resistant bacteria mean an over reliance on carbapenem antibiotics (e.g. Meropenem); this has led to a rapid rise in carbapenemase producing Enterobacteriaceae. Not only are there no new antibiotics becoming available to treat these resistant bacteria, carbapenems also predispose to CDAD. Ultimately CDAD rates will increase while our ability to treat resistant infections decreases.

The current strategy of restricting antibiotics is storing up a problem for the future. Restrictive antibiotic guidelines put a strong selective pressure on bacteria that are far better at evolving than humans. Controlling CDAD in the environment may be a better long-term solution even though this proves harder to implement.

Doctor A examines Patient W and diagnoses CDAD. He wrongly uses alcohol gel to clean his hands (alcohol gel does not kill spores △). Doctor A should have used soap and water and isolated patient W

Doctor A correctly gives Ciprofloxacin to Patient Z. Patient Z acquires *Clostridium difficile* spores from the environment, which exploit the niche left by Ciprofloxacin leading to Patient Z developing CDAD

Patient W has CDAD but is not isolated in a side room

Patient Z is in renal failure, has a catheter associated UTI with *Pseudomonas* and a severe Penicillin allergy

Doctor B's Patient

Doctor B's Patient

Doctor A transmits a few *Clostridium difficile* spores to Patient X via his hands but there is no niche for the spores to exploit. Patient X is at risk of becoming a carrier of *Clostridium difficile*

Doctor A does not transmit *Clostridium difficile* spores to Patient Y. Even though Patient Y is on predisposing antibiotics they do not develop CDAD because they have not acquired the bacteria

Patient X with asthma is examined, there is no need for antibiotics

Patient Y with community acquired pneumonia is on Co-amoxiclav and Clarithromycin

Doctor A washes his hands at the sink with soap and water removing the *Clostridium difficile* spores

The development of CDAD is often multi-factorial and there are many predisposing factors but ultimately the patient has to acquire the bacterium *Clostridium difficile* before they can develop CDAD or become a carrier of *Clostridium difficile*.

The root cause for CDAD in Patient Z is failure to isolate Patient W in a side room NOT the antibiotic Ciprofloxacin

Diarrhoea and Vomiting (D&V)

Diarrhoea and vomiting is not a common cause of mortality amongst most people, however the old and frail or immunodeficient can die. The microorganisms that cause diarrhoea and vomiting are so infectious they easily spread around healthcare settings unless precautions are taken. The majority of cases are caused by viruses such as *Norovirus* and *Rotavirus*.

Mode of Transmission
- Faecal-oral spread. In a patient with *Norovirus* each gram of stool contains approximately 10-100 million infectious doses of virus

Incubation Period
- *Norovirus* - 24-48 hours
- *Rotavirus* - 24-72 hours

Period of Communicability
- Up to 48 hours after symptoms resolve
- Virus is often still detectable at low levels in stool after symptoms resolve, so ongoing effective hand hygiene is essential

Best Practice Control Measures

Hand hygiene	With soap and water, alcohol gel is **NOT** effective
PPE	See section – Infection Control, Personal Protective Equipment Remove **ALL** PPE before leaving room
Isolation	Side room preferably with own toilet facility
Ward closure	Only after advice from the Infection Control Team (ICT) and only if insufficient number of side rooms to isolate cases
Staffing	If ward closed, access to ward for essential staff only Symptomatic staff must not return to work until 48 hours after last episode of diarrhoea or vomiting
Environmental decontamination	Deep cleaning of the clinical area daily and after patient is discharged
Patient care	Accurate recording of symptoms Stool sample for testing under advice from ICT Do not prescribe anti-motility agents If patients require investigations in other departments, inform those departments of patient's condition in advance Patient should be last on a list and deep cleaning commence after patient's departure

Hints and Tips
Even with the very best cleaning regimens, a patient with diarrhoea will put their normal gastrointestinal flora into the environment whatever the cause of their diarrhoea. This can include Enterobacteriaceae, *Enterococcus* spp. and *Pseudomonas* spp. even though these are not causes of diarrhoea. If patients with diarrhoea due to the same cause (e.g. *Norovirus* or CDAD) were kept together in the same clinical area (cohorted) transfer of normal gastrointestinal flora will occur between patients. If one patient has antibiotic resistant bacteria in their normal flora e.g. GRE, then all cohorted patients will eventually acquire the antibiotic resistant bacteria. Therefore cohorting patients should be avoided, source isolation is best practice.

Multiple Antibiotic Resistant Gram-negative Bacteria

Increasing antibiotic resistance in Gram-negative bacteria is making initial antibiotic choice more difficult and therefore mortality is rising. Currently there are few new anti-Gram-negative antibiotics being developed by the pharmaceutical industry.

There are 3 main groups of multiple antibiotic resistant Gram-negative bacteria:
- Enterobacteriaceae with ESBL, AmpC or carbapenemase enzymes – including *Escherichia coli*, *Klebsiella* spp., *Enterobacter cloacae*, *Citrobacter freundii*, *Morganella morganii*, *Serratia marcescens*
- *Acinetobacter* spp. – resistant to aminoglycoside antibiotics as well as occasionally carbapenems and Colistin
- *Pseudomonas* spp. – resistant to combinations of Ceftazidime, Piptazobactam, carbapenems, aminoglycosides and quinolones

Mode of Transmission
- Transmission can occur via hands or via faecal-oral colonisation.

Incubation Period
- Many Gram-negative bacteria are able to colonise people. Once the microorganism is part of the patient's normal flora it can potentially cause infection and be spread to others at any time. The majority of infections with Gram-negative bacteria follow previous colonisation.

Period of Communicability
- Potential cross-infection can occur at any time whilst the patient remains colonised with the resistant bacteria. However, risk is highest with environmental contamination e.g. during outbreaks of diarrhoea.

Best Practice Control Measures

Careful antibiotic prescribing	Certain antibiotics have been implicated in the selection of antibiotic resistant Gram-negative bacteria e.g. Ciprofloxacin and the Beta-lactam-Beta-lactamase inhibitor combination antibiotics such as Co-amoxiclav and Piptazobactam
Hand hygiene	With soap and water or alcohol hand gel
PPE	See section – Infection Control, Personal Protective Equipment Remove **ALL** PPE before leaving room
Isolation	Side room preferably with own toilet facility
Environmental decontamination	Deep cleaning of the clinical area daily and after patient is discharged

Carbapenemases
Strains of *Klebsiella* spp. and *Escherichia coli* are now regularly isolated which are resistant to the carbapenem antibiotics. A carbapenemase is any Beta-lactamase enzyme that:
- Can breakdown carbapenem antibiotics
- Gives resistance to **ALL** of the Beta-lactam antibiotics such as the penicillins and cephalosporins
- Is often associated with other genes giving resistance to other antibiotics such as the quinolones and aminoglycosides

Carbapenemases are important because the carbapenems (Ertapenem, Meropenem, Imipenem and Doripenem) are often seen as the last line of antibiotics in the fight against infections with Gram-negative bacteria. Carbapenem resistance is not associated with a specific infection but rather with a diverse clinical spectrum of diseases. Infections due to bacteria with these enzymes have a very high mortality in excess of 50%.

The genes which encode these enzymes are usually located on a mobile genetic element such as a plasmid and therefore have the potential to spread between bacterial species. The most important currently are known as the "Big Five":
- *Klebsiella pneumoniae* carbapenemase (KPC)
- New Delhi metallo-beta-lactamase (NDM)
- Verona integron-encoded metallo-beta-lactamase (VIM)
- Imipenem metallo-beta-lactamase (IMP)
- Oxacillin carbapenemases (OXA)

Treatment of Patients with Infections
Most carbapenemase-producing bacteria remain susceptible to: Polymyxins e.g. Colistin, Tigecycline, Nitrofurantoin and Fosfomycin. The current recommendations for the treatment of patients with severe infections caused by carbapenemase producing bacteria are combinations of antibiotics: Colistin **PLUS** carbapenem, Colistin **PLUS** Tigecycline or Colistin **PLUS** aminoglycoside.

Patient Screening
On admission to hospital, patients will be classified as either:
1) NOT infected or colonised (no further action required)
2) CONFIRMED (infection or colonisation)
3) SUSPECTED (infection or colonisation)

How to Screen for Carbapenemase–Producing Bacteria
- Rectal charcoal swab with visible faecal material **OR** stool sample
- **PLUS** charcoal swab from any wound and device-related site if hospitalised within the previous 12 months in a country with a high prevalence of carbapenemase producing bacteria

CONFIRMED
- Patients who have a positive microbiological culture for carbapenemase producing bacteria from a clinical specimen or screening test at any stage during their admission to any hospital

SUSPECTED
- Patients who have been an inpatient in a hospital abroad
- **OR** been an inpatient in a UK hospital known to have had problems with spread of carbapenemase-producing Enterobacteriaceae
- **OR** previously been colonised or had an infection with a carbapenemase producing Enterobacteriaceae
- **OR** had close contact with a person who has been colonised or had an infection with a carbapenemase producing Enterobacteriaceae

Screening	Send weekly screening samples
Careful antibiotic prescribing	If patient has an infection seek specialist advice from a Microbiologist or Infectious Diseases Physician
Hand hygiene	With soap and water or alcohol hand gel
Personal Protective Equipment	See section – Infection Control, Personal Protective Equipment Remove **ALL** PPE before leaving room
Isolation	Side room preferably with own toilet facility for duration of hospital stay
Environmental decontamination	Deep cleaning of the clinical area daily and after patient discharge

Patients with **CONFIRMED** infections or colonisation who have 3 negative screening samples should **ONLY** be moved out of isolation if there is a serious risk to their health from remaining in isolation. This is because the screening tests are not perfect and even if negative now previously positive patients can become positive again, especially if given antibiotics. If in doubt discuss with the Infection Control Team.

Contact Screening and Management
If a patient has not been isolated in a side room and is found to have a carbapenemase-producing bacterium then all contacts within the bays or wards in which they have been should also be screened. This **DOES NOT** include household contacts or members of hospital staff.

All contacts should be isolated or cohorted together whilst awaiting results of screening samples if possible. If initial screening tests are negative they should have repeat screening samples sent on day 2 and day 4 and if they remain negative in all three samples they can then be managed as normal and the isolation or cohorting relaxed.

If a contact tests positive then they should be managed as a **CONFIRMED** infection or colonisation **AND** all of their contacts should be screened.

No further management is recommended after the patient is discharged from hospital although nursing care facilities would be recommended to consider the risk of transmission within their environments.

The patient and their General Practitioner should be made aware of the patient's status so that if they are re-admitted to hospital the hospital is made aware of their status.

Warning
In 2015, 25% of pork and poultry meat on sale in China were found to contain Enterobacteriaceae resistant to Colistin. The Colistin resistance was encoded by a gene in a plasmid (which can transfer to other bacteria) called MCR-1. With MCR-1 mother nature now has all she needs to create bacteria, such as *E. coli,* which are resistant to **ALL** antibiotics currently used to treat infections. Complete resistance occurred in a patient from the USA who had surgery in India in 2017.

New Antibiotics for Treating Resistant Gram-negative Bacteria

New antibiotics for the treatment of antibiotic resistant Gram-negative bacteria can be split into:
- **Combinations** of existing beta-lactams with beta-lactamase inhibitors e.g. Ceftolozane + Tazobactam, Ceftazidime + Avibactam, Meropenem + Vaborbactam, Imipenem + Relebactam and Aztreonam + Avibactam
- **New versions** of old antibiotics that aren't beta-lactams e.g. Eravacycline, Plazomicin and Cefiderocol.

Spectrum of activity of "new" antibiotics

✓ = active   ?= partial/unreliable activity   - = inactive

Antibiotic	Enterobacteriaceae (e.g. *E. coli, Klebsiella* spp.)					Pseudomonas spp.		Acinetobacter spp.
	ESBL	AmpC	KPC	OXA-48	NDM	Efflux	AmpC	
Ceftolozane + Tazobactam	✓	?	-	?	-	✓	✓	-
Ceftazidime + Avibactam	✓	✓	✓	✓	-	?	✓	-
Meropenem + Vaborbactam	✓	✓	✓	-	-	-	✓	?
Imipenem + Relebactam	✓	✓	✓	-	-	✓	✓	?
Aztreonam + Avibactam	✓	✓	✓	✓	✓	-	?	-
Eravacycline	✓	✓	✓	✓	✓	-	-	✓
Plazomicin	✓	✓	✓	✓	-	?	?	?
Cefiderocol	✓	✓	✓	✓	✓	✓	✓	✓

Note: As of November 2018 only Ceftolozane + Tazobactam and Ceftazidime + Avibactam are routinely available in the UK.

Meticillin Resistant *Staphylococcus aureus* (MRSA)

MRSA is *Staphylococcus aureus* that has acquired resistance to the antibiotic Meticillin. **REMEMBER** MRSA is resistant to all of the Beta-lactam antibiotics in common use: Flucloxacillin, Co-amoxiclav, Piptazobactam, cephalosporins and carbapenems. Although hospitals and the Department of Health concentrate on MRSA figures, 3% of the population carry MRSA as part of the normal flora in their nose and 30% of the population carry Meticillin sensitive *Staphylococcus aureus* (MSSA) as part of their normal flora.

Mode of Transmission
- MRSA is usually transmitted between patients on the hands of healthcare staff or on contaminated equipment (fomites).

Incubation Period
- MRSA is able to colonise people. Once the microorganism is part of the patient's normal flora it can potentially cause infection and be spread to others at any time. Most MRSA infections follow previous colonisation.

Period of Communicability
- Potential cross-infection can occur at any time whilst the patient remains colonised with the resistant bacteria. However risk, is highest when patients have skin diseases that allow heavy shedding of bacteria e.g. eczema, psoriasis.

Screening
Current UK practice is to screen all previously positive patients and all new patients admitted to high-risk units including:

- Vascular surgery
- Neurosurgery
- Cardiothoracic surgery
- Orthopaedics and trauma
- Critical care (ICU, HDU, SCBU)
- Renal dialysis
- Haematology and oncology
- Coronary Care

Body sites to screen include:
- Nose and groin
- Umbilicus in neonates
- Wounds – any breach in skin including IV catheter sites (separate swab for each site or you risk transmitting bacteria)
- Urine if patient catheterised
- Sputum if productive cough

Suppression Therapy

All cases	Nasal ointment: Mupirocin 2% (Bactroban®) applied to inside of the nose 3x/day for 5 days Alternative Naseptin® (Chlorhexidine **PLUS** Neomycin) 4x/day for 10 days
PLUS For adults	Body and hair wash: 4% Chlorhexidine 1x/day for 5 days Alternative Octenisan® wash 1x/day for 5 days

Patients should be re-screened 48 hours after MRSA suppression therapy has stopped. If the patient remains positive continue to manage as MRSA positive. If the patient tests negative, rescreen at 48 hourly intervals until 3 negative screens at which point the patient is considered MRSA-free. If any of these screens are positive then continue to manage the patient as MRSA positive.

Careful antibiotic prescribing	Avoid using Beta-lactam antibiotics on their own for infections where *Staphylococcus aureus* is a potential pathogen and ensure the use of an antibiotic that is active against MRSA
Hand hygiene	With soap and water or alcohol gel
PPE	See section – Infection Control, Personal Protective Equipment Remove **ALL** PPE before leaving room
Isolation	Side room preferably with own toilet facility
Environmental decontamination	Change laundry daily after bathing Deep cleaning of the clinical area daily and after patient is discharged
Patient care	If patients require investigations in other departments, inform those departments of patient's condition in advance Patient should be last on a list and deep cleaning commence after patient's departure

Myth

MRSA is more transmissible than MSSA. **FALSE** – MRSA and MSSA are just as easily transmitted. The only difference is that MRSA is resistant to the Beta-lactam antibiotics, which have traditionally been used to treat infections caused by *Staphylococcus aureus*.

MRSA was identified as an infection control target because it has an easily recognisable antibiotic sensitivity pattern, which allowed descriptive epidemiology to show to whom and where it had been transmitted. This, in turn, allowed infection control strategies to be formulated to prevent transmission. MSSA could not be used because 30% of the population carry different strains as part of their normal flora; it is impossible to distinguish between these strains based on sensitivity patterns.

Infection control policies concentrate on important communicable infections but they do not always concentrate on **ALL** the transmissible microorganisms. There is always a danger that Department of Health targets might take precedence over microbiological priorities. The most transmissible microorganisms that worry Microbiologists, due to their potential to cause outbreaks, are currently (in order of concern):
1. **High mortality respiratory or droplet spread infections** e.g. Viral Haemorrhagic Fever (VHF), Severe Acute Respiratory Syndrome (SARS), pandemic influenza and MDR and XDR tuberculosis
2. **Respiratory viruses** e.g. seasonal influenza, RSV and *Adenovirus*
3. **Droplet spread viruses** e.g. Measles and Chicken Pox (VZV)
4. **Gastroenteritis** e.g. *Norovirus*, *Rotavirus* and *Clostridium difficile*
5. **Respiratory bacteria** e.g. *M. tuberculosis* and *N. meningitidis*
6. **Resistant bacteria** e.g. MRSA, GRE, antibiotic resistant Gram-negative bacteria

MRSA is not the only infection control concern; good infection control practices (hand washing, PPE, isolation and deep cleaning) should be taken with **ALL** patients.

Panton-Valentine Leukocidin (PVL) Positive *Staphylococcus aureus*

PVL positive *Staphylococcus aureus* is a *S. aureus* that produces the toxin PVL. The toxin may be a defence mechanism used by the bacteria against the host's immune system as it breaks down white blood cells and increases the virulence of these bacteria.

Of the 30% of the population who have *S. aureus* as part of their normal flora, approximately 2% have bacteria that can produce PVL toxin.

PVL positive *S. aureus* often cause recurrent and severe skin and soft tissue infections such as boils and carbuncles, but occasionally they are implicated in more severe infections such as necrotising pneumonia, which has a 75% mortality rate.

PVL positive *S. aureus* can be either MRSA or MSSA. It is difficult to predict which will produce PVL toxin except on the basis of a clinical history of recurrent skin and soft tissue infections.

The normal treatment for PVL positive *S. aureus* is with antibiotics that have the ability to switch off toxin production such as Clindamycin and Linezolid.

> **Warning**
> There is increasing evidence that the use of cell wall active agents, such as the Beta-lactams (Flucloxacillin, Co-amoxiclav, Piptazobactam, cephalosporins and carbapenems), to treat PVL positive *S. aureus*, causes increased toxin production by the bacteria. One theory for this is that if bacterial survival is threatened the bacteria's "immune response" is to increase PVL toxin production. Another theory is that by lysing the bacterial cell the contents of the cell will be released including toxin. Whatever the reason, PVL positive patients treated with Beta-lactams often become more unwell despite apparent antibiotic sensitivity on laboratory testing (in vitro).

Mode of Transmission
- PVL positive *S. aureus* appears to be more capable of transferring between people than normal *S. aureus*, even though this is not a Department of Health target. As a result, "closed" communities are at risk of PVL positive *S. aureus* outbreaks, e.g. military personnel, sports teams, prisons and nurseries. PVL positive *S. aureus* is usually transmitted between patients on the hands of healthcare staff or on contaminated equipment (fomites).

Incubation Period
- Many PVL positive *S. aureus* are able to colonise people. Once the microorganism is part of the patient's normal flora it can potentially cause infection and be spread to others at any time. The majority of infections with PVL positive *S. aureus* follow previous colonisation.

Period of Communicability
- Potential cross-infection can occur at any time whilst the patient remains colonised with the resistant bacteria. However, risk is highest when patients have skin diseases that allow heavy shedding of bacteria e.g. eczema, psoriasis.

Screening
- Public Health England recommend screening close contacts of patients with proven PVL positive strains of *S. aureus* and offering both the patient and their contacts topical suppression. This is similar to the process used for MRSA.

Body sites to screen include:
- Nose
- Groin
- Throat

Suppression Therapy

All cases	Nasal ointment: Mupirocin 2% (Bactroban®) applied to inside of the nose 3x/day for 5 days Alternative Naseptin® (Chlorhexidine **PLUS** Neomycin) 4x/day for 10 days
PLUS For adults	Body and hair wash: 4% Chlorhexidine 1x/day for 5 days Alternative Octenisan® wash 1x/day for 5 days

Patients should be re-screened 48 hours after suppression therapy has stopped. If the patient remains positive continue to manage as PVL positive. If the patient tests negative, rescreen at 48 hourly intervals until 3 negative screens at which point the patient may be considered PVL-free. If any of these screens are positive then continue to manage the patient as PVL positive.

Best Practice Control Measures

Careful antibiotic prescribing	Use Clindamycin or Linezolid to treat proven infections
Hand hygiene	With soap and water or alcohol gel
PPE	See section – Infection Control, Personal Protective Equipment Remove **ALL** PPE before leaving room
Isolation	Side room
Environmental decontamination	Change laundry daily after bathing Deep cleaning of the clinical area daily and after patient is discharged
Patient care	If patients require investigations in other departments, inform those departments of patient's condition in advance Patient should be last on a list and deep cleaning commence after patient's departure

Glycopeptide Resistant *Enterococcus* (GRE) is often also referred to as Vancomycin Resistant *Enterococcus* (VRE) as the glycopeptide antibiotics include Vancomycin as well as Teicoplanin. Enterococci are part of the normal bowel flora of most people. They are relatively less virulent than other bacteria and do not often cause infections. So why do Infection Control Teams and Microbiologists pay particular attention to bacteria like GRE? The answer is because of the way the bacteria gained the resistance to the glycopeptide antibiotics rather than the bacteria themselves.

Warning
Enterococci became resistant to glycopeptides by acquiring a new gene, the GRE gene called vanA, which changed the structure of the *Enterococcus* spp. cell wall.

The GRE gene can potentially be transferred from GRE into other bacteria such as *Staphylococcus aureus* or *Streptococcus pneumoniae*. Consider how dangerous it would be if the GRE gene entered MRSA, resulting in the creation of Glycopeptide resistant *S. aureus* (GRSA). GRSA, unlike GRE, would cause many infections, some of which would be life-threatening. The presence of the GRE gene in GRSA would mean that regular antibiotics could not be used, resulting in an increased number of patient deaths. GRSA has already been reported. This is why Microbiologists worry about GRE.

Fortunately, the GRE gene is only transferable from certain species of GRE, in particular Glycopeptide Resistant *Enterococcus faecium* and *Enterococcus faecalis*. In these species, the GRE gene is on a transposon, a piece of genetic material that can readily transfer between bacteria of the same species and sometimes bacteria of different species (see section – Antibiotics, How is Antibiotic Resistance Spread?).

There are some species of GRE (*Enterococcus casseliflavus* and *Enterococcus gallinarum*) in which the GRE gene is part of the chromosome and not on a transposon. This form of GRE gene cannot be transferred to other bacteria. Seeing these bacteria on a report is of less concern as they rarely cause serious infections and cannot transfer their resistance. Microbiologists are less concerned about these types of GRE.

Mode of Transmission
- Transmission can occur via hands or via faecal-oral spread.

Incubation Period
- Many GRE are able to colonise people. Once the microorganism is part of the patient's normal flora it can potentially cause infection and be spread to others at any time. The majority of infections with GRE follow previous colonisation.

Period of Communicability
- Potential cross-infection can occur at any time whilst the patient remains colonised with the resistant bacteria. However, risk will be highest when environmental contamination from gastrointestinal carriage is highest e.g. during periods of diarrhoea.

Careful antibiotic prescribing	Certain combinations of antibiotics have been implicated in the selection of GRE. In particular, combinations of glycopeptides with cephalosporins or fluoroquinolones (to which Enterococci are inherently resistant).
Hand hygiene	With soap and water or alcohol hand gel
PPE	See section – Infection Control, Personal Protective Equipment Remove **ALL** PPE before leaving room
Isolation	Side room preferably with own toilet facility
Environmental decontamination	Deep cleaning of the clinical area daily and after patient is discharged
Patient care	If patients require investigations in other departments, inform those departments of patient's condition in advance Patient should be last on a list and deep cleaning commence after patient's departure

<u>Viral Haemorrhagic Fever (VHF)</u>

In terms of Infection control, patients with Viral Haemorrhagic Fever (VHF) are the highest priority for isolation. However, for most hospitals the priority is to transfer the patient to a specialist High Level Isolation Unit (HLIU) rather than isolate them within the local hospital. In the UK the HLIU is at the Royal Free Hospital NHS Trust in London.

Viral Haemorrhagic Fevers are rare in the UK and usually only occur in travellers, or contact with travellers, to endemic parts of the world such as Central and West Africa, South America, the Middle East and Eastern Europe. A single UK acquired case has occurred in a laboratory worker who sustained a needlestick injury from a patient with VHF.

The most important viral haemorrhagic fevers are:
- Lassa fever
- Marburg
- Ebola
- Crimean-Congo haemorrhagic fever

Warning
All Viral Haemorrhagic Fevers are infection control emergencies that have a high mortality rate, both in patients and the staff who look after these patients.

Clinical Features
VHFs usually begin with sudden onset:
- Fever
- Headache
- Joint and muscle pains
- Sore throat
- Weakness
- Diarrhoea and vomiting

Later signs are:
- Rash
- Haemorrhages

Mode of Transmission
- Direct or indirect with specific vectors in the country of origin:
  - Lassa fever (rats)
  - Ebola and Marburg (bats and monkeys)
  - Crimean-Congo haemorrhagic fever (ticks)
- Person-to-person from exposure to infected body fluids

Incubation Period
- 3-21 days but normally 7-10 days

Period of Communicability
- It is not known when a patient with VHF first becomes infectious
- Normally, the virus is first detected in body fluids when the patient becomes febrile
- It is not known for certain how long the body fluids remain infectious

Assessment of Risk

In **ALL SUSPECTED CASES** an Infectious Diseases Physician or Microbiologist should be called to assess for risk; risk assessment is a legal requirement in the UK.

Low possibility of VHF	Temperature ≥37.5 ˚C **PLUS** been in endemic area within 21 days of onset of illness
Possibility of VHF	Previously low possibility **PLUS** fever that does not settle within 72 hours **OR** Previously low possibility **PLUS** organ failure **AND/OR** haemorrhage **AND/OR** uncontrolled vomiting
High possibility of VHF	Temperature ≥37.5 ˚C **PLUS** been in endemic area within 21 days of onset of illness **PLUS** answers "yes" to **ONE** of the following questions: 1. Travelled to an area with a current VHF outbreak 2. Lived or worked in basic rural conditions where Lassa is endemic 3. Visited caves/mines or had contact with primates, antelopes or bats in an area where Ebola or Marburg are endemic 4. Travelled to an area where Crimean-Congo is endemic and sustained a tick bite, crushed a tick with bare hands, or had close involvement with animal slaughter **OR** Temperature ≥37.5 °C **PLUS** contact with known **OR** strongly suspected case of VHF **OR** their body fluids including handling clinical specimens

Investigations

In the UK, the Infectious Diseases Physician or Microbiologist will discuss VHF testing with the National Imported Fever Service based at Porton Down on 0844 7788990. Ward staff should not call this service directly.

Sample requirements include **ALL** of the below:
- 4.5ml* serum in red or yellow vacutainer tube
- 4.5ml* whole blood in purple EDTA vacutainer tube
- 20-25ml urine in a sterile universal

Note: *For children a minimum of 1ml can be sent however it will not have an extended imported fever screen in the event the VHF test is negative and the diagnosis is still unclear. Send >1ml if possible.

Urgent results are usually available within 4-6 hours of arrival in the testing laboratory. A positive malaria test **DOES NOT** exclude the diagnosis of VHF; dual infection can occur.

If a patient tests positive for VHF then they should be transferred to an HLIU; in the UK this is located at the Royal Free London NHS Foundation Trust, contact the oncall Infectious Diseases Consultant on 0207 7940500.
IMPORTANT No further tests should be carried out locally unless they would be immediately life-saving.

Control Measures

Low Possibility of VHF – only admit if necessary	
Public health	Notify Consultant in Communicable Disease Control for Public Health England
Isolation	If patient already admitted, transfer to or keep in a single occupancy room with own toilet facility Door to be kept closed If available use a negative pressure room
Hand hygiene	Soap and water or alcohol hand gel
PPE	Use gloves, plastic aprons, fluid repellent surgical face mask and visor **AT ALL TIMES** **PLUS** FFP3 respirator face masks for aerosol-generating procedures* Remove **ALL** PPE before leaving room
Laboratory tests	No specimens should be sent to the laboratory without prior discussion with the Microbiologist Minimum tests can be carried out at containment level 2 in closed analysers or in containment level 3 for open tests e.g. malaria screen
Staff	Restrict the number of staff who have contact with patient to essential staff only Compile a list of all staff in contact with the case, which should be retained by Occupational Health Department
Environmental decontamination	Deep clean clinical area daily by nursing staff caring for patient and after patient is discharged All waste to be treated as infected and disposed of by incineration

*Aerosol-generating procedures include:
- Endotracheal intubation
- Bronchoscopy
- Airway suctioning
- Positive pressure ventilation via a face mask
- High frequency oscillatory ventilation
- Central line insertion
- Diagnostic sputum induction

Possibility OR High Possibility of VHF	
Transfer patient	**DO NOT ADMIT THE PATIENT INTO THE HOSPITAL** Admit or transfer the patient to an HLIU in a Category III ambulance (the ambulance service needs to be notified of the possible diagnosis)
Public health	Notify Consultant in Communicable Disease Control for Public Health England
Transfer patient	If bleeding, diarrhoea or vomiting discuss with HLIU about transferring patient in a Category III ambulance (the ambulance service needs to be notified of the possible diagnosis)
Isolation	If patient already admitted, transfer to or keep in a single occupancy room with own toilet facility and transfer to HLIU as soon as possible Door to be kept closed If available use a negative pressure room
Hand hygiene	Soap and water or alcohol hand gel
PPE	If fever only: Use gloves, plastic aprons, fluid repellent surgical face mask and visor **AT ALL TIMES** **PLUS** FFP3 respirator face masks for aerosol-generating procedures* If bleeding, diarrhoea or vomiting: Use double gloves with extra-long cuffs, surgical cap, full length plastic endoscopy apron over a fluid repellent disposable gown or suit, FFP3 respirator face mask and visor and wellington boots **AT ALL TIMES** Remove **ALL** PPE before leaving room
Laboratory tests	No specimens should be sent to the laboratory without prior discussion with the Microbiologist Minimum tests can be carried out at containment level 2 in closed analysers or in containment level 3 for open tests e.g. malaria screen Further precautions as per local laboratory protocols
Staff	Restrict the number of staff who have contact with patient to essential staff only Use buddy system: two staff members in full PPE inside the room with third staff member outside but in full PPE to assist if necessary and a fourth staff member to observe practice and maintain staff safety and compliance with infection control practice Compile a list of all staff in contact with the case, which should be retained by Occupational Health Department
Environmental decontamination	Deep clean clinical area daily by nursing staff caring for patient and after patient is discharged All waste to be treated as infected and disposed of by incineration

Management of Staff in Contact with VHF

The ICT will determine who is responsible for the assessment, categorisation and management of staff contacts. Each potential contact should be individually assessed for risk of exposure and categorised as per the table below. If required a designated Monitoring Officer will be assigned for the staff member.

Risk category	Description	Advice
Category 0	No contact with Ebola case	• Reassure
Category 1 (very low risk)	No direct contact with patient or body fluids within 21 days including household contact whilst patient asymptomatic	• Reassure • If feeling unwell take temperature, if ≥37.5 ˚C telephone normal medical services • No restrictions on activity or travel
Category 2 (low risk)	Direct contact with symptomatic patient (e.g. household contact) with no contact with body fluids, routine medical or nursing care, handling of laboratory specimens; but used appropriate PPE	• Reassure • Self-monitor temperature twice daily and for other symptoms for 21 days from last exposure • If temperature ≥37.5 ˚C or other symptoms contact designated Monitoring Officer • No restriction on travel • Postpone non-essential medical or dental treatment
Category 3 (high risk)	Unprotected exposure of skin or mucus membranes to potentially infected body fluids including: household contact with body fluids, inappropriate PPE, handling of laboratory specimens without precautions, needlestick injury, kissing or sexual contact within 3 months of patient recovery	• Daily temperature monitoring and report **ALL** recordings to designated Monitoring Officer • If symptoms develop inform designated Monitoring Officer immediately • Local travel only • If healthcare worker no patient contact for 21 days • Postpone non-essential medical or dental treatment • Do not share toothbrushes or razors • Barrier contraception or avoid unprotected sex for 21 days

<u>Needlestick Injuries</u>

The term "needlestick injury" once described when a needle unintentionally punctured a person's skin. However, the term has become used to include any situation where one person is unintentionally exposed to another person's body fluids (e.g. blood, urine or sputum) which may contain a transmissible microorganism. The main microorganisms of concern are those commonly referred to as blood-borne viruses (BBV): *Hepatitis B Virus*, *Hepatitis C Virus* and *Human Immunodeficiency Virus*.:

Mode of Transmission

The most common mechanisms of exposure are through inoculation with a sharp object such as a hypodermic needle (true needlestick injury) and splashes to mucous membranes. The main risk is transmission of *Hepatitis B Virus*, although most patients and staff are more concerned about HIV even though the risk is much lower.

The risk of infection following injection of blood through a hypodermic needle is of the order of:

Hepatitis B: 1 in 3   **Hepatitis C:**   1 in 30   **HIV:**   1 in 300

Management of Needlestick Injury

If a member of staff receives a needlestick injury they should have someone to help them manage the situation objectively. This is usually:

Normal Hours   Occupational Health or Genitourinary Medicine

Out of Hours   A&E doctor or a senior doctor within their own team

Management is based on type of exposure, likelihood of contamination and potential microorganism. The recipient is the person who sustains the injury and the donor is the person whose body fluid is received.

Hepatitis B Virus (HBV)

Healthcare staff should have been vaccinated against *Hepatitis B Virus* and know their status. Non-significant exposure includes no significant risk e.g. a sterile needle, or recipient not exposed to any body fluids.

HBV Non-significant Exposure

Recipients HBV status	Action
≤1 dose HBV vaccine	Initiate HBV vaccination full course
≥2 doses HBV vaccine pre-exposure (anti-HBs unknown)	Finish course of HBV vaccine
Known vaccine responder (anti-HBs >10mIU/ml)	Consider 1 booster dose of HBV vaccine
Known vaccine non-responder (anti-HBs <10mIU/ml)	Consider 1 booster dose of HBV vaccine

HBV Significant Exposure

Management of significant exposure is based upon the recipient's immune status and the donor's infectivity or risk of having hepatitis B.
- **HBIG** = Hepatitis B immunoglobulin
- **Accelerated course of HBV vaccine** = dose given immediately followed by further doses at one and two months.

Recipient's HBV status	Donor's HBsAg Status		
	+ve	Unknown	−ve
≤1 dose HBV vaccine	HBIG x1 **PLUS** Accelerated course of HBV vaccine	Accelerated course of HBV vaccine	Initiate HBV vaccination full course
≥2 doses HBV vaccine pre-exposure (anti-HBs unknown)	1 dose of HBV vaccine and finish course	1 dose of HBV vaccine and finish course	Finish course of HBV vaccine
Known vaccine responder (anti-HBs >10mIU/ml)	1 booster dose of HBV vaccine if last dose ≥1 year ago	1 booster dose of HBV vaccine if last dose ≥1 year ago	Consider 1 booster dose of HBV vaccine
Known vaccine non-responder (anti-HBs <10mIU/ml)	HBIG x1 **PLUS** Consider 1 booster dose of HBV vaccine **PLUS** give 2nd dose of HBIG one month later	HBIG x1 **PLUS** Consider 1 booster dose of HBV vaccine **PLUS** give 2nd dose of HBIG one month later	Consider 1 booster dose of HBV vaccine

Adapted from: Public Health Laboratory Service Hepatitis Subcommittee (1992)

Hepatitis C Virus (HCV)
Test donor for HCV. Send recipient's serum to the laboratory for saving in case later testing required. HCV infection can present months to years after exposure. There is no specific treatment for acute exposure to HCV.

Human Immunodeficiency Virus (HIV)
Post-Exposure Prophylaxis (PEP) should ideally be started within 1 hour of potential exposure to HIV; it is not effective if given more than 72 hours after exposure. PEP should not be given lightly, assess the risk of HIV exposure against the potential serious side effects e.g. convulsions, liver failure, lactic acidosis and bone marrow failure. If given then an HIV test must be taken prior to starting and the recipient should be referred to GUM or Infectious Diseases at the earliest opportunity.

PEP is recommended when the risk of transmission is greater than 1 in 1,000 and could be considered when the risk is up to 1 in 10,000. Risk of HIV transmission = Risk source HIV positive x Risk of exposure. Fortunately, the British Association of Sexual Health & HIV (BASHH) has done the maths!

The calculated transmission risks in the UK for certain situations are:

Type of exposure	Unknown HIV status of donor			Known HIV positive donor
	Donor has no specific risk factors	Donor from Sub-Saharan Africa	Donor IVDU	
Blood transfusion	1 in 20,000	n/a	n/a	9 in 10
Needlestick injury	1 in 70,000	1 in 5,000	1 in 40,000	1 in 300
Splash to mucous membrane	1 in 35,000	1 in 2,500	1 in 20,000	1 in 150

The current PEP recommendations in the UK are:

Type of exposure	Donor HIV positive		Unknown HIV status of donor	
	Viral load detected	**Viral load NOT detected**	**Low HIV prevalence**	**High HIV prevalence***
Splash to mucous membrane	Consider	Not recommended	Not recommended	Consider
Needlestick injury (in the community)	n/a	n/a	Not recommended	Consider
Bite	Not recommended	Not recommended	Not recommended	Not recommended

Note: * IVDU, Sub-Saharan African, Men who have sex with men, Eastern European

The current recommended PEP in the UK is:
Truvada (Tenofovir-Emtricitabine) 1 tablet OD
PLUS Raltegravir 1 tablet BD

Total Duration
28 days

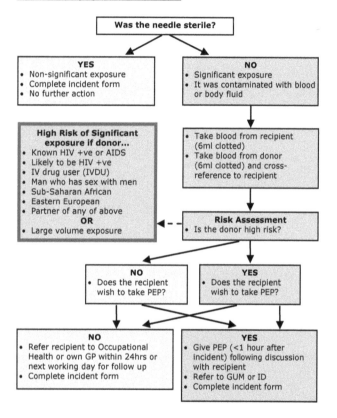

Was the needle sterile?

YES
- Non-significant exposure
- Complete incident form
- No further action

NO
- Significant exposure
- It was contaminated with blood or body fluid

High Risk of Significant exposure if donor...
- Known HIV +ve or AIDS
- Likely to be HIV +ve
- IV drug user (IVDU)
- Man who has sex with men
- Sub-Saharan African
- Eastern European
- Partner of any of above
  OR
- Large volume exposure

- Take blood from recipient (6ml clotted)
- Take blood from donor (6ml clotted) and cross-reference to recipient

Risk Assessment
- Is the donor high risk?

NO
- Does the recipient wish to take PEP?

YES
- Does the recipient wish to take PEP?

NO
- Refer recipient to Occupational Health or own GP within 24hrs or next working day for follow up
- Complete incident form

YES
- Give PEP (<1 hour after incident) following discussion with recipient
- Refer to GUM or ID
- Complete incident form

<u>Outbreaks</u>

Definition of an outbreak: two or more cases of infection associated in **time**, **place** or **person OR** a **single case** of a rare infection occurring out of context, or of significant clinical or political magnitude. Examples of outbreaks:

- **Time** – 2 patients on the same operating list developing MRSA wound infections post-operatively
  - Cause may be a problem with theatre ventilation, failure of instrument sterilisation, poor surgical practice or post-operative wound care
- **Place** – 2 patients on same ward develop CDAD with same strain of *Clostridium difficile*
  - Cause may be failure to isolate first patient, inadequate environmental cleaning, poor hand hygiene, insufficient staffing
- **Person** – 2 patients on different wards at different times develop Influenza after being treated by the same Physiotherapist
  - Cause may be Physiotherapist with *Influenza Virus* infection, insufficient staffing to support sick leave, failure to vaccinate staff
- **Single case** – patient in hospital for 2 weeks develops Legionellosis (incubation period 2-10 days)
  - Cause may be failure to control levels of *Legionella pneumophila* in hospital water supply according to UK national legislation meaning other patients at risk and hospital legally responsible for infection and if patient dies corporate manslaughter charges may follow

Investigating an outbreak

Every member of staff has a responsibility to cooperate and assist in the investigation and management of an outbreak when requested by the Infection Control Team (ICT)
- Is this an outbreak? (see definition above)
- Put in place interim control measures to protect patients
- ICT call an outbreak meeting
  - Establish case definition; what is the outbreak about?
  - Confirm cases are real; do they meet the case definition?
  - Confirm outbreak and determine extent; look for additional cases
  - Examine descriptive epidemiological features of the cases to look for common factors
  - Generate hypothesis as to potential cause of outbreak
- Investigate hypothesis
  - Patient, staff or environmental screening, coordinated by ICT
- Implement control measures
  - Need for additional resources, clinical, laboratory or allied health professional staff
  - Close beds or wards, cohorting/isolation facilities, transfer patients
  - Review potentially implicated medications
  - Environmental cleaning, additional domestic support
  - Secondment of appropriate area link-professional to ICT
- Communication
  - With patients and relatives, staff and the press
- Write a report to ensure lessons are learnt to prevent repeat outbreak

Clinical Scenarios

What do Junior Doctors need to be able to do?

1. Take a clinical history
2. Perform a clinical examination and elicit relevant clinical signs
3. Recognise sick patients
4. Implement emergency care for sick patients
5. Formulate a differential diagnosis
6. Investigate a differential diagnosis
7. Prescribe appropriately and safely
8. Monitor and review patients appropriately and effectively
9. Prevent transmission of infection between patients
10. Recognise their own limitations and when they need to ask for help

Common Mistake

When faced with a patient with an infection it is tempting to start treatment for all of the potential causes of that infection. **This is a mistake.** Like any other drugs, antibiotics have side-effects and these can adversely influence patient care.

If a patient already has failure of one organ system, either due to the infection or a pre-existing clinical condition, then drug-inducing another organ failure may lead to end-of-life care. In this situation the infection didn't kill the patient, the treatment did!

Example:

A patient with chronic lymphocytic leukaemia (CLL), a long-term haematological condition, is admitted to the Critical Care Unit with severe community acquired pneumonia and respiratory failure. They now have two organs failing, lungs and bone marrow. They are treated with IV Co-amoxiclav and Clarithromycin but because they have CLL they are also given liposomal Amphotericin B just in case they have a rare fungal infection and IV Ganciclovir because they might just have CMV pneumonitis. Both additional agents are nephrotoxic and the patient develops severe renal failure. A discussion is had with the family and as the patient now has 3 organs failing a decision is made to start end-of-life care and the patient dies. Did the patient die from pneumonia or multi-organ failure due to unnecessary antibiotics?

When deciding whether to start an antibiotic consider the likelihood of the infection you are thinking of treating and the potential consequences of any side-effects or complications. If you still have a good reason to prescribe then go ahead, otherwise wait.

Respiratory
Infections

Community Acquired Pneumonia (CAP)

Community acquired pneumonia (CAP) is an acute infection of lung tissue with onset outside of hospital or within 48 hours of admission to hospital.

The NICE guidelines suggest that patients from nursing homes should be treated as CAP, however this disregards the level of care the resident is receiving. Some would argue that those who receive a level of nursing care equivalent to that received in hospital should be treated as hospital acquired pneumonia rather than CAP because they have a different normal flora (see section – Basic Concepts, Bacterial Flora in a Normal Person in a Hospital or Long-term Care Facility).

The British Thoracic Society Definitions for diagnosis are:

In community	• Cough **PLUS** one other lower respiratory tract symptom • New focal chest signs on examination • One systemic symptom • No other explanation
In hospital (<48 hours)	• Symptoms and signs consistent with pneumonia • New chest X-ray shadowing

Clinical Features

Respiratory symptoms and signs	Systemic symptoms

• Cough
• Shortness of breath
• Purulent sputum
• Chest pain
• Chest signs of consolidation
  – Reduced chest movement
  – Dull percussion
  – Bronchial breathing
  – Increased tactile vocal fremitus
    and vocal resonance
	• Fever
	• Sweats
	• Shivers
	• Aches
	• Pains

Children
• Fever • Increased respiratory rate • Cough • Recession • Chest pain or pain referred to abdomen

Common Mistake
Some doctors diagnose pneumonia on the basis of hearing crackles on auscultation of the chest. **This is a mistake.** Crackles in the chest generally indicate heart failure or fibrosis but not pneumonia, especially in the elderly.

Assessment of Severity
Score = 1 each per criterion e.g. **C** + **R** + **>65** = 3

C =	Confusion (new)
U =	Urea >7mmol/L
R =	Respiratory Rate >30/min
B =	Blood pressure <90mmHg systolic **OR** ≤ 60mmHg diastolic
65 =	Age >65 years

CURB-65	0-1	Can often be discharged on oral antibiotics
CURB-65	2	Usually require observation in hospital
CURB-65	3-5	Admit to hospital

In primary care the CURB-65 score can be modified to a **CRB-65** score (without urea) to assess risk of death and whether to admit to hospital:

CRB-65	0	1% mortality, manage at home
CRB-65	1-2	1-10% mortality, consider admitting to hospital
CRB-65	3-4	>10% mortality, admit to hospital

When CURB-65 was introduced (1996) elderly care in the UK was >65 years old; an age previously associated with worsening health. Frailty, rather than age, may now be a better indicator as CURB-65 overestimates severity in some otherwise healthy over 65 year olds e.g. some 70 year olds are treated with IV antibiotics when they should really be given orals and sent home.

Hints and Tips
CURB-65 can underestimate severity in young patients (<30 years) as they don't often become confused or drop their blood pressure, even when very unwell. Young patients with severe pneumonia often do not score more than 2 in the CURB-65 scoring system. Try using just "CURB" to assess severity in young patients.

C =	Confusion (new)
U =	Urea >7mmol/L
R =	Respiratory Rate >30/min
B =	Blood pressure <90mmHg systolic **OR** ≤ 60mmHg diastolic

Change the score by 1 less point to give a better assessment of severity in young patients i.e. 2-4 requires admission to hospital instead of 3-5.

CURB	0	Can often be discharged on oral antibiotics
CURB	1	Usually require observation in hospital
CURB	2-4	Admit to hospital

Causes

Common	• *Streptococcus pneumoniae* • *Haemophilus influenzae* • *Staphylococcus aureus* • *Mycoplasma pneumoniae* • *Legionella pneumophila* (especially if travelled) • *Chlamydophila pneumoniae* • Viral e.g. *Influenza Virus, Parainfluenza Virus, Respiratory Syncytial Virus* (RSV), *Adenovirus*
If history of COPD	As above plus: • *Pseudomonas aeruginosa*
Aspiration	As above plus: • Anaerobes e.g. *Bacteroides* spp., *Fusobacterium* spp.
Zoonotic	• *Chlamydophila psittaci* (from parrots and budgerigars)
Empyema	• *Staphylococcus aureus* • *Streptococcus pneumoniae* • *Streptococcus anginosus* group • Anaerobes e.g. *Bacteroides* spp., *Fusobacterium* spp.

Warning
Two conditions which are often missed and are not covered by the normal antibiotics used to treat community acquired pneumonia are:
Tuberculosis – consider in patients from endemic countries, returned travellers or contacts of people with tuberculosis.
Pneumocystis Pneumonia (PCP) – consider in patients with HIV infection or those who have risk factors for HIV infection.

Myth
Doctors traditionally refer to "atypical pneumonia" however, **this is a poor term**. "Atypical pneumonia" is pneumonia caused by bacteria that cannot easily be grown in a microbiology laboratory e.g. *Mycoplasma pneumoniae* and *Chlamydophila pneumoniae*. It was the Victorians that first coined the phrase as they could not identify these bacteria. However, with modern methods "atypical pneumonia" bacteria were identified and found to be common causes of pneumonia and hence the term "atypical" is highly misleading. Clinically there is no difference between how different bacterial pneumonias present. The conditions should be called "mycoplasmal pneumonia" or "chlamydial pneumonia" etc. just like we use staphylococcal pneumonia or streptococcal pneumonia.

"Atypical" as a term should really be abolished and "non-culturable", for example, should be used. Non-culturable is used throughout this book.

Investigations

Sputum	• Low sensitivity; approximately 50% • Will grow upper respiratory tract bacteria, which may or may not be the cause of CAP • Microscopy and culture for acid fast bacilli in tuberculosis • PCR for *M. pneumoniae* and *Chlamydophila* spp. as well as respiratory viruses
Viral throat swab	• PCR for respiratory viruses
Blood cultures	• Positive in ≤ 25% of cases
Urine antigens	• *Streptococcus pneumoniae* • *Legionella pneumophila* serogroup 1
Blood	• Serology in paired samples 10-14 days apart, complement fixation tests for *Chlamydophila* spp., *Mycoplasma* spp., viruses
Bronchoalveolar Lavage (BAL)	• Bypasses upper respiratory tract flora • Can be directed or non-directed • Especially useful for tuberculosis and PCP • PCR for *M. pneumoniae* and *Chlamydophila* spp.
Tap pleural effusion	• For microscopy, culture and sensitivity • Empyema = pH <7.2, glucose <2.2mol/L, LDH >1000IU/L

Treatment

If CURB-65 score 0-2	
1st line	PO Amoxicillin **PLUS** PO Clarithromycin (if *Mycoplasma* spp. or *Chlamydophila* spp. suspected)
2nd line (if 1st line contraindicated)	PO Doxycycline **OR** PO Levofloxacin

If CURB-65 score 3-5	
1st line	IV Co-amoxiclav **PLUS** IV Clarithromycin
2nd line (if 1st line contraindicated)	IV Teicoplanin **OR** IV Vancomycin **PLUS** PO or IV Levofloxacin
If MRSA positive	**ADD** IV Teicoplanin **OR** IV Vancomycin

If history of COPD	
1st line	IV Piptazobactam
2nd line (if 1st line contraindicated)	IV Meropenem
If MRSA positive	**ADD** IV Teicoplanin **OR** IV Vancomycin

If Legionella pneumophila	
1st line	PO or IV Levofloxacin
2nd line (if 1st line contraindicated)	PO Azithromycin

Community acquired aspiration pneumonia	
1st line	IV Co-amoxiclav
2nd line (if 1st line contraindicated)	IV Teicoplanin **OR** IV Vancomycin **PLUS** IV Ciprofloxacin **PLUS** IV Metronidazole
If MRSA positive	**ADD** IV Teicoplanin **OR** IV Vancomycin

Children	
1st line	PO or IV Co-amoxiclav
2nd line (if 1st line contraindicated)	PO or IV Clarithromycin
If MRSA positive	**ADD** IV Teicoplanin **OR** IV Vancomycin

Total Duration
5-7 days
Legionella pneumonia: 7-10 days (14-21 days if immunosuppressed)
Empyema requires drainage and 2-4 weeks total treatment

Dosing
See section - Antibiotics, Empirical Antibiotic Guidelines.

Prognosis and Complications
Mortality is dependent on CURB-65 score:

CURB-65	**0-1**	<3%
CURB-65	**2**	9%
CURB-65	**3-5**	15-40%

Up to 40% of patients with *Streptococcus pneumoniae* reactivate *Herpes Simplex Virus* (HSV) leading to cold sores.

Hints and Tips
It is important to explain to patients that it takes time to fully recover from an episode of pneumonia.
For most patients the following time scale should apply:
- 1 week – fever settles
- 4 weeks – chest pain and sputum production reduces
- 6 weeks – cough and shortness of breath reduces, if symptoms persist consider alternative diagnosis e.g. malignancy
- 3 months – all symptoms resolve, may still experience tiredness
- 6 months – back to normal

Prophylaxis and Prevention
No role for antibiotics to prevent recurrence
Vaccine against *Streptococcus pneumoniae*:
- 23-valent (adults) covers approximately 96% of pneumonia strains but not active in <2 year olds
- 13-valent (children) covers approximately 90% of pneumonia strains
- Vaccination of children reduces exposure and hence infection in adults by decreasing reservoir of bacteria in community

Aspiration Pneumonia

Aspiration pneumonia should not be considered as a standalone diagnosis in terms of the bacteria likely to cause the condition. Instead it is better to consider the environment the patient is in, community or hospital, as the normal flora they aspirate will be different. This is why community acquired aspiration pneumonia should be treated with antibiotics that cover bacteria found in the community environment, and hospital acquired aspiration pneumonia should be treated with antibiotics that cover bacteria found in the hospital environment.

For patients who aspirated while in the community (see section – Clinical Scenarios, Community Acquired Pneumonia).
For patients who aspirated more than 48 hours after admission or who are from long-term care facilities (see section - Clinical Scenarios, Hospital Acquired Pneumonia).

Myth
Some doctors believe that aspiration pneumonia (either community acquired or hospital acquired) requires treating with Metronidazole in addition to other antibiotics in order to cover anaerobic bacteria. **FALSE** - Co-amoxiclav, Piptazobactam and Meropenem all provide excellent anaerobic cover and do not require the addition of Metronidazole.

Hospital Acquired Pneumonia (HAP)

Hospital acquired pneumonia (HAP) is a respiratory infection developing >48 hours after hospital admission and that was not incubating at the time of admission.

Clinical Features
- Fever >38.3°C
- Purulent sputum
- New or persistent infiltrates on chest X-ray, which cannot be explained by another reason
- Increasing oxygen requirement
- Leucocytosis >10x10^9/L or leucopaenia <4x10^9/L

Causes

Early ≤4 days after admission	• *Streptococcus pneumoniae* • *Haemophilus influenzae* • *Staphylococcus aureus* • *Moraxella catarrhalis* • Viral e.g. *Respiratory Syncytial Virus* (RSV), *Rhinovirus, Influenza Virus*
Late >4 days after admission	As above plus: • *Pseudomonas aeruginosa*
Aspiration Pneumonia	As above plus: • Anaerobes e.g. *Bacteroides* spp., *Fusobacterium* spp.

Investigations
- Sputum culture may help identify the causative microorganism, but may only isolate upper respiratory tract normal flora
- If there are systemic symptoms consider taking blood cultures

Treatment
This is usually based upon local epidemiology and risk of complications of therapy such as *Clostridium difficile* associated diarrhoea. Children, interestingly, rarely get HAP and specific treatment guidelines are not included here.

Early ≤ 4 days	
1st line	PO or IV Co-amoxiclav
2nd line (if 1st line contraindicated)	PO or IV Levofloxacin
If MRSA positive	**ADD** IV Teicoplanin **OR** IV Vancomycin

Late >4 days	
1st line	IV Piptazobactam
2nd line (if 1st line contraindicated)	IV Teicoplanin **OR** IV Vancomycin **PLUS** PO **OR** IV Ciprofloxacin
If MRSA positive	**ADD** IV Teicoplanin **OR** IV Vancomycin

Hospital acquired aspiration pneumonia	
1st line	IV Piptazobactam
2nd line (if 1st line contraindicated)	IV Teicoplanin **OR** IV Vancomycin **PLUS** IV Ciprofloxacin **PLUS** IV Metronidazole
If MRSA positive	**ADD** IV Teicoplanin **OR** IV Vancomycin

Common Mistake
It is often believed that antibiotics for hospital acquired pneumonia (HAP) are "better" than antibiotics for community acquired pneumonia (CAP). **They are not**. Antibiotics are chosen to treat the likely causes of each infection. HAP and CAP are different clinical conditions with different causal bacteria; patients in hospitals and the community have different "normal flora" (see sections – Basic Concepts, Bacteria Flora in a Normal Person in the Community and Basic Concepts, Bacteria Flora in a Normal Person in a Hospital or Long-term Care Facility).

For example, a patient with CAP is started on Co-amoxiclav and Clarithromycin but does not show immediate improvement. The doctor "escalates" the patient to Piptazobactam (often used in hospital guidelines to treat HAP) thinking this is better. This is usually a mistake. The doctor has swapped good antibiotic cover for all the community microorganisms including non-culturable bacteria, for a narrower spectrum antibiotic, Piptazobactam. The patient may no longer be being treated for their pneumonia if it is caused by *Mycoplasma pneumoniae*, *Legionella pneumophila* or *Chlamydophila pneumoniae*.

So HAP guidelines in some respects actually reduce antibiotic cover. Knowing which bacteria are **not likely** and which are **more likely** in HAP enables the hospital guidelines to limit antibiotic choices to those specifically targeted against the causes rather than using broad spectrum antibiotics, which may lead to resistance. HAP guidelines are therefore not an escalation process for CAP.

Total Duration
5-7 days

Dosing
See section - Antibiotics, Empirical Antibiotic Guidelines.

Prognosis and Complications
Mortality up to 30% depending on underlying co-morbidities.

Ventilator Associated Pneumonia (VAP)

Ventilator associated pneumonia (VAP) is pneumonia developing >48 hours after implementing endotracheal intubation or mechanical ventilation, which was not present before intubation.

Clinical Features
- Patient mechanically ventilated for ≥ 48 hours **PLUS**
- New or worsening pulmonary infiltrates on chest X-ray **PLUS**
- Raised WBC **PLUS**
- Growth of a pathogenic bacterium at significant levels from a lower respiratory tract sample (aspiration or BAL)

Causes

Common	• *Staphylococcus aureus* (MSSA and MRSA) • *Streptococcus pneumoniae* • *Haemophilus influenzae* • *Pseudomonas* spp. • Enterobacteriaceae e.g. *Escherichia coli*, *Klebsiella* spp., *Enterobacter* spp., *Serratia marcescens*

Investigations
- Endotracheal secretions – culture and sensitivity indicates what a patient is colonised with, not necessarily what is causing the infection
- Bronchoalveolar lavage (BAL) - either directed or non-directed, bypassing upper respiratory tract flora, sampling directly from the lung
- Blood cultures – if systemic signs of infection

Treatment

1st line	IV Piptazobactam
2nd line (if 1st line contraindicated)	IV Teicoplanin **OR** IV Vancomycin **PLUS** IV Ciprofloxacin
If MRSA positive	**ADD** IV Teicoplanin **OR** IV Vancomycin

Total Duration
5-7 days

Dosing
See section - Antibiotics, Empirical Antibiotic Guidelines.

> **Warning**
> Critical Care Units may have problems with specific bacteria, e.g. *Acinetobacter* spp., so be aware of your own unit's guidelines.

Prognosis and Complications
25-75% mortality depending on underlying co-morbidities and infection with antibiotic resistant bacteria.

Prophylaxis and Prevention
- Regular suctioning of pooled secretions in upper respiratory tract
- Sterile water for mouth washes
- Effective hand hygiene

Infective Exacerbation of COPD

Infective exacerbation of COPD is the term used for worsening respiratory function in patients known to have chronic obstructive pulmonary disease (COPD).

Clinical Features
- Increasing shortness of breath
- Increasingly purulent sputum
- Increasing amount of sputum
- Chest X-ray **DOES NOT** show changes indicative of pneumonia; if it does then treat for pneumonia not infective exacerbation of COPD

Causes

Viral	• *Respiratory Syncytial Virus* (RSV) • *Rhinovirus* • *Influenza Virus* • *Parainfluenza Virus* • *Adenovirus*
Bacterial	• *Streptococcus pneumoniae* • *Staphylococcus aureus* • *Haemophilus influenzae* • *Moraxella catarrhalis*

Investigations
- Sputum culture may help identify the causative microorganism, but may only isolate upper respiratory tract normal flora

Treatment

1st line	PO Amoxicillin
2nd line (if 1st line contraindicated)	PO Clarithromycin **OR** PO Doxycycline

Total Duration
5-7 days

Dosing
See section - Antibiotics, Empirical Antibiotic Guidelines.

Prognosis and Complications
Most patients get better with treatment.

Prophylaxis and Prevention
Prophylactic antibiotics should be avoided; although they may reduce the frequency of exacerbations ultimately they tend to lead to increasingly resistant bacteria within the patient's normal flora. This results in increasingly difficult-to-treat infections with a higher mortality.

Acute Bronchitis

Inflammation or irritation of the main airways, the bronchi, of the lungs.

Clinical Features
- Cough
- Shortness of breath
- Wheeze
- Malaise
- Chest X-ray **DOES NOT** show changes indicative of pneumonia; if it does then treat for pneumonia not acute bronchitis

Causes

Viral	• *Respiratory Syncytial Virus* (RSV) • *Rhinovirus* • *Influenza Virus* • *Parainfluenza Virus* • *Adenovirus*

Investigations
- Viral nose and throat swabs may identify the cause but investigations not normally required

Treatment
Antibiotics are not normally indicated. Antibiotics may be prescribed if patient at risk of developing pneumonia e.g. >80 years old, immunosuppressed, COPD or severe heart failure.

1st line	PO Amoxicillin
2nd line (if 1st line contraindicated)	PO Clarithromycin **OR** PO Doxycycline

Total Duration
5-7 days

Dosing
See section - Antibiotics, Empirical Antibiotic Guidelines.

Prognosis and Complications
Most patients get better without treatment.
Antibiotics decrease the duration of cough by half a day but have no impact on mortality or morbidity, therefore their use needs to be balanced against the risk of side effects and possible adverse events.

Upper Respiratory Tract Infection (URTI)

Upper respiratory tract infection (URTI) is a non-specific term used to describe a group of infections with a mixture of similar symptoms and hence why the term URTI was probably coined to keep it simple. These conditions are primarily caused by viruses and are self-limiting. Patients often call these conditions, "The Common Cold", "Flu" or "Sore Throat".

Clinical Features
- Rhinorrhoea
- Sore throat
- Fever
- Headache
- Dry cough
- Lethargy

Causes

Coryza Laryngitis Pharyngitis Rhinitis	Common viruses: • *Rhinovirus* • *Adenovirus* • *Human Metapneumovirus* • *Respiratory Syncytial Virus* (RSV) • *Parainfluenza Virus* • *Influenza Virus*

Investigations
Clinical diagnosis, no formal investigations required.

Treatment
Supportive treatment only (antipyretics and adequate hydration).

Influenza

Influenza is an acute viral infection of the respiratory tract, spread by droplets and aerosols.

Clinical Features
In order to meet a clinical diagnosis of influenza the patient has to fit the diagnostic criteria of:
- Temperature >38°C **OR** history of fever within 7 days
- **PLUS** ≥ 2 "flu-like" symptoms – cough, sore throat, rhinorrhoea, headache, malaise, myalgia or arthralgia

> **Myth**
> Men think their flu is worse than women, so called "man flu". **FALSE** - Influenza in men and women is caused by the same viruses; women just seem to cope better...

Causes
Influenza is always caused by the *Influenza Virus*, there are 3 types:

Influenza A	Common seasonal influenza Can cause epidemics and pandemics
Influenza B	Common seasonal influenza Can cause epidemics but not pandemics
Influenza C	Usually sporadic Does not cause epidemics or pandemics
"Swine Flu" and "Bird Flu"	These are layman terms for *Influenza A Virus*. Swine Flu is *Influenza A Virus* in pigs and Bird Flu is *Influenza A Virus* in birds. *Influenza A Virus* in humans is still just *Influenza A Virus*

Investigations
- Nose and throat viral swabs (green viral swab) for PCR

Treatment
If patients are well enough they should **NOT** be admitted into hospital in order to prevent exposing other patients to the virus. Treatment is mainly supportive (antipyretics and adequate hydration), however if in high risk groups (see below) specific treatment should be started within 48 hours:

1st line	PO Oseltamivir
2nd line (if 1st line contraindicated)	Inhaled Zanamivir*

Note: *Zanamivir is available as an IV and nebulised preparation but these are both currently unlicensed in the UK and available on a compassionate use named patient basis only for those in whom inhaled Zanamivir cannot be given.

> **Warning**
> Rates of Oseltamivir resistance in *Influenza A Virus* are increasing. The risk is highest in the H1N1 type rather than others e.g. H3N2. As a result, if a severely immunosuppressed patient (see below, High Risk Groups - Immunodeficient) is diagnosed with influenza when the dominant strain circulating in the population is H1N1 then Zanamivir should be used first line rather than Oseltamivir.

High Risk Groups
- Pregnant or up to 2 weeks postpartum
- Children <6 months old
- Morbidly obese BMI >40
- Age >65
- Diabetes mellitus
- Chronic cardiac, renal, pulmonary, hepatic or neurological condition
- Immunodeficient
  - >40mg Prednisolone per day or equivalent
  - Primary immunodeficiency
  - On immunosuppressive treatment or within 6 months of treatment
  - Bone marrow transplant recipients on immunosuppressive treatment or within 12 months of treatment
  - Patients with current graft vs. host disease
  - HIV positive patients with CD4 <200/mm^3

Total Duration
5 days
If on AICU or immunodeficient give 14 days as often there is prolonged secretion of the virus

Dosing
See section - Antibiotics, Empirical Antibiotic Guidelines.

Prognosis and Complications
Mortality usually <0.5%.
Secondary bacterial pneumonia (CAP or HAP) can occur, causing mortality to increase; 20% of secondary bacterial pneumonias are caused by *Staphylococcus aureus*.

Prophylaxis and Prevention
For high risk groups above give Post-Exposure Prophylaxis with Oseltamivir or Zanamivir within 48 hours of exposure.

Low risk of Oseltamivir resistance (e.g. H3N2)	PO Oseltamivir 75mg OD for 10 days
High risk of (e.g. H1N1) **OR** known resistance to Oseltamivir in severely immunosuppressed patients	Inhaled Zanamivir 10mg OD for 10 days

Infection Control Precautions
See section – Infection Control, Influenza.

Tuberculosis (TB)

Tuberculosis (TB) is a bacterial infection caused by any of the 5 species of mycobacterium from the group of bacteria known as the *Mycobacterium tuberculosis* (MTB) complex. Tuberculosis is more common in developing countries and countries where healthcare services have broken down due to political turmoil e.g. Eastern Europe and the former Soviet States.

Clinical Features
90% of primary infections are asymptomatic.

Common	
Pulmonary	• Fever • Cough • Weight loss • Night sweats • Rigors • Pleuritic pain
Variations	
Disseminated (Miliary) or Extra-pulmonary	• Pericardial effusion – shortness of breath • Lymphadenopathy • Gastrointestinal disturbance • Genitourinary – symptoms of UTI • Skin lesions • Osteomyelitis • Septic arthritis • Meningitis • Brain abscess

Causes

MTB Complex includes	
Common	• *Mycobacterium tuberculosis* • *Mycobacterium bovis*
Uncommon	• *Mycobacterium africanum* • *Mycobacterium microti* • *Mycobacterium ulcerans*

Investigations

Mantoux Test	• Skin test for which the size of reaction is related to likelihood of disease
Sputum (3 deep cough samples including 1 early morning sample)	• Microscopy for acid fast bacilli using Ziehl-Neelsen stain • Liquid culture – takes up to 42 days, but MTB usually grows within 14 days
Bronchoalveolar lavage (BAL)	• Microscopy for acid fast bacilli using Ziehl-Neelsen stain • Liquid culture – takes up to 42 days, but MTB usually grows within 14 days
Gastric lavage (consider 3 samples in children if unable to cough sputum)	• Microscopy for acid fast bacilli using Ziehl-Neelsen stain • Liquid culture – takes up to 42 days, but MTB usually grows within 14 days

Biopsy or needle aspiration (**DO NOT** send in formalin)	• Microscopy for acid fast bacilli using Ziehl-Neelsen stain • Liquid culture – takes up to 42 days, but MTB usually grows within 14 days
TB Blood culture	• Specific sample bottle usually acquired from microbiology laboratory
Molecular detection	• High specificity up to 90% • Low sensitivity 60% due to small numbers of bacteria present in specimens • Usually reserved for confirming identification after culture and detecting resistance to Rifampicin
Interferon gamma release assays (IGRAs)	• e.g. T spot, Quantiferon • Highly specific to MTB complex • Does not cross-react with BCG vaccination • Does not distinguish active from latent disease • Can give false negative results in immunodeficient patients
Adenosine deaminase	• Can be performed on any fluid from normally sterile sites, most commonly pleural fluid • >40U/L is suggestive of tuberculosis

Treatment

Pulmonary and Extra-pulmonary (not meningitis)	2 months daily quadruple therapy (PO Isoniazid, PO Rifampicin, PO Pyrazinamide and PO Ethambutol) **THEN** 4 months of daily PO Isoniazid and PO Rifampicin
Meningitis	2 months daily quadruple therapy (PO Isoniazid, PO Rifampicin, PO Pyrazinamide and PO Ethambutol) **THEN** 10 months of daily PO Isoniazid and PO Rifampicin
Other agents active against TB used in 2nd line treatments	• Fluoroquinolones (See section – Antibiotics, Ciprofloxacin and Levofloxacin) • Aminoglycosides (See section – Antibiotics, Gentamicin, Amikacin and Tobramycin) • Bedaquiline, Delamanid • Para-aminosalicylic acid, Capreomycin, Cycloserine, Ethionamide, Thiacetazone

Warning
Some antibiotics commonly used to treat other types of infections can inhibit the growth of *Mycobacteria* spp. making cultures negative e.g. aminoglycosides, fluoroquinolones, carbapenems, Co-amoxiclav and Linezolid. Where possible take samples before starting antibiotics or at least within 7 days.

Prognosis and Complications

There is a risk of reactivation after primary infection:

- 5-10% reactivation risk during patient's lifetime even with a normal immune system
- 5-10% reactivation risk yearly with HIV co-infection

Mortality

4% with treatment.

Prophylaxis and Prevention

Treatment of latent infection	
Following exposure to tuberculosis or Positive Mantoux or Positive IGRA with normal chest X-ray	PO Isoniazid daily for 6 months **OR** PO Isoniazid daily for 3 months **PLUS** PO Rifampicin daily for 3 months

Infection Control Precautions

See section – Infection Control, Tuberculosis.

Multidrug Resistant TB (MDR TB) and Extensively Drug Resistant TB (XDR TB)

Multidrug resistant TB (MDR TB) and extensively drug resistant TB (XDR TB) are an emerging problem. The long length of treatment (6 months pulmonary or 12 months meningitis) causes problems with patient compliance and resulting incomplete treatment is in part responsible for the antibiotic resistance in multidrug resistant TB (MDR TB). In the same way, incomplete treatment of MDR TB is partly responsible for extensively drug resistant TB (XDR TB).

Definition of Resistant TB
MDR TB - Resistant to Isoniazid and Rifampicin
XDR TB - Resistant to Isoniazid, Rifampicin, fluoroquinolones and aminoglycosides

Risk Factors for MDR TB in the UK
- Previous TB treatment
- Current TB treatment failure
- Contact with patient with known MDR TB
- HIV co-infection
- London resident
- Male aged 25-44
- Travel to or from a country with known MDR TB

In the UK in 2015 approximately 1.4% of newly diagnosed TB and 5.7% of reactivated TB was MDR TB, however in Eastern Europe and Central Asia 20% of new TB and 50% of relapsed TB were MDR TB.

Treatment
Treatment of MDR and XDR TB should be guided by a Physician experienced in the management of MDR and XDR TB. Treatment is individualised, based upon sensitivity testing, to include at least 5 active antimicrobials for a total duration of 18-24 months. Drugs used include aminoglycosides, fluoroquinolones, Ethionamide, Cycloserine, Para-aminosalicylic acid as well as any remaining active first line agents.

There are two new antimicrobials available for the treatment of XDR TB, Bedaquiline and Delamanid.

Mortality
25% for MDR TB
50% for XDR TB

Infection Control Precautions
See section – Infection Control, Multidrug Resistant Tuberculosis.

Head and Neck Infections

Otitis Media

Otitis media is an infection of the middle ear.

Clinical Features
- Pain
- Discharge
- Decreased hearing
- Fever
- Loss of balance
- Erythema of the tympanic membrane

For Chronic Otitis Media
Symptoms present for ≥ 6 weeks with associated discharge.

Causes

Acute	• *Streptococcus pneumoniae* • *Haemophilus influenzae* • Group A Beta-haemolytic *Streptococcus* (*Streptococcus pyogenes*) • *Moraxella catarrhalis* • Viral e.g. *Respiratory Syncytial Virus* (RSV), *Rhinovirus, Influenza Virus* ,
Chronic	Often mixed microorganisms: • *Streptococcus pneumoniae* • *Haemophilus influenzae* • *Staphylococcus aureus* • Anaerobes • *Pseudomonas aeruginosa* (uncommon)

Investigations
- If severe, send discharge for culture and sensitivity

Treatment

Acute	
1st line	PO Amoxicillin
2nd line (if 1st line contraindicated)	PO Clarithromycin
Chronic	
1st line	PO Co-amoxiclav (**BEWARE** no *Pseudomonas aeruginosa* cover)
2nd line (if 1st line contraindicated) or *Pseudomonas* spp.	PO Levofloxacin

Total Duration
Acute: 5 days
Chronic: 4 weeks

Dosing
See section - Antibiotics, Empirical Antibiotic Guidelines.

Prognosis and Complications
Most patients get better with treatment, but risk of hearing loss if not adequately treated.

<u>Otitis Externa</u>

Otitis externa is an acute infection of the skin of the pinna and auditory canal.

Clinical Features
- Spreading erythema of pinna and auditory canal
- Acute inflammation – pain, redness, heat, swelling and loss of function

For Malignant Otitis Externa (Rare)
More common in elderly, diabetes mellitus and immunodeficiency as well as following piercing of the helix (cartilage) of the ear
- Necrosis of tissue and bone
- Severe pain and tenderness with discharge
- Systemic symptoms such as fever, chills, rigors

Causes

Common	• *Staphylococcus aureus* • Beta-haemolytic *Streptococcus* (Groups A, C and G)
Malignant Otitis Externa	• *Pseudomonas aeruginosa*

Myth
Pseudomonas aeruginosa is a very common cause of otitis externa **FALSE**
P. aeruginosa is a rare cause of otitis externa usually associated with an underlying illness such as diabetes mellitus or immunosuppression as well as specific patients e.g. swimmers. *P. aeruginosa* colonises warm moist sites, e.g. an inflamed external auditory meatus, therefore it grows from ear swabs even when not causing infection.

Investigations
- If severe, send discharge for culture and sensitivity

For Malignant Otitis Externa
- Swab discharge for culture and sensitivity
- Pus or tissue for culture and sensitivity
- Blood cultures

Treatment

1st line	TOP 2% Acetic Acid TDS
2nd line (if 1st line contraindicated)	TOP Neomycin Sulphate + Corticosteroid TDS

If antibiotics are required:

1st line	PO Flucloxacillin
2nd line (if 1st line contraindicated)	PO Erythromycin **OR** PO Doxycycline
If MRSA positive	IV Teicoplanin **OR** IV Vancomycin
Malignant Otitis Externa	IV Piptazobactam **OR** PO or IV Ciprofloxacin

Total Duration
7-10 days
Malignant otitis externa: 4-6 weeks

Dosing
See section - Antibiotics, Empirical Antibiotic Guidelines.

Prognosis and Complications
Most patients get better with treatment, but malignant otitis externa can be life-threatening.

There are a number of common infections that can affect the eye or its
surrounding structures:
- **Blepharitis** – inflammation of the eyelid
- **Conjunctivitis** – inflammation of the conjunctiva
- **Keratitis** – inflammation of the cornea, more common in contact lens
  wearers
- **Endophthalmitis** – inflammation of the ocular cavity including the aqueous
  and vitreous humours. Usually secondary to trauma or surgery

Clinical Features

Blepharitis	• Mild pain • Redness • Purulent discharge
Conjunctivitis	• Mild pain or itching • Redness • Purulent discharge • Conjunctival oedema and haemorrhage
Keratitis	• Rapid onset of pain • Redness • Photophobia • Corneal clouding • Corneal defects • Hypopyon (pus inside the anterior chamber) • Decreased visual acuity
Endophthalmitis	• Usually secondary to trauma or surgery • Rapid onset of severe pain • Redness • Discharge • Photophobia • Swelling of the eyelid • Decreased visual acuity

Causes

Blepharitis	• *Staphylococcus aureus*
Conjunctivitis	• Viral e.g. *Adenovirus, Influenza Virus, Enterovirus* • *Chlamydia* spp. • *Staphylococcus aureus* • *Streptococcus pneumoniae* • *Haemophilus influenzae* • *Moraxella catarrhalis* • *Neisseria gonorrhoeae* • *Pseudomonas aeruginosa* (especially in contact lens wearers)
Keratitis	As for conjunctivitis plus: • *Streptococcus* spp. • Fungi – *Fusarium* spp., *Aspergillus* spp.
Endophthalmitis	As for keratitis plus: • Enterobacteriaceae • Anaerobes • Fungi – *Candida* spp.

Investigations
- Viral swab for PCR
- Chlamydia swab for PCR
- Bacterial swab for culture and sensitivity
- If severe, send discharge for microscopy, culture and sensitivity
- Keratitis often requires a corneal scrape by an Ophthalmologist for microscopy, culture and sensitivity
- Endophthalmitis often requires intravitreal sampling by an Ophthalmologist for microscopy, culture and sensitivity

Treatment
Keratitis and endophthalmitis are emergencies that require specialist management by an Ophthalmologist in order to prevent loss of sight.

Blepharitis	TOP Chloramphenicol 1% eye ointment QDS
Bacterial conjunctivitis	TOP Chloramphenicol 0.5% eye ointment QDS If *Pseudomonas* spp. suspected: **ADD** Levofloxacin 0.5% eye drops 2 hourly for 2 days **THEN** QDS
Chlamydial conjunctivitis	PO Erythromycin 500mg QDS
Gonococcal conjunctivitis	IV Ceftriaxone
Bacterial keratitis	**SEEK SPECIALIST OPHTHALMOLOGY ADVICE** Levofloxacin 0.5% eye drops hourly (day and night) for 2 days **THEN** hourly during the day for 3 days **THEN** QDS
Endophthalmitis	**SEEK SPECIALIST OPHTHALMOLOGY ADVICE** Intravitreal antibiotics required

Total Duration
Blepharitis: 2 weeks
Bacterial conjunctivitis: 1 week
Chlamydial conjunctivitis: 2 weeks
Gonococcal conjunctivitis: 24 hours (3 days if corneal involvement)
Keratitis and Endophthalmitis: seek specialist Ophthalmology advice

Prognosis and Complications
- Blepharitis very rarely progresses to orbital cellulitis.
- Keratitis can progress to corneal perforation or visual loss.
- Endophthalmitis can rapidly progress to visual loss without appropriate treatment.

Orbital Cellulitis

Orbital cellulitis is an acute infection of the contents of the orbit. Infection of the skin around the eye anterior to the orbital septum should be treated as normal cellulitis.

Clinical Features
- Fever
- Rhinorrhoea
- Headache

- Pain on moving eye
- Reduced eye movement
- Eyelid oedema
- Pain and tenderness over the eye

Causes
Usually presents as a secondary infection from an infected sinus e.g. paranasal, ethmoid, frontal. Occasionally secondary to trauma, otitis media and dental infections.

Common	• *Staphylococcus aureus* • Group A Beta-haemolytic *Streptococcus* (*Streptococcus pyogenes*) • *Streptococcus pneumoniae*
Uncommon	• Gram-negative bacteria if chronic sinusitis • Fungal e.g. *Aspergillus* spp., *Mucor* spp.

Investigations
- Pus or tissue for microscopy, culture and sensitivity
- Blood cultures

Treatment

1st line	IV Cefotaxime **OR** IV Ceftriaxone **PLUS** IV Metronidazole
2nd line (if 1st line contraindicated)	IV Meropenem **OR** IV Ciprofloxacin **PLUS** IV Clindamycin
If MRSA positive	**ADD** IV Teicoplanin **OR** IV Vancomycin
If fungal	IV Liposomal Amphotericin (e.g. AmBisome) **OR** PO Posaconazole

Total Duration
7-10 days

Dosing
See section - Antibiotics, Empirical Antibiotic Guidelines.

Prognosis and Complications
- Risk of visual loss
- Extension into the cavernous sinus causing thrombosis and death
  - Signs of cavernous sinus thrombosis
    - Headache
    - Eye pain
    - Neck stiffness
    - Reduced consciousness
- Other complications include meningitis and cerebral abscess

Sinusitis

Sinusitis is inflammation of the paranasal sinuses. Blocked drainage of secretions leads to increased numbers of bacteria from the upper respiratory tract and hence increased inflammation. Symptoms can be acute (<4 weeks duration) or chronic (≥4 weeks duration).

Clinical Features
- Fever
- Facial pain
- Discharge from sinuses
- Post-nasal drip and unpleasant taste in mouth

Causes

Viral	• *Rhinovirus* • *Influenza Virus* • *Parainfluenza Virus* • *Adenovirus*
Bacteria	Often mixed microorganisms: • *Streptococcus pneumoniae* • *Staphylococcus aureus* • *Haemophilus influenzae* • Alpha-haemolytic *Streptococcus* spp. • *Moraxella catarrhalis* • Anaerobes

Investigations
- Usually a clinical diagnosis
- If pus drained then send for culture and sensitivity

Treatment

Acute	
1st line	PO Amoxicillin
2nd line (if 1st line contraindicated)	PO Doxycycline
Chronic	
1st line	PO Co-amoxiclav
2nd line (if 1st line contraindicated)	PO Levofloxacin **PLUS** PO Metronidazole

Total Duration
Acute: 10 days
Chronic: 3-4 weeks

Dosing
See section - Antibiotics, Empirical Antibiotic Guidelines.

Prognosis and Complications
Spontaneous resolution in 2/3 of patients. Complications are rare but can be severe:
- Orbital cellulitis
- Brain abscess
- Meningitis
- Cavernous sinus thrombosis
- Subdural empyema

Prophylaxis and Prevention
No role for antibiotics to prevent recurrence.

<u>Tonsillitis</u>

Tonsillitis is inflammation of the glandular tissue of the oropharynx.

Clinical Features
- Pain
- Fever
- Swelling
- Tonsillar pus

Causes

Common	• Viruses – *Adenovirus, Respiratory Syncytial Virus* (RSV), *Parainfluenza Virus* • Beta-haemolytic *Streptococcus* (Groups A, C and G) • Anaerobes – *Fusobacterium* spp.

Investigations
- Throat swab for culture and sensitivity

Centor Score and FeverPAIN Score
Clinical criteria can be used to estimate the percentage of patients who have *S. pyogenes* (Group A Beta-haemolytic *Streptococcus*) and who therefore should be given antibiotics. These include the Centor and FeverPAIN scores.

Centor	FeverPAIN
Score 1 point for each of the following (total 0-4): • Tonsillar exudates • Tender anterior cervical lymphadenopathy • Fever by history • Absence of cough	Score 1 point for each of the following (total 0-5): • **Fever** over 38°C. • **P**urulence (pharyngeal/tonsillar exudate). • **A**ttend rapidly (3 days or less) • **I**nflamed tonsils (severe) • **N**o cough or coryza

Centor Score Interpretation

Centor Score	Patients with *S. pyogenes*	Recommendation
0	0%	No test, no treatment
1	7%	No test, no treatment
2	21%	Throat swab or rapid antigen test. Treat if positive
3	38%	Treat if throat swab or rapid antigen test positive or treat empirically if tests not available
4	57%	Treat empirically

FeverPAIN Score Interpretation

FeverPAIN Score	Patients with *S. pyogenes*	Recommendation
0	0%	No test, no treatment
1	13-18%	Throat swab or rapid antigen test. Treat if positive
2-3	34-40%	Treat if throat swab or rapid antigen test positive or treat empirically if tests not available
4-5	62-65%	Treat empirically

Treatment
Treatment is usually only indicated for tonsillitis caused by Group A Beta-haemolytic *Streptococcus*, and so should only be started if the throat swab is culture positive or high Centor or FeverPAIN score. Treatment aims to eliminate carriage and reduce the incidence of complications including local abscesses, rheumatic fever and glomerulonephritis.

1st line	PO Phenoxymethylpenicillin (Penicillin V)
2nd line (if 1st line contraindicated)	PO Clarithromycin

Total Duration
10 days

Dosing
See section - Antibiotics, Empirical Antibiotic Guidelines.

Prognosis and Complications
Group A Beta-haemolytic streptococcal disease can result in rheumatic fever and glomerulonephritis following acute infection, however these are rare in the UK.

> **Warning**
> *Fusobacterium necrophorum* can cause a severe infection of the structures of the neck, including the carotid artery, called Lemierre's Syndrome. This can then spread to cause cavernous sinus thrombosis or anaerobic pneumonia (known as necrobacillosis). This life-threatening infection requires treatment with IV Benzylpenicillin **PLUS** Metronidazole.

Prophylaxis and Prevention
Patients with severe, recurrent tonsillitis may undergo tonsillectomy to prevent recurrence.

Rheumatic Fever and Rheumatic Heart Disease

Rheumatic fever may occur 1-5 weeks after tonsillitis or upper respiratory tract infection in 3% of untreated patients. Treatment reduces the incidence of rheumatic heart disease and long-term cardiac problems.

Jones Criteria

The diagnosis of rheumatic fever is based upon the Jones criteria and requires evidence of preceding Group A Beta-haemolytic *Streptococcus* infection by positive culture or elevated or rising Anti-Streptolysin O Titre (ASOT) **PLUS** 2 major **OR** 1 major and 2 minor criteria.

Major Criteria	Minor Criteria
• Carditis • Polyarthritis • Chorea • Erythema marginatum • Subcutaneous nodules	• Arthralgia • Fever • Elevated ESR or CRP • Prolonged PR interval on ECG

Prophylaxis and Prevention

Patients who have had one episode of rheumatic fever should be given long-term antibiotics to prevent further cases as these can lead to progressive cardiac damage.

Prophylactic Antibiotics	
Lifelong antibiotics	1st Line PO Penicillin V 250-500mg BD 2nd Line PO Erythromycin 250-500mg OD

Glomerulonephritis

The exact incidence of glomerulonephritis after tonsillitis or upper respiratory tract infection is unclear, although if the strain of Group A Beta-haemolytic *Streptococcus* is definitely nephrotoxigenic then the attack rate is 10-15% within 3 weeks. Of those affected, 10% go on to have severe renal failure and hypertension.

> **Warning**
>
> In any unvaccinated patient with a severe sore throat, painful cervical lymphadenopathy, neck swelling and difficulty breathing, consider a potential diagnosis of **diphtheria**, caused by the bacterium *Corynebacterium diphtheriae*.
>
> Diphtheria is a **medical emergency**. Patients have asymmetrical adherent greyish white pharyngeal membranes with surrounding inflammation which may extend into the trachea and cause airway obstruction. Diphtheria can also cause myocarditis.
>
> **Diphtheria is highly contagious; strict infection control is required.**
>
> Treatment of diphtheria should be under the supervision of a Microbiologist or Infectious Diseases Physician and an Anaesthetist as it requires airway protection, antitoxin and antibiotics. Diphtheria is fortunately rare in the UK however cases are still seen in patients, usually from Eastern Europe and the former Soviet Union.

Urogenital Infections

Urinary Tract Infection (UTI)

Urinary tract infection (UTI) is infection of the urinary tract by microorganisms which normally originate in the gastrointestinal tract and ascend into the urinary tract. It is important to distinguish between uncomplicated and complicated UTIs as the length of treatment differs.

- **Uncomplicated UTI** is an infection in a structurally and functionally normal urinary tract
- **Complicated UTI** is an infection in a structurally and / or functionally abnormal urinary tract
  - UTIs in men, pregnancy and children are also **ALL** complicated

Catheter-associated UTIs have similar symptoms to uncomplicated or complicated UTIs but different causes and so need different treatment.

Urethral syndrome is a form of UTI that only occurs in women and is characterised by urgency and pain on passing urine. It is important to make the distinction of urethral syndrome from other types of UTI because although the causes are the same, the treatment is different.

Clinical Features
- Frequency
- Urgency
- Incontinence
- Dysuria
- Nocturia
- Polyuria
- Hesitancy
- Suprapubic pain
- Loin-to-groin pain e.g. flank and back
- Fever or chills
- Rigors
- Sepsis

Causes

Common	• *Escherichia coli* • *Proteus* spp. • *Klebsiella* spp. • *Enterobacter* spp.
Pregnancy	As above plus: • *Staphylococcus saprophyticus*
Catheter-associated	As for common plus: • *Pseudomonas* spp. • *Enterococcus* spp. • *Staphylococcus aureus* • *Candida* spp.

> **Hints and Tips**
> *Proteus* spp. are strongly associated with urinary tract stones because they break down urea into ammonia, which alkalinises urine and facilitates stone formation. A patient with *Proteus* spp. in their blood culture due to a UTI should be investigated for urinary tract stones.

> **Warning**
> *Staphylococcus aureus* is not normally a cause of uncatheterised UTI
> - In men who are not catheterised, investigations should focus on systemic *S. aureus* infection e.g. infective endocarditis, septic arthritis and osteomyelitis
> - In women it is usually a contaminant from the perineum

Investigations

- Urine microscopy, culture and sensitivity: Mid-stream urine (MSU), clean catch urine or supra-pubic aspirate (SPA)
- Urine dipstick (bacterial nitrites **PLUS** leucocytes)
  - Negative Predictive Value (NPV) ≈ 97% **CAN** rule out UTI
  - Positive Predictive Value (PPV) ≈ 60% **CANNOT** prove UTI
  - NPV (72%) and PPV (92%) in women <65 years old with cloudy urine **PLUS** ≥2 of:
    - ○ Moderate-severe dysuria
    - ○ Nocturia
    - ○ Smelly urine
- Blood cultures if systemic symptoms

Treatment
Antibiotics do not work for **urethral syndrome** because the antibiotics do not stay in the urethra long enough to be effective. Treatment is to increase fluid intake to flush bacteria out of the urethra.

UTI (Uncomplicated & Complicated)	
1st line	PO Trimethoprim
2nd line (if 1st line contraindicated)	PO Nitrofurantoin **OR** PO Pivmecillinam Hydrochloride **OR** PO Fosfomycin
Pregnancy	PO Cefalexin

Pyelonephritis	
1st line	PO Co-amoxiclav **OR** IV Gentamicin
2nd line (if 1st line contraindicated)	PO or IV Ciprofloxacin
Pregnancy	IV Cefuroxime

Warning
Antibiotic treatment of UTIs is becoming increasingly challenging. Approximately 6% of community acquired UTIs in the UK are now caused by bacteria producing Extended-Spectrum Beta-Lactamases (ESBL).

Risk factors for ESBL-positive *Escherichia coli* infection include:
- Recurrent UTIs
- Previous treatment with Ciprofloxacin
- Previous infection with ESBL-positive *E. coli*

ESBLs are associated with resistance to the majority of oral antibiotics. Fosfomycin and Pivmecillinam Hydrochloride are old antibiotics making a comeback as they are active against these bacteria; otherwise the alternative treatment is IV Meropenem or IV Temocillin.

Fosfomycin
Uncomplicated UTI (women only): 3g stat
Complicated UTI: 3g stat **PLUS** 3g 3 days later

Pivmecillinam Hydrochloride
Uncomplicated UTI: 400mg TDS 3 days

Total Duration
Uncomplicated UTI (women only): 3 days
Complicated UTI (including pregnancy): 7 days
Pyelonephritis: 7 days
Pyelonephritis in pregnancy: 14 days

Dosing
See section - Antibiotics, Empirical Antibiotic Guidelines.

Prognosis and Complications
UTI can result in impairment of renal function, especially in young children with recurrent infections and vesico-ureteric reflux.

Prophylaxis and Prevention
Prophylactic antibiotics are used in children who experience recurrent UTIs in order to try and preserve renal function.

Adult patients who have 2 confirmed UTIs in 6 months or ≥3 UTIs in a year may benefit from antibiotics to aid healing of the bladder. Advise about maintaining hydration and post coital voiding as appropriate before considering antibiotic prophylaxis.

Prophylactic Antibiotics	
1st line	Self-administered or standby antibiotics (see UTI treatment above) **OR** Post-coital antibiotics: • Trimethoprim 200mg stat **OR** • Nitrofurantoin 100mg stat **OR** • Pivmecillinam Hydrochloride 200mg stat
2nd line (if 1st line unsuccessful)	Prophylaxis with 3-6 months of: • Trimethoprim 200mg nocté **OR** • Nitrofurantoin 100mg nocté **OR** • Pivmecillinam Hydrochloride 200mg nocté **OR** • Methenamine Hippurate 1g BD

Examples of Urology Requests, Results and Interpretations

Clinical Details on the request form:
Fever, supra-pubic pain and incontinence
Result

Specimen	Urine
Appearance	-
Microscopy	WBCs >100x10^6/L No epithelial cells
Culture	Escherichia coli

How is this Interpreted?
The high WBC count (>100x10^6/L) shows there is inflammation in the urinary tract. The absence of epithelial cells indicates that the urine sample has not been in contact with the skin of the perineum and is therefore not likely to be contaminated with skin flora. *E. coli* is one of the bacteria expected to be grown from a patient with a UTI. In the presence of the urinary tract symptoms in the clinical details this result confirms a diagnosis of UTI in this patient.

Clinical Details on the request form:
Acute confusion in an elderly patient
Result

Specimen	Urine
Appearance	-
Microscopy	WBCs <10x10^6/L No epithelial cells
Culture	Escherichia coli

How is this Interpreted?
The absence of WBCs (<10x10^6/L) shows there is no evidence of inflammation in the urinary tract. Even though there are no epithelial cells to indicate contact with the skin of the perineum the growth of *E. coli* in the absence of inflammation represents contamination and not infection. Another reason for the acute confusion should be sought.

Clinical Details on the request form:
Fever, rigors, tachycardia
Result

Specimen	Urine
Appearance	-
Microscopy	WBCs >100x10^6/L Epithelial cells ++
Culture	Escherichia coli

How is this Interpreted?
The presence of WBCs (>100x10^6/L) shows possible inflammation in the urinary tract, however there is also evidence that the urine has been in contact with the skin of the perineum from the presence of epithelial cells. Although *E. coli* is a common cause of UTI the possibility of contamination (epithelial cells ++) in this sample means that it is impossible to say if the patient's symptoms are due to a UTI. Even if the patient does have a UTI, it is not possible to determine if the UTI is due to the *E. coli*, which could have been picked up from the perineum and grown instead of the true cause. This is an unhelpful result, and is due to the fact that the sample has not been taken carefully, and has been in contact with the perineum.

Prostatitis

Prostatitis is an acute infection of the prostate. The condition can be chronic if present for >3 months or recurrent episodes occur with the same bacteria over a 3 month period or more.

Clinical Features
- Dysuria (difficulty passing urine)
- Frequency
- Urinary tract obstruction secondary to swelling
- Abdominal pain
- Tender prostate on examination

Causes

Common	• *Escherichia coli* • *Klebsiella* spp. • *Enterobacter* spp. • *Proteus mirabilis* • *Enterococcus* spp.

Hints and Tips
The same Gram-negative bacteria that cause urinary tract infections are also the common causes of prostatitis. Clinical examination and the history should be used to differentiate prostatitis from UTI although they can present in a very similar manner making the diagnosis difficult. Recurrent UTIs in a man that do not respond to antibiotics may actually be prostatitis. This requires a long course of treatment with an antibiotic that can get into the prostate.

Investigations
- Urine for microscopy, culture and sensitivity
- Raised Prostate Specific Antigen in 60% of acute prostatitis
- Prostatic discharge not usually taken as there is a risk of inducing sepsis through prostatic massage

Treatment
Only certain antibiotics get into the prostate to sufficiently treat prostatitis so treatment is limited, especially in antibiotic resistance. See section – Antibiotics, Table of Antibiotics Tissue Penetration

1st line	PO Ciprofloxacin
2nd line (if 1st line contraindicated)	PO Trimethoprim

Total Duration
Acute: 28 days
Chronic: 1-3 months

Dosing
See section - Antibiotics, Empirical Antibiotic Guidelines.

Prognosis and Complications
Complications include chronic infection (5%) or abscess formation (2%).

Sexually transmitted diseases (STDs) are infections transmitted person-to-person through sexual intercourse. Patients with one STD should be tested for other STDs. STDs include: syphilis, chlamydia, gonorrhoea, genital herpes, non-gonococcal urethritis (rarely symptomatic in women), blood-borne viruses and pelvic inflammatory disease (PID) - an acute infection of the female upper genital tract. PID is an infection in women caused by the vaginal flora ascending to infect any of the pelvic contents; it is not necessarily an STD although it is considered here for simplicity. PID includes endometritis, salpingitis, parametritis, oophoritis, tubo-ovarian abscess and pelvic peritonitis.

> **Common Mistake**
> The very young to the very old can present with STDs. Doctors sometimes avoid taking a sexual history for fear of offending the patient. **This is a mistake.** If asked in a sensitive manner, patients are rarely offended. If an STD is suspected take a sexual history to assess the risk of infection; it's less embarrassing to ask the questions than to miss a treatable infection.

Clinical Features

Male	• May be asymptomatic • Urethral discharge • Dysuria • Balanoposthitis (inflammation of the glans and foreskin)
Female	• May be asymptomatic • Vaginal discharge • Abdominal pain • Dysuria • Uterine bleeding • Infertility • Fever • Pruritis • Fitz-Hugh-Curtis Syndrome (right upper quadrant pain associated with perihepatitis)

Syphilis is described as **early** or **late** depending on how soon after acquiring the infection it presents. Early syphilis presents ≤2 years (usually primary or secondary) and late syphilis presents >2 years (usually secondary or tertiary).

Syphilis (early ≤2 years or late >2 years)	
Primary (infection at the point of inoculation)	• Chancre (painless swelling or punched out ulcer with regional lymphadenopathy)
Secondary (infection has spread from the primary site)	• Usually rash **PLUS** lymphadenopathy but can mimic any other infection • Raised mucous patches (usually in the mouth) and condylomata lata (highly infectious painless wart-like lesions on warm moist sites e.g. genitals and perineal skin) • Rare - meningitis or cranial nerve palsy, uveitis, optic neuropathy, keratitis or retinal necrosis

Tertiary (infection has spread from the primary or secondary site)	Symptoms usually present 20-40 years after initial infection: • Gummatous (granulomatous lesions with central necrosis usually on skin or bones) • Cardiovascular (inflammation of the ascending aorta) • Neurological arteritis (leading to CVA), progressive cognitive decline (leading to dementia), tabes dorsalis (sensory ataxia, nerve pain, pupil abnormalities, absent reflexes and loss of proprioception)

Causes

Syphilis	• *Treponema pallidum*
Chlamydia	• *Chlamydia trachomatis*
Gonorrhoea	• *Neisseria gonorrhoeae*
Genital Herpes	• *Herpes Simplex Virus* (HSV)
Non-Gonococcal Urethritis	• *Chlamydia trachomatis* • *Mycoplasma genitalium* • *Ureaplasma* spp. • *Trichomonas vaginalis* • *Adenovirus* • *Herpes Simplex Virus* (HSV)
Blood-borne Viruses	• *Hepatitis B Virus* • *Hepatitis C Virus* • *Human Immunodeficiency Virus* (HIV)
Pelvic Inflammatory Disease (PID)	Can be any of the above or polymicrobial with enteric flora

Investigations

No test is 100% sensitive or specific for STDs. Nucleic acid amplification tests (NAATs) are the test of choice for gonorrhoea and chlamydia. Culture can also be performed to obtain antibiotic sensitivities for *Neisseria gonorrhoeae*.
• Men
  – First pass urine for NAATs (urine held for ≥1 hour before taking sample of the first part of the urine stream)
  – Urethral or meatal swab for culture for *Neisseria gonorrhoeae*
• Women
  – Vulvovaginal or endocervical swabs for NAATs and culture for *Neisseria gonorrhoeae*
  – For PID send urethral or vaginal discharge for culture and sensitivity
• Anterior urethral smear or first pass urine for quantification of neutrophil polymorphs
• Viral swab for HSV (green viral swab)
• Blood for syphilis serology, hepatitis B, C and HIV

Syphilis Serology
It is important to be able to interpret the different syphilis serology tests, in combination, to establish if there is active or recent infection, evidence of past infection or false positive results.

The serology tests are:
- Non-treponemal
  - Rapid Plasma Reagin (RPR)
- Treponemal
  - *T. pallidum* enzyme immunoassay (EIA)
  - *T. pallidum* particle agglutination assay (TPPA)

Result	Interpretation	What it really means...
EIA negative	No evidence of treponemal infection	Not syphilis If high risk of recent infection within the past 4 weeks then repeat in 2-4 weeks
EIA positive TPPA positive RPR negative or positive ≤16	Consistent with treponemal infection at some time	Previous or recent syphilis. Repeat test with second sample to confirm result.
EIA positive TPPA positive RPR positive >16	Consistent with recent or active treponemal infection	Recent or active syphilis Repeat test with second sample to confirm result
EIA positive **confirmed** in second assay TPPA negative RPR positive (any value)	Consistent with treponemal infection at some time	Previous or recent syphilis A positive EIA and RPR but a negative TPPA should be automatically tested in the laboratory using a 2nd EIA or IgG immunoblot test. The 2nd EIA is confirmatory
EIA positive **not confirmed** in second assay TPPA negative RPR positive (any value)	EIA and RPR likely to be false positives. Treponemal infection unlikely but please repeat to confirm	Syphilis unlikely A single test for treponemal antibody/antigen that does not confirm in 2 further tests is likely to be a false positive and in this context the positive RPR is not diagnostic of treponemal infection If result changes in repeat sample then interpret the repeat result If result in repeat sample remains unchanged then interpret as no evidence of past or present treponemal infection
EIA positive TPPA negative RPR negative	No evidence of past or present treponemal infection	Likely false positive EIA test. If high risk* of recent infection within the past 4 weeks then repeat after 2-4 weeks

Note: *High risk = sexual activity with possible or probable exposure to syphilis

Treatment

Patients being treated for STDs should be advised to avoid sexual intercourse until after treatment completed **OR** 7 days after Azithromycin.

Syphilis	
Early (present ≤2 years)	IM Benzathine penicillin 2.4MU single dose **OR** IM Procaine penicillin 600,000 unit OD for 10 days **OR** PO Doxycycline 100mg BD for 14 days **OR** IM Ceftriaxone 500mg OD for 10 days
Late (present >2 years) Gummatous Cardiovascular	IM Benzathine penicillin 2.4MU 1 dose per week for 3 weeks **OR** IM Procaine penicillin 600,000 unit OD for 14 days **OR** PO Doxycycline 100mg BD for 28 days
Late (present >2 years) Neurological	IV Benzylpenicillin 1.8-2.4g 4 hourly for 14 days **OR** PO Doxycycline 100mg BD for 28 days **OR** IV or IM Ceftriaxone 2g OD for 10-14 days

Note: monitor RPR/VDRL at 3, 6 and 12 months and **THEN** 6 monthly until negative **OR** low and unchanged over 12 months; if ≥4-fold increase consider treatment failure or reinfection.

Chlamydia	
1st line	PO Doxycycline 100mg BD for 7 days **OR** PO Azithromycin 1g single dose
2nd line (if 1st line contraindicated)	PO Erythromycin 500mg BD 10-14 days

Note: Test of cure is not normally recommended in chlamydia; however patients' ≤25 years old should be retested in 3-6 months to look for reinfection.

Gonorrhoea	
1st line	IM Ceftriaxone 500mg single dose **PLUS** PO Azithromycin 1g single dose
2nd line (if 1st line contraindicated)	PO Azithromycin 2g single dose **OR** PO Ciprofloxacin 500mg single dose

Note: Test of cure is recommended in all cases of gonorrhoea either with culture at 72 hours post treatment (if still symptomatic) or with NAATs 2 weeks post treatment (if asymptomatic).

Genital Herpes	
1st line	Not normally treated, as acute exacerbations are self-limiting Genital Herpes cannot be completely cured If extensive painful ulceration, treat with PO Aciclovir 400mg TDS for 5 days or IV Aciclovir 5mg/kg TDS for 5 days

Non-Gonococcal Urethritis (NOT *Mycoplasma genitalium*)	
1st line	PO Doxycycline 100mg BD for 7 days
2nd line (if 1st line contraindicated)	PO Azithromycin 1g stat

Non-Gonococcal Urethritis (DUE TO *Mycoplasma genitalium*)	
1st line	PO Doxycycline 100mg BD for 7 days **THEN** PO Azithromycin 1g stat **THEN** 500mg OD for 2 days
2nd line (if 1st line contraindicated)	PO Moxifloxacin 400mg OD for 14 days

Blood-borne Viruses
See sections – Clinical Scenarios, Hepatitis and Clinical Scenarios, *Human Immunodeficiency Virus* (HIV and AIDS)

Pelvic Inflammatory Disease (PID)	
1st line Mild (Outpatient)	IM Ceftriaxone stat **PLUS** PO Doxycycline for 14 days **PLUS** PO Metronidazole for 5 days
2nd line Mild (Outpatient)	PO Ofloxacin for 14 days **PLUS** PO Metronidazole for 5 days
1st line Severe (Inpatient)	IV Ceftriaxone, treat until afebrile for 48 hours **PLUS** PO Doxycycline for 14 days **PLUS** PO or IV Metronidazole for 5 days
2nd line Severe (if 1st line contraindicated)	IV Clindamycin **PLUS** IV Gentamicin, treat until afebrile for 48 hours **THEN** Doxycycline **AND** Metronidazole as above 1st line Mild

Note: PID dosing, see section - Antibiotics, Empirical Antibiotic Guidelines

Prognosis and Complications

- Men – STDs can progress to epididymo-orchitis, prostatitis and reactive arthritis (Reiter's syndrome)
- Women – STDS can progress to salpingitis or pelvic inflammatory disease with resultant infertility or ectopic pregnancy, and reactive arthritis (Reiter's syndrome)
- *Neisseria gonorrhoeae* disseminates in 1% of genital infections to cause rash, fever, septic arthritis and sepsis
- Tertiary syphilis or reactivation of syphilis is rare but can occur up to 20 years after primary infection
- PID can lead to infertility, ectopic pregnancies and chronic pelvic pain

Prophylaxis and Prevention

Contact tracing and treatment to prevent further transmission of STDs, via the Genitourinary Medicine (GUM) service.

Skin, Soft Tissue, Bone and Joint Infections

<u>Cellulitis</u>

Cellulitis is an acute infection of the skin and subcutaneous tissues.

Clinical Features
- Spreading erythema
- Acute inflammation – pain, redness, heat, swelling and loss of function
- Systemic symptoms – fever, tachycardia, hypotension

> **Warning**
> If erythema is rapidly progressive, pain is out of proportion to clinical
> signs or cellulitis is present in children who have Chicken Pox (Varicella
> Zoster) then consider necrotising fasciitis. **This is an emergency**, (see
> section – Emergencies, Necrotising Fasciitis).

> **Common Mistake**
> Erythema, as a symptom of chronic lymphoedema, is often thought to be
> cellulitis. **This is a mistake.** The changes are not due to infection and do
> not respond to antibiotic treatment. This is a particularly common mistake
> with bilateral lower limb changes. Bilateral cellulitis is very rare but
> bilateral oedema secondary to heart failure is common and does not
> respond to antibiotic treatment.

Causes

Common	• *Staphylococcus aureus* • Beta-haemolytic *Streptococcus* (Groups A, C and G)
Diabetics or Vascular Insufficiency	• *Staphylococcus aureus* • Beta-haemolytic *Streptococcus* (Groups A, B, C and G) • Gram-negative bacteria e.g. *Pseudomonas aeruginosa* • Anaerobes e.g. *Clostridium* spp.
Returned Travellers	• *Staphylococcus aureus* • Beta-haemolytic *Streptococcus* (Groups A, C and G) • Opportunists e.g. *Aeromonas* spp., *Vibrio vulnificus*

Investigations
- Usually a clinical diagnosis
- If broken skin consider taking skin swabs after removing overlying slough
- If systemic symptoms consider taking blood cultures

> **Myth**
> If you grow bacteria from a wound then you must treat with antibiotics.
> **FALSE** - Ulcers and pressure sores become colonised with enteric bacteria
> (e.g. *Escherichia coli*, *Pseudomonas* spp. and *Enterococcus* spp.). The
> growth of these types of bacteria from broken areas of skin suggests they
> have become part of the normal flora and are not causing infection. They
> do not usually need treating.

Treatment

1st line	PO or IV Flucloxacillin
2nd line (if 1st line contraindicated)	PO Erythromycin **OR** PO Clindamycin **OR** IV Teicoplanin **OR** IV Vancomycin
If diabetic /vascular	**ADD** PO or IV Metronidazole **PLUS** IV Gentamicin if *Pseudomonas* spp.
If MRSA positive	IV Teicoplanin **OR** IV Vancomycin

Total Duration
10-14 days

Dosing
See section - Antibiotics, Empirical Antibiotic Guidelines.

Common Mistake
Some doctors treat cellulitis with Flucloxacillin in patients colonised with MRSA. **This is a mistake.** Cellulitis is commonly caused by *S. aureus*. If the patient is a carrier of MRSA then the cellulitis will be caused by MRSA as this is the patient's normal flora. MRSA is resistant to most Beta-lactam antibiotics including Flucloxacillin. Cellulitis caused by MRSA should be treated with glycopeptides, oxazolidinones, tetracyclines or aminoglycosides.

Normal Antibiotic Sensitivity of MRSA

Sensitive	Usually Sensitive	Resistant
• Glycopeptides e.g. Teicoplanin • Oxazolidinones e.g. Linezolid	• Tetracyclines e.g. Doxycycline • Aminoglycosides e.g. Gentamicin	• **MOST** Beta-lactam antibiotics • Quinolones e.g. Ciprofloxacin • Macrolides e.g. Erythromycin • Lincosamides e.g. Clindamycin

Prognosis and Complications
Most patients get better with treatment.

Prophylaxis and Prevention
No role for antibiotics to prevent recurrence.

Hints and Tips
Some patients with "recurrent" cellulitis in a limb with lymphoedema may benefit from a prolonged course of PO Doxycycline, PO Penicillin V or PO Erythromycin for 1 month to prevent recurrence, as in this case the "recurrence" is usually a failure to eradicate the original infection in the lymphoedematous limb.

In a few rare instances, low dose PO Penicillin V (250-500mg BD) or PO Erythromycin (250-500mg OD) for 1-2 years may reduce the incidence of true recurrent cellulitis.

Bites

Bites can either be from a human or an animal. Microbiologically, human bites are worse than cat bites, which in turn are worse than dog bites. Human bites are dirtier than other types of bites although cat bites often have a narrow entrance that closes rapidly leaving an anaerobic environment in which bacteria can proliferate.

Clinical Features
- Spreading erythema
- Acute inflammation – pain, redness, heat, swelling and loss of function
- Abscess
- Pus or serosanguinous discharge

Causes
Infection is usually polymicrobial and caused by the oral flora of whatever or whoever bit the patient. Secondary infections can occur with the normal causes of cellulitis.

Animal	• *Pasteurella multocida* • *Capnocytophaga canimorsus* • *Bacteroides* spp. • *Fusobacterium* spp.
Human	• *Staphylococcus aureus* • *Streptococcus* spp. • *Haemophilus* spp. • *Eikenella* spp. • *Bacteroides* spp. • *Fusobacterium* spp.

Investigations
- Usually a clinical diagnosis
- If broken skin consider taking skin swabs
- If fluid discharge send for microscopy, culture and sensitivity
- If systemic symptoms consider taking blood cultures

> **Common Mistake**
> Some doctors treat the human bite but sometimes forget potential blood-borne virus exposure to hepatitis B, hepatitis C and HIV . **This is a mistake.** Consideration should be given to Post-Exposure Prophylaxis (PEP) for bites from a carrier of these viruses (see section – Infection Control, Needlestick Injuries).

Treatment
Wounds should be irrigated with sterile water and any foreign material removed e.g. broken teeth.
If possible, do not initially close the wound as this can worsen anaerobic infection. Consider waiting 24-48 hours or allow to heal by secondary intention.

1st line	PO Co-amoxiclav
2nd line (if 1st line contraindicated)	PO Doxycycline **PLUS** PO Metronidazole

Total Duration
10-14 days

Dosing
See section - Antibiotics, Empirical Antibiotic Guidelines.

Other considerations
- Tetanus booster if soil has contaminated the wound or there is devascularised tissue
- Consider rabies vaccination in returned traveller

Prognosis and Complications
Complications include retained foreign body, septic arthritis, abscess, osteomyelitis, tendonitis, bacteraemia and fractures.

Rabies
Rabies is a severe viral encephalitis that is almost always fatal even with treatment. Rabies can be transmitted via the saliva of infected mammals including dogs, cats, bats and other wild animals, normally through a bite. The incubation period for rabies can vary from a few days to over 19 years depending on what part of the body was bitten, the severity of the bite and the strain of *Rabies Virus*.

The best way of preventing rabies, other than not being bitten, is to be vaccinated against *Rabies Virus*.

In the event of a bite from an animal, a risk assessment for potential rabies exposure should be undertaken and Post-Exposure Prophylaxis (PEP) be given based on this risk assessment. In the UK there is no risk of rabies from any animal **other than bats**. If in doubt seek expert advice. In the UK the best source of advice is the consultant on duty for rabies advice at the Viral Reference Department at Public Health England Colindale, telephone number 020 8327 6017, who will also arrange rabies immunoglobulin if it is required.

Rabies Risk Assessment Considers
- The geographical location where the bite occurred e.g. is the country rabies free, low risk or high risk
- The type of exposure e.g. no contact, minimal contact, bites
- The immune status of the person receiving the bite e.g. non-immune, partially vaccinated, fully vaccinated. If there is any doubt about the patient's immune status then treat them as non-immune.

Post-Exposure Prophylaxis (PEP)
- No risk country or low risk exposure = no PEP
- Fully immunised = 2 doses of rabies vaccine
- Low risk country, none immune = 5 doses of rabies vaccine
- High risk country, high risk exposure, non-immune = 5 doses of rabies vaccine **PLUS** rabies immunoglobulin

The sooner PEP can be given the more likely it is to be effective at preventing infection.

Infected Burns, Skin Grafts and Post-Operative Wounds

Infected burns, skin grafts and post-operative wounds are included together as the approach to their management is the same. All represent acute inflammation of tissue around broken areas of skin.

Clinical Features
- Pain, swelling, erythema
- Increasingly purulent discharge
- Systemic signs - fever, sepsis

Causes

Common	- *Staphylococcus aureus*(MSSA and MRSA) - Beta-haemolytic *Streptococcus* (Groups A, C and G)
Occasional	- Gram-negative bacteria e.g. Enterobacteriaceae, *Pseudomonas aeruginosa* - Anaerobes e.g. *Clostridium* spp.

Myth
Some doctors believe that if bacteria are grown from an area of broken skin it must be infected. **FALSE** - This is often not the case because any area of broken skin will rapidly become colonised by bacteria including those normally regarded as bowel flora (e.g. *Escherichia coli*, *Pseudomonas* spp. and *Enterococcus* spp.). In addition, many ulcers contain dead tissue (slough), which is often mistaken for pus but is in fact just detached tissue. Infected areas of broken skin show signs of acute inflammation – pain, erythema, swelling as well as purulent discharge. Without these signs the growth of bacteria indicates colonisation not infection and does not require treatment with antibiotics.

Investigations
- Infection of a skin wound is a clinical diagnosis based on the presence of inflammation
- Swabs may be helpful but only after removing overlying slough
- If systemic symptoms consider taking blood cultures

Treatment
If there is an abscess present, consider incision and drainage.

1st line	PO or IV Flucloxacillin **PLUS** IV Gentamicin if *Pseudomonas* spp. present
2nd line (if 1st line contraindicated)	IV Teicoplanin **OR** IV Vancomycin **PLUS** IV Gentamicin if *Pseudomonas* spp. present
If diabetic /vascular	**ADD** Metronidazole
If MRSA positive	IV Teicoplanin **OR** IV Vancomycin **PLUS** IV Gentamicin if *Pseudomonas* spp. present

Total Duration
7 days

Dosing
See section - Antibiotics, Empirical Antibiotic Guidelines.

Prognosis and Complications
Most patients get better with treatment, but underlying skin defects may take longer to heal.

Prophylaxis and Prevention
If post-operative wounds are devascularised, consider giving 5 days of IV Benzylpenicillin **PLUS** IV Metronidazole to prevent anaerobic infection including *Clostridium perfringens* gas gangrene, a form of necrotising fasciitis.

Intravascular Device Associated Infection

Intravascular device associated infection is an infection due to the presence of an intravascular catheter.

Types of Intravascular Device

Peripheral Venous Catheter	Short-term intravascular access, often known as a cannula
Peripheral Arterial Catheter	Short-term intra-arterial access for measuring cardiopulmonary status of critically ill patients
Short-term Central Venous Catheter (CVC)	Inserted into the jugular or subclavian veins with the end of the catheter in the superior vena cava
Peripherally Inserted Central Catheter (PICC)	Inserted into a peripheral vein with the end of the catheter in the superior vena cava
Long-term Central Venous Catheter (CVC)	Surgically implanted CVC tunnelling under the skin before entering into a large blood vessel, usually the subclavian vein e.g. Broviac, Groshong, Hickman catheters
Totally Implanted Catheter	Surgically inserted with a subcutaneous port, accessible through a self-sealing septum via a needle through the skin e.g. Portacath

Clinical Features

- Fever and rigors (especially when the IV device is used)
- Erythema
- Pain at exit or tunnel site
- Discharge from exit site

MILD (localised symptoms)
MODERATE - SEVERE (systemic symptoms)

Types of Infection

Phlebitis	Inflammation along the tract of the catheterised blood vessel
Exit site infection	Inflammation of the skin <2cm from where the IV catheter exits the body; often associated with pain, discharge, fever
Tunnel infection	Inflammation >2cm from the catheter exit site along the subcutaneous tract of a tunnelled CVC
Pocket infection	Inflammation of the subcutaneous pocket of a totally implantable device
IV catheter-associated bloodstream infection	Bacteraemia or fungaemia as a result of an infected IV catheter

Causes

Common	• *Staphylococcus aureus* (MSSA and MRSA) • Coagulase negative *Staphylococcus* spp.
Sepsis or Neutropaenia or AICU / HDU patients	• *Staphylococcus aureus* (MSSA and MRSA) • Enterobacteriaceae e.g. *Klebsiella* spp., *Enterobacter* spp., *Serratia marcescens* • *Pseudomonas aeruginosa* • *Enterococcus* spp. • *Candida* spp.

Investigations

- Culture of catheter tip if infection suspected
  - Do not routinely send catheter tip unless infection suspected
- Blood cultures from both CVC and peripheral blood vessel (taken and sent at the same time = "Paired")
  - "Paired" - comparison of "time to positivity" between CVC and peripheral samples can help distinguish CVC infection from other infections. If the same volume of blood is incubated in the same conditions, and the CVC blood culture is positive >2 hours before peripheral, this suggests CVC infection
- If Coagulase negative *Staphylococcus* spp. isolated from blood cultures, repeat blood cultures and **ONLY** treat if repeat cultures also positive

Myth

Some doctors believe if bacteria are cultured from a CVC tip it is always significant. **FALSE** - Many CVC tips are contaminated with skin bacteria on removal. Most microbiology laboratories do not use methods capable of differentiating contamination from infection because these are technically demanding and time consuming. An IV catheter related infection cannot be diagnosed purely on the basis of the culture result. However, the antibiotic sensitivity of the microorganism grown from the catheter tip of a patient who has a suspected CVC infection can help guide treatment.

Treatment

First line treatment is removal of the intravascular catheter.

Peripheral Catheter Infection e.g. cannula	**MILD**: PO Doxycycline **MODERATE - SEVERE**: IV Teicoplanin **OR** IV Vancomycin
Bacterial CVC Infection	IV Teicoplanin **OR** IV Vancomycin **PLUS** IV Gentamicin
Candida CVC Infection	IV Caspofungin **PLUS** Change all IV lines and repeat blood cultures after 48 hours to ensure suppression of infection

Total Duration

7 days
If blood culture positive: 7-14 days

Dosing

See section - Antibiotics, Empirical Antibiotic Guidelines.

Prognosis and Complications

Staphylococcus aureus bacteraemia has 20% mortality even with treatment. Mortality increases depending on underlying co-morbidities and any resulting complications. Development of infective endocarditis following bacteraemia has 100% mortality if untreated.

Prophylaxis and Prevention

No role for antibiotics to prevent occurrence.

Osteomyelitis

Osteomyelitis is an infection of bone causing progressive bone destruction.

Clinical Features
- Pain
- Fever
- Swelling of overlying soft tissue
- Systemic symptoms e.g. fever, sepsis

Causes
Entry of bacteria into bone can either be haematogenous, via the bloodstream from a distant source such as a UTI, or by direct inoculation from trauma or surgery.

Common	• *Staphylococcus aureus* • Beta-haemolytic *Streptococcus* (Groups A, C and G)
If diabetic / elderly	• *Staphylococcus aureus* • Beta-haemolytic *Streptococcus* (Groups A, B, C and G) • Enterobacteriaceae e.g. *Escherichia coli, Klebsiella* spp.
Secondary to trauma	As above plus: • Anaerobes e.g. *Clostridium* spp.

Investigations
- Haematology and Biochemistry
- Raised white blood cell count, Erythrocyte Sedimentation Rate (ESR) and C-Reactive Protein (CRP)
- Blood cultures
- Bone biopsy
  - For microscopy, culture and sensitivity
  - Preferably before antibiotics are started, but do not delay antibiotics unnecessarily
- **DO NOT** send swabs of pus. Some Orthopaedic Surgeons have a habit of going in to bones and joints and washing out copious amounts of pus and only sending a swab! Send pus or tissue in a sterile universal (see section – Microbiology, How to Take Microbiology Specimens)

Treatment

Remove prosthetic material, if possible. Bacteria form biofilms on prosthetic material and this makes these types of infections very resistant to treatment.

1st line	IV Flucloxacillin **PLUS** PO Fusidic Acid
2nd line (if 1st line contraindicated)	IV Teicoplanin **OR** IV Vancomycin **PLUS** PO Fusidic Acid
If diabetic /elderly	IV Ceftriaxone
If MRSA positive	IV Teicoplanin **OR** Vancomycin **PLUS** PO Fusidic Acid
If Traumatic injury	**ADD** IV Metronidazole

Total Duration

6 weeks (at least 2-4 weeks intravenously).

Dosing

See section - Antibiotics, Empirical Antibiotic Guidelines.

Prognosis and Complications

Most patients get better with treatment, however a small number will go on to develop chronic infection or permanent damage to the bone with associated deformity.

Prophylaxis and Prevention

No role for antibiotics to prevent recurrence.

<u>**Septic Arthritis**</u>

Septic arthritis is inflammation of the joint space due to infection, which can occur in both native and prosthetic joints.

Clinical Features
- Pain, particularly on movement of the joint
- Fever in 60-80% of patients
- Swelling of joint
- Systemic symptoms e.g. fever, sepsis

Definition of Prosthetic Joint Infection
- Presence of a sinus tract that communicates with prosthesis
- Intra-operative tissue histology showing acute inflammation
- Joint pus with no other aetiology
- Positive culture from pre-operative arthrocentesis **OR** ≥2 intra-operative samples growing the same bacteria

Causes
Entry of bacteria into the joint can either be haematogenous, via the bloodstream from another source such as a UTI, or by direct inoculation from trauma or surgery.

Native Joint	
Common	• *Staphylococcus aureus* • Beta-haemolytic *Streptococcus* (Groups A, C and G)
Children	• *Staphylococcus aureus* • Beta-haemolytic *Streptococcus* (Groups A, C and G) • *Kingella kingae* • *Streptococcus pneumoniae* • *Haemophilus influenzae* type b (Hib)
If diabetic / elderly	• *Staphylococcus aureus* • Beta-haemolytic *Streptococcus* (Groups A, B, C and G) • Enterobacteriaceae e.g. *Escherichia coli*, *Klebsiella* spp.
Sickle Cell	As for common plus: • *Salmonella* spp.
Following bites	As for common plus: • *Pasteurella multocida* • *Capnocytophaga canimorsus* • *Eikenella corrodens*

Prosthetic Joint	
Acute or early presentation (days to weeks)	• *Staphylococcus aureus* • Beta-haemolytic *Streptococcus* (Groups A, B, C and G) • Enterobacteriaceae e.g. *Escherichia coli*, *Klebsiella* spp.
Chronic or late presentation (months to years)	• Coagulase negative *Staphylococcus* spp. • *Corynebacterium* spp. • *Cutibacterium* spp.

Investigations

- Haematology and Biochemistry
  - Raised white blood cell count, Erythrocyte Sedimentation Rate (ESR) and C-Reactive Protein (CRP)
- Blood cultures
- Synovial Fluid in purple EDTA vacutainer
  - For microscopy, culture and sensitivity
  - Preferably before antibiotics are started, but do not delay antibiotics unnecessarily
  - Raised white blood cell count
  - Gram stain positive in 50% of cases
  - Culture positive in 80-90% of cases
- Swabs are not suitable as they should not be Gram stained

Additional for Suspected Prosthetic Joint Infection

- Patients should be antibiotic free for ≥2 weeks prior to excision of prosthesis to enhance yield of microorganisms on culture
- Consider pre-operative diagnostic arthrocentesis for total white blood cell count (WBC) and percentage neutrophil count (if no inflammatory arthropathy) **PLUS** culture
- Intra-operative 5-6 peri-prosthetic samples for culture

On the Horizon

There is increasing evidence that a simple colorimetric strip test for leucocyte esterase (an enzyme produced by white blood cells and therefore a marker for inflammation) in synovial fluid is of value in diagnosing prosthetic joint infections. This is a simple "dipstick" type test which could be used in the operating theatre to help guide treatment. Studies suggest the positive predictive value is almost 100% and the negative predictive value is 93%. It is probable that these will become part of standard practice in the near future.

Interpretation of Diagnostic Arthrocentesis

Procedure	Result suggestive of infection
Total Knee Arthroplasty (1-3 months post implantation)	>27,800 WBC/µL >89% neutrophils
Total Knee Arthroplasty (>3 months post implantation)	>1700 WBC/µL >65% neutrophils
Total Hip Arthroplasty	>4200 WBC/µL

Empirical Treatment
Urgent drainage of the joint space and removal of prosthetic material if possible. Bacteria form biofilms on prosthetic material and this makes these types of infections very resistant to treatment. Ideally patients should be antibiotic free for at least 2 weeks prior to excision of old prosthesis in order to enhance the yield of microorganisms on culture.

Native Joint	
1st line	PO or IV Flucloxacillin **PLUS** PO Fusidic Acid
2nd line (if 1st line contraindicated)	IV Teicoplanin **OR** IV Vancomycin **PLUS** PO Fusidic Acid
Children	IV Ceftriaxone
If diabetic / elderly	IV Ceftriaxone
If MRSA positive	IV Teicoplanin **OR** IV Vancomycin **PLUS** PO Fusidic Acid
Sickle cell	IV Ceftriaxone
Following Bites	IV Co-amoxiclav

Prosthetic Joint	
1st line	IV Teicoplanin **OR** IV Vancomycin **PLUS** PO Rifampicin
2nd line (if 1st line contraindicated)	IV Daptomycin **PLUS** PO Rifampicin

Total Duration
Native joint: 6 weeks (at least 2-4 weeks intravenous)
Prosthetic joint: 3 months (normally 6 weeks intravenous)

Dosing
See section - Antibiotics, Empirical Antibiotic Guidelines.

Definitive Treatment

1 Stage Revision (Usually occurs inadvertently when what is thought to be aseptic loosening turns out to be infection)	
Staphylococcus aureus	2-6 weeks pathogen specific IV antibiotic **PLUS** PO Rifampicin (If Rifampicin cannot be used give 4-6 weeks IV therapy) **THEN** Oral companion therapy to total of 3 months treatment
Other bacteria	4-6 weeks pathogen specific IV **OR** highly bioavailable oral antibiotic

2 Stage Revision
(Patient should be off antibiotic for 2-8 weeks prior to 2nd stage procedure)

Staphylococcus aureus	4-6 weeks pathogen specific IV antibiotic **OR** highly bioavailable oral antibiotic **PLUS** PO Rifampicin
Other bacteria	4-6 weeks pathogen specific IV **OR** highly bioavailable oral antibiotic

Debridement and Retention of Prosthesis
(If no sinus, <30 days post op or <3 weeks after onset of symptoms)

Staphylococcus aureus (Total Hip, Elbow, Shoulder or Ankle Arthroplasty)	2-6 weeks pathogen specific IV antibiotic **PLUS** PO Rifampicin (If Rifampicin cannot be used give 4-6 weeks IV therapy) **THEN** Oral companion therapy to total of 3 months treatment
Staphylococcus aureus (Total Knee Arthroplasty)	2-6 weeks pathogen specific IV antibiotic **PLUS** PO Rifampicin (If Rifampicin cannot be used give 4-6 weeks IV therapy) **THEN** Oral companion therapy to total of 6 months treatment
Other bacteria	4-6 weeks pathogen specific IV **OR** highly bioavailable oral antibiotic

Permanent Resection Arthroplasty

Staphylococcus aureus	4-6 weeks pathogen specific IV antibiotic **OR** highly bioavailable oral antibiotic **PLUS** PO Rifampicin
Other bacteria	4-6 weeks pathogen specific IV **OR** highly bioavailable oral antibiotic

Staphylococcus aureus (MSSA)

1st line	IV Flucloxacillin 2g 4-6 hourly **PLUS** PO Rifampicin 300-450mg BD
2nd line (if 1st line contraindicated)	IV Ceftriaxone 1-2g OD **OR** IV Vancomycin 15mg/kg BD **OR** IV Daptomycin 6mg/kg OD **PLUS** PO Rifampicin 300-450mg BD
Potential oral companion therapy	PO Rifampicin 300-450mg BD **PLUS** PO Ciprofloxacin 750mg BD **OR** PO Levofloxacin 500mg BD **OR** PO Flucloxacillin 500mg-1g QDS **OR** PO Doxycycline 100mg BD **OR** PO Cephalosporin

Staphylococcus aureus (MRSA)	
1st line	IV Vancomycin 15mg/kg BD **PLUS** PO Rifampicin 300-450mg BD
2nd line (if 1st line contraindicated)	IV Daptomycin 6mg/kg OD **OR** IV/PO Linezolid 600mg BD **PLUS** PO Rifampicin 300-450mg BD
Potential oral companion therapy	PO Rifampicin 300-450mg BD **PLUS** PO Ciprofloxacin 750mg BD **OR** PO Levofloxacin 500mg BD **OR** PO Doxycycline 100mg BD **OR** PO Co-trimoxazole 960mg BD

Beta-haemolytic Streptococcus (Groups A, B, C, G)	
1st line	IV Benzylpenicillin 2.4g 4 hourly
2nd line (if 1st line contraindicated)	IV Ceftriaxone 1-2g OD **OR** IV Vancomycin 15mg/kg BD

Enterococcus spp.	
1st line	IV Vancomycin 15mg/kg BD
2nd line (if 1st line contraindicated)	IV Daptomycin 6mg/kg OD **OR** IV/PO Linezolid 600mg BD

Enterobacteriaceae	
1st line	IV Ceftriaxone 1-2g OD
2nd line (if 1st line contraindicated)	IV Ciprofloxacin 400mg TDS **OR** PO Ciprofloxacin 750mg BD **OR** IV Ertapenem 1g OD

Pseudomonas aeruginosa	
1st line	IV Meropenem 1g TDS
2nd line (if 1st line contraindicated)	IV Ciprofloxacin 400mg TDS **OR** PO Ciprofloxacin 750mg BD **OR** IV Ceftazidime 2g TDS

Amputation	
If all infected material removed	24-48 hours pathogen specific IV **OR** highly bioavailable oral antibiotic

Chronic Suppression Therapy	
All bacteria	Oral companion **OR** pathogen specific oral antibiotic therapy
If unable to remove all infected material	4-6 weeks pathogen specific IV **OR** highly bioavailable oral antibiotic

Prognosis and Complications
Prosthetic joints are unlikely to respond to antibiotics alone without removal of the prosthesis.

Prophylaxis and Prevention
No role for antibiotics to prevent recurrence.

174

Gastrointestinal Infections

<u>Gastroenteritis and Diarrhoea and Vomiting (D&V)</u>

Gastroenteritis is inflammation of the stomach and small intestine causing ≥3 liquid or loose stools/diarrhoea in 24 hours with or without vomiting.

Clinical Features
- Liquid or loose stool, which takes the shape of the container it is put in (types 5-7 on the Bristol Stool Chart, see Appendix 2)
- Vomiting
- Speed of onset related to infectious cause
  - Minutes to hours caused by pre-formed toxin
  - Hours to days caused by viruses and bacteria
- Systemic symptoms, fever, sweats, chills, aches and pains, caused by *Campylobacter* spp., typhoid and paratyphoid
- Chronic symptoms (>2 weeks) commonly caused by parasites

Causes

Common	
Pre-formed toxin	• *Staphylococcus aureus* • *Bacillus cereus* • *Clostridium perfringens*
Viruses	• *Norovirus* • *Rotavirus* • *Adenovirus*
Bacteria	• *Campylobacter* spp. • *Shigella* spp. • *Salmonella* spp. • *Escherichia coli*, including O157 • *Clostridium difficile*
Parasites	• *Cryptosporidium* spp. • *Giardia lamblia*

Returned travellers	
Bacteria	As above plus: • *Vibrio cholerae* • *Vibrio parahaemolyticus* • *Salmonella typhi* (typhoid) • *Salmonella paratyphi* (paratyphoid)

Investigations
- Stool
  - Culture or PCR for bacteria
  - Toxin testing for *Clostridium difficile*
  - Antigen testing or PCR for viruses
  - Microscopy is not routinely performed: request ova, cysts and parasites (OCP) only if these are clinically suspected
    - PCR for *Cryptosporidium* spp. and *Giardia lamblia* if available

Common Mistake
Some doctors believe that antibiotics should be used to treat gastroenteritis. **This is a mistake.** In fact antibiotics can potentially make some infections worse e.g. antibiotics can increase toxin production in *Escherichia coli* O157 leading to increased risk of Haemolytic Uraemic Syndrome.

Treatment

Supportive treatment only (adequate hydration) in patients with a normal immune system except for:

- *Clostridium difficile* (see section – Clinical Scenarios, *Clostridium difficile* Associated Disease)
- Typhoid and paratyphoid
- *Giardia lamblia*

Typhoid or Paratyphoid	IV Ceftriaxone 2g OD 10-14 days **OR** PO Ciprofloxacin 500mg BD 7-10 days **OR** PO Azithromycin 1g OD 5-7 days
Giardia lamblia	PO Metronidazole 400mg TDS 5-10 days

Note: these are specific treatment durations for these particular clinical scenarios

> **Warning**
> Ciprofloxacin should not be used to treat typhoid or paratyphoid unless the bacteria are shown to be sensitive on laboratory testing because 60% of typhoid and 85% of paratyphoid are now resistant to Ciprofloxacin. Ceftriaxone should be used empirically until antibiotic sensitivities are known.
>
> **Note:** patients' temperatures take longer to settle on Ceftriaxone (up to 7 days)...allow time for the Ceftriaxone to work.

Dosing
See section - Antibiotics, Empirical Antibiotic Guidelines.

Prognosis and Complications
It is estimated that one in every 1,000 campylobacter infections (treated or untreated) leads to Guillain-Barre syndrome 1-3 weeks after infection (this equates to up to 40% of Guillain-Barre syndrome cases).

Prophylaxis and Prevention
Vaccinate against *Rotavirus* as part of the primary course of childhood immunisations.

Most bacterial causes of gastroenteritis e.g. *Campylobacter* spp., *Shigella* spp., *Salmonella* spp. and *Escherichia coli* O157 are Notifiable Infectious Diseases (see section – Microbiology, Notifiable Infectious Diseases in the UK).

Infection Control Precautions
See section – Infection Control, Diarrhoea and Vomiting.

> **Warning**
> Do not routinely cohort patients with diarrhoea and vomiting, as patients may also be carriers of other enteric bacteria, which are more likely to spread if the patient has D&V e.g. ESBL-positive *Escherichia coli* and GRE.

Clostridium difficile Associated Disease (CDAD)

Clostridium difficile Associated Disease (CDAD) is the most common cause of antibiotic associated diarrhoea. Symptoms present 5-10 days after starting antibiotics. Up to 3% of the population are asymptomatic carriers of *Clostridium difficile* and although they have no symptoms they represent an infection control issue as they can spread the infection.

Diagnosis of CDAD
- One or more episodes of stool loose enough to take the shape of the container (types 5-7 on the Bristol Stool Chart, see Appendix 2)
  - **PLUS** not attributable to another cause including medicines
  - **PLUS** a positive laboratory test for *Clostridium difficile* toxin
  - **OR** evidence of pseudomembranous colitis on endoscopy

Risk Factors for Severe Disease:
- Age >85 years
- Temperature >38.5°C
- Increasing creatinine >50% over baseline
- Signs of colitis
- Colonic dilatation
- Immunosuppressed
- Admission to an Intensive Care Unit
- White blood cell count >15 x 10^9/L **OR** <1.5 x 10^9/L
- Hypotension

Clinical Features
- Diarrhoea
- Nausea
- Dehydration
- Abdominal pain
- Fever
- Bowel perforation
- Toxic megacolon (>6cm diameter with no obstruction)

> **Warning**
> Certain antibiotics are regarded as high-risk for predisposing to *Clostridium difficile* and should be used with caution.
> **REMEMBER the "4Cs":**
> - **C**ephalosporins
> - **C**iprofloxacin (and other quinolones)
> - **C**lindamycin
> - **C**o-amoxiclav

Causes
CDAD is caused by toxins produced by the bacterium *Clostridium difficile*

Investigations
- Stool (liquid stool only) 2-stage test taking 3-4 hours and performed daily by laboratories
  - All inpatients >2 years old, with a liquid stool sample
  - All outpatients >65 years old, with a liquid stool sample
  - Outpatients under 65 years old, with a liquid stool sample, if specifically requested
- Sampling to test for cure is not required; 50% of successfully treated patients have positive tests up to 6 weeks after infection has cleared

Microbiology laboratories cannot test for *Clostridium difficile* toxin in children under 2 years old. **FALSE** - Laboratories can do this test but the results would be meaningless, as almost all babies are temporarily colonised with *Clostridium difficile* in their guts. This gradually disappears as they get older. Under 2 year olds are not clinically affected by this colonisation because they do not have gastrointestinal receptors for the toxin.

Treatment

Stop the offending antibiotic. If the patient still requires treatment for another infection then discuss the options with a Microbiologist and consider continuing *Clostridium difficile* treatment for 1 week beyond stopping the other antibiotics. Severe and critically ill patients need an urgent surgical review.

Initial Episode of Infection	
Mild/Moderate	PO Metronidazole 500mg TDS
Severe	PO Vancomycin 125mg QDS **IF NO RESPONSE** PO Vancomycin 500mg QDS
Critically Ill	PO Vancomycin 500mg QDS **PLUS** IV Metronidazole 500mg TDS

Recurrent Infection	
1st Recurrence	As for Mild/Moderate or Severe above
2nd Recurrence	PO Vancomycin 125mg QDS for 14 days **THEN** BD for 7 days **THEN** OD for 7 days **THEN** Alternate days for 7 days **THEN** every 3 days for 14 days **OR** PO Fidaxomicin 200mg BD for 10 days
Further recurrences	PO Fidaxomicin 200mg BD for 10 days (if not previously used) **OR** PO Vancomycin 125mg QDS for 14 days **THEN** PO Rifaximin 400mg TDS for 10 days **OR** Faecal bacteriotherapy

Antibiotics that **DO NOT** normally predispose to CDAD:
- IV Piptazobactam
- PO Doxycycline
- IV Benzylpenicillin
- IV Vancomycin
- IV Teicoplanin
- IV Temocillin
- IV Gentamicin

Faecal Bacteriotherapy

Faecal bacteriotherapy, also known as "faecal transplantation", involves replacement of the colonic contents with stool containing normal flora from a donor. Donors are screened for various infections prior to donation; samples are held frozen in a "faeces donor bank" up until they are required. Faecal bacteriotherapy has a 94% cure rate in pseudomembranous colitis caused by *Clostridium difficile*. The lack of widespread adoption in the NHS, even though it is approved by the National Institute for Health and Care Excellence (NICE), is related to the social and medical stigmatisation associated with the concept of deliberately introducing someone else's faeces into another person.

Common Mistake

Some doctors assume that treatment with PO Vancomycin should be converted to IV when treating CDAD in patients who are "Nil By Mouth". **This is a mistake.** IV Vancomycin does not get into the gut lumen and therefore has no activity in CDAD. If it is not possible to give an oral or nasogastric antibiotic the patient should be discussed with a Microbiologist or Gastroenterologist.

Total Duration
Initial Episode: 14 days
Recurrent Infections: as stated in treatment table

Dosing
See section - Antibiotics, Empirical Antibiotic Guidelines.

Prognosis and Complications
90% of patients with CDAD respond to treatment. However, 20-30% of these have recurrent infection. These patients should be retreated or offered faecal bacteriotherapy which has a 94% cure rate in pseudomembranous colitis. The mortality from toxic megacolon is 64%.

Prophylaxis and Prevention
Clostridium difficile can exist as both spores and vegetative bacteria and therefore can survive drying. The bacteria can persist in the environment for a long time and hence the need for deep cleaning between patients. Environmental control is the best way to prevent CDAD.

Infection Control Precautions
See section – Infection Control, *Clostridium difficile* Associated Disease.

On the Horizon
Ribaxamase® is an oral Ambler Class A beta-lactamase enzyme active against penicillins and cephalosporins (including 3rd generation or extended spectrum e.g. Ceftriaxone). Its purpose is to "mop up" any IV penicillin or cephalosporin that "spills" over into the gut. Ribaxamase® prevents disruption of the normal gut flora, whilst still allowing systemic activity of the beta-lactam. This reduces the risk of *Clostridium difficile* Associated Disease and selective pressure driving antibiotic resistance. It is expected that other oral enzymes will be produced in the future to protect the normal gut flora from other classes of antibiotics.

Necrotising Pancreatitis

Pancreatitis is inflammation of the pancreas; commonly caused by gallstones and alcohol consumption. When the pancreas becomes inflamed digestive enzymes leak out and start to "digest" the surrounding tissues causing further inflammation. Pancreatitis and necrotising pancreatitis are not infections; however dead pancreatic tissue can become infected leading to infected necrotising pancreatitis. **Note:** Less than 20% of patients with pancreatitis have necrotising pancreatitis; only 6% of patients with pancreatitis have infected necrotising pancreatitis.

Clinical features
- Central upper abdominal pain radiating to the back
- Fever
- Tachycardia
- Hypotension
- Tachypnoea
- Shock and multi-organ failure

Causes

Infected necrotising pancreatitis	Often mixed microorganisms: • Enterobacteriaceae e.g. *Escherichia coli*, *Klebsiella* spp., *Enterobacter* spp., *Proteus* spp. • *Enterococcus* spp. • Anaerobes e.g. *Bacteroides* spp., *Clostridium* spp., *Fusobacterium* spp.

Investigations
- Serum amylase or lipase (enzymes released from damaged pancreas)
- Blood cultures
- CT abdomen
- Fine needle aspiration of necrotic pancreas for microscopy and culture

Treatment
Antibiotics are only indicated if the necrotic pancreas is infected. Consider necrosectomy if no clear improvement at 2 weeks.

1st line	IV Piptazobactam
2nd line (if 1st line contraindicated)	IV Ciprofloxacin **PLUS** IV Metronidazole

Total Duration
2 weeks

Dosing
See section – Antibiotics, Empirical Antibiotic Guidelines

Prognosis and Complications
Untreated infected necrotising pancreatitis has a mortality of 70% whereas antibiotics reduce this to 12%

Prophylaxis and Prevention
No role for antibiotics to prevent infection of necrotic pancreas

<u>Cholecystitis and Cholangitis</u>

Acute cholecystitis is inflammation of the gallbladder, usually secondary to cystic duct obstruction.

Acute cholangitis is inflammation of the biliary tree due to obstruction of the common bile duct.

Clinical Features

Cholecystitis	• Fever • Nausea • Right upper quadrant or epigastric pain and tenderness
Cholangitis	• Charcot's Triad – fever + right upper quadrant pain + jaundice (present in 85% of patients) • Right upper quadrant or epigastric pain and tenderness • Sepsis

Causes

Cholecystitis and Cholangitis	Often mixed microorganisms: • Enterobacteriaceae e.g. *Escherichia coli*, *Klebsiella* spp., *Enterobacter* spp., *Proteus* spp. • *Enterococcus* spp. • Anaerobes e.g. *Bacteroides* spp., *Clostridium* spp., *Fusobacterium* spp.

Investigations
- Blood cultures
  - Positive in 50% of cases
  - Cholecystitis and cholangitis are usually polymicrobial. Even if a single predominant bacterium is grown, it is important to treat this as a mixed infection
- Bile for culture and sensitivity
- Abdominal ultrasound scans are diagnostic in 90% of cases

Treatment
Patients may require surgical decompression of the biliary tree, especially with cholangitis.

1st line	IV Amoxicillin **PLUS** IV Gentamicin **PLUS** IV Metronidazole
2nd line (if 1st line contraindicated)	IV Teicoplanin **OR** IV Vancomycin **PLUS** IV Gentamicin **PLUS** IV Metronidazole

Total Duration
5-7 days

Dosing
See section - Antibiotics, Empirical Antibiotic Guidelines.

Prognosis and Complications
Complications occur in 10-15% of patients with cholecystitis:
- Gallbladder empyema
- Emphysematous cholecystitis
- Gallbladder perforation leading to peritonitis
- Pericholecystic abscess
- Intra-abdominal abscess
- Cholangitis (following cholecystitis)
- Liver abscess
- Pancreatitis
- Bacteraemia

Prophylaxis and Prevention
No role for antibiotics to prevent recurrence.

Peritonitis

Primary Peritonitis is inflammation of the peritoneum due to infection unrelated to other intra-abdominal abnormalities. Bacteria spread from the gastrointestinal tract via the lymphatics, blood or occasionally via translocation across the gut mucosal wall. In women, spread can also be via the fallopian tubes. Patients with cirrhosis and/or ascites are most at risk.

Secondary peritonitis is inflammation of the peritoneum as a result of a breach in a mucosal barrier leading to gastrointestinal or genitourinary flora entering the peritoneal cavity. The common reasons for secondary peritonitis are perforation of an intra-abdominal viscus e.g. appendicitis or following surgery.

Clinical Features
- Abdominal tenderness and/or guarding
- Hyperthermia **OR** hypothermia
- Increased respiratory rate
- Fever
- Increased heart rate
- Hypotension

Causes

Primary Peritonitis	
Common	• Enteric bacteria (70% of patients) e.g. *Escherichia coli*, *Klebsiella* spp., *Enterococcus* spp., *Streptococcus* spp.
Uncommon	• *Mycobacterium tuberculosis* • *Streptococcus pneumoniae* (associated with HIV infection) • *Neisseria gonorrhoeae* • *Chlamydia trachomatis*

Secondary Peritonitis	
Common	• Usually polymicrobial including Enterobacteriaceae, *Enterococcus* spp., *Streptococcus* spp., anaerobes and occasionally *Candida* spp.

Investigations
- Peritoneal fluid for microscopy, culture and sensitivity
- Gram stain is positive in 40% of cases
- White blood cell count >250/µL is significantly raised and suggests infection (sensitivity 86%, specificity 98%)
- Blood cultures
  - Positive in 1/3 patients
- Peritonitis is usually polymicrobial. Even if a single predominant bacterium is grown, it is important to treat this as a mixed infection

Treatment
All patients with peritoneal fluid white blood cell counts >250/µL or positive Gram stains should be treated empirically until culture results are known. If the patient has perforated an intra-abdominal viscus then the main treatment is surgery.

Primary peritonitis	
1st line	IV Co-amoxiclav **PLUS** IV Gentamicin
2nd line (if 1st line contraindicated)	IV Teicoplanin **OR** IV Vancomycin **PLUS** IV Gentamicin **PLUS** IV Metronidazole

Secondary peritonitis	
1st line	IV Piptazobactam **PLUS** IV Gentamicin
2nd line (if 1st line contraindicated)	IV Teicoplanin **OR** IV Vancomycin **PLUS** IV Gentamicin **PLUS** IV Metronidazole

Total Duration
5-7 days

Dosing
See section - Antibiotics, Empirical Antibiotic Guidelines.

Prognosis and Complications
Mortality depends on underlying co-morbidities but can be as high as 60% if there is established infection and organ failure secondary to sepsis.

Prophylaxis and Prevention
In primary peritonitis, antibiotic prophylaxis decreases the frequency of infection in patients with cirrhosis and ascites who have had a previous episode of peritonitis.

1st line	PO Co-trimoxazole
2nd line (if 1st line contraindicated)	PO Ciprofloxacin

In secondary peritonitis, antibiotics should be given to cover clean-contaminated or contaminated surgery. Contaminated surgery has a post-operative infection rate of 30-40%; antibiotics reduce this to 4-8%. Clean-contaminated surgery is where the surgeon will be entering a non-sterile site such as the bowel e.g. appendicectomy. Contaminated surgery is where there are faeces in the peritoneum or a penetrating injury.

> **Warning**
> Perforation of an intra-abdominal viscus can give rise to a form of necrotising fasciitis called "synergistic gangrene". This is a severe soft tissue infection cause by mixed bacteria and is a surgical emergency (see section – Emergencies, Necrotising Fasciitis).

Viral Hepatitis

Viral hepatitis is inflammation of the liver as a result of a viral infection. Treatment depends on the infectious cause and whether it is acute or chronic. Acute hepatitis is hepatitis for <6 months. Chronic hepatitis is hepatitis for ≥6 months; hepatitis B is persistence of hepatitis B surface antigen (HBsAg) in blood and hepatitis C is persistence of viral RNA in blood. Remember there are other causes of hepatitis, such as therapeutic drugs, alcohol and drug misuse, autoimmune and metabolic diseases.

Clinical Features

Acute (<6 months)	• Can be asymptomatic • Anorexia • Malaise • Right upper quadrant pain • Jaundice • Liver failure
Chronic (>6 months)	As for acute plus: • Weight loss • Abdominal distension • Confusion • Signs of liver failure

Causes

Acute	• *Hepatitis A Virus* • *Hepatitis B Virus* (+/- *Hepatitis D Virus*) • *Hepatitis C Virus* • *Hepatitis E Virus* • *Epstein Barr Virus* (EBV) • *Cytomegalovirus* (CMV)
Chronic	• *Hepatitis B Virus* (+/- *Hepatitis D Virus*) • *Hepatitis C Virus* • *Hepatitis E Virus*

- *Hepatitis B Virus*, *Hepatitis C Virus* and *Hepatitis D Virus* are viruses transmissible through blood and body fluids
- *Hepatitis A Virus* and *Hepatitis E Virus* are transmitted via the faecal-oral route
- CMV and EBV are regarded as "kissing contact" viruses transmissible through close contact with mucosal membranes

> **Warning**
> If your patient did not have hepatitis on admission and now has symptoms it is unlikely that they have acquired an infectious cause as an inpatient. It is more likely that they have been given a therapeutic drug that has caused the hepatitis. Many drugs such as pain killers, anticonvulsants, statins and even the oral contraceptive pill can do this as well as antibiotics.

Investigations
- Biochemistry
  - Raised ALT and AST
  - Often raised bilirubin
- Serology
  - *Hepatitis A Virus* (anti-HAV IgM)
  - *Hepatitis B Virus* (HBsAg, anti-HBs, anti-HBc and IgM anti-HBc)
  - *Hepatitis C Virus* (anti-HCV)
  - *Hepatitis D Virus* (anti-HDV IgM) only if hepatitis B positive
  - *Hepatitis E Virus* (anti-HEV IgM and IgG)
  - EBV (IgM and IgG)
  - CMV (IgM and IgG)

An IgM antibody positive test for *Hepatitis A Virus*, EBV and CMV indicates that the patient has an acute infection (see section – Microbiology, How to Interpret Microbiology Results – Serology and Virology). Hepatitis B and hepatitis C serology, however, can be confusing because there are multiple different antibody, antigen and molecular tests. It is important to be able to interpret these results in combination in order to establish if there is acute infection, chronic infection, evidence of past infection or even immunity due to vaccination.

Interpretation of Serology for Hepatitis B

Test	Result	Interpretation
HBsAg Anti-HBc Anti-HBs	Negative Negative Negative	No evidence of infection **OR** immunity
HBsAg Anti-HBc Anti-HBs	Negative Positive Positive	Evidence of past infection with subsequent immunity
HBsAg Anti-HBc Anti-HBs	Negative Negative Positive	No evidence of infection but immune due to vaccination
HBsAg Anti-HBc IgM Anti-HBc Anti-HBs	Positive Positive Positive Negative	Acute infection
HBsAg Anti-HBc IgM anti-HBc Anti-HBs	Positive Positive Negative Negative	Chronic infection
HBsAg Anti-HBc Anti-HBs	Negative Positive Negative	Discuss with Gastroenterologist or Microbiologist 4 possible interpretations: • Resolved infection (most common) • False positive anti-HBc therefore susceptible to infection • Low level chronic infection • Resolving acute infection

HBsAg = Hepatitis B surface antigen (evidence of acute or chronic hepatitis, patient is infectious).

Anti-HBc = Total Hepatitis B core antibody (appears at the onset of symptoms and persists for life, evidence of active or past infection).

IgM anti-HBc = IgM specific Hepatitis B core antibody (evidence of acute infection **NOT** positive in chronic infection).

Anti-HBs = Hepatitis B surface antibody (part of the normal immune response to hepatitis B or the vaccine; evidence of immunisation or past infection. **NOT** positive in acute or chronic infection, as the infection has now resolved).

Interpretation of Serology for Hepatitis C

The investigation of possible HCV infection depends on whether acute or chronic infection is suspected, and involves a combination of an IgG antibody test (anti-HCV) and viral RNA PCR (PCR). A positive IgG antibody means the infection has been present for 8 to 24 weeks; a positive RNA PCR means the virus is replicating and confirms active infection. The table below show how to interpret the results of these two tests and when to repeat the tests. If HCV infection is diagnosed the next step is to perform genotyping on the virus as this dictates how the infection is treated.

Infection	Initial Tests	Explanation	Test 4 weekly until 12 weeks	Explanation	Test at 24 weeks	Explanation
Acute	PCR −ve anti-HCV −ve	No evidence of HCV infection Repeat in 12 weeks to confirm	PCR −ve anti-HCV −ve	No evidence of HCV infection	-	-
	PCR +ve anti-HCV −ve	Acute HCV infection likely Repeat at 4, 8 and 12 weeks	PCR −ve anti-HCV +ve	Clearance of HCV infection	PCR −ve anti-HCV +ve	Clearance of HCV infection
			PCR +ve anti-HCV +ve **OR** viral load does not drop by 2 log10 at week 4	Chronic HCV infection likely Repeat in 12 weeks to confirm	PCR +ve anti-HCV +ve	Chronic HCV infection
Chronic	PCR +ve anti-HCV +ve	Acute or chronic HCV infection Repeat in 12 weeks to confirm	PCR −ve anti-HCV +ve	Clearance of HCV infection	-	-
			PCR +ve anti-HCV +ve **OR** viral load does not drop by 2 log10 at week 4	Chronic HCV infection	-	-

There is no specific treatment for viral hepatitis caused by *Hepatitis A Virus*, *Hepatitis E Virus*, CMV and EBV. *Hepatitis D Virus* is treated by treating *Hepatitis B Virus*.

The treatment of hepatitis B and C requires specialist advice from a Gastroenterologist. Treatment courses last for months and can be poorly tolerated by patients due to side effects. Patients with hepatitis B, C or D should be advised to avoid unprotected sexual intercourse until after successful treatment.

Hepatitis B	
Acute	No treatment 90% of acute hepatitis resolves spontaneously, reactivation can occur but is rare and usually triggered by immunosuppressive therapy
Acute with severe liver failure	PO Lamivudine
Chronic and asymptomatic	No treatment Treatment may start when there is evidence of liver damage (raised ALT) to prevent cirrhosis and hepatocellular carcinoma
Chronic with raised ALT	PO Nucleoside inhibitors e.g. Lamivudine, Tenofovir or Entecavir **PLUS** SC PegIFN

Treatment of Hepatitis C

Treatment of hepatitis C depends on the stage of liver disease and the Genotype of *Hepatitis C Virus*. Hepatitis C is divided into six genotypes with many subtypes. Most infections in the UK are genotypes 1, 2 or 3. Treatment is with a combination of Direct Acting Antivirals (DAA) which act on HCV-encoded non-structural proteins that are vital to the replication of the virus. They include proteases, nucleoside and non-nucleoside inhibitors, and NS5A protein inhibitors. The aim of treatment is a sustained virological response (SVR) when the DAA is stopped, essentially curing the patient. SVR is defined as an undetectable RNA level 12 weeks following the completion of therapy.

Some experts recommend waiting to see if the patient will clear their HCV infection themselves before starting treatment however there is increasing evidence that early treatment has a higher success rate of achieving an SVR than waiting to see if the patient is going to develop chronic infection. If the patient fails to drop their HCV viral load on PCR at 4 weeks or if they still have detectable viral load at 12 weeks then the British HIV Association (BHIVA) recommend that they should start treatment.

Hints and Tips
Hepatitis C Virus can become resistant to antivirals during treatment. However, on stopping treatment this reverses back to sensitive "wild-type". Restarting treatment does not trigger resistance again because HCV is an RNA virus and cannot store the resistance genes.

Hepatitis C			
Stage of liver disease	Genotype	1st line treatment	Duration
Non-cirrhotic	1a	Sofosbuvir **PLUS** Ledipasvir	8-12 weeks
	1b	Sofosbuvir **PLUS** Ledipasvir	8-12 weeks
	2	Sofosbuvir **PLUS** Velpatasvir	12 weeks
	3	Sofosbuvir **PLUS** Velpatasvir	12 weeks
	4	Grazoprevir **PLUS** Elbasvir	12 weeks
	5/6	Sofosbuvir **PLUS** Velpatasvir	12 weeks
Compensated cirrhosis	1a	Sofosbuvir **PLUS** Ledipasvir	12 weeks
	1b	Sofosbuvir **PLUS** Ledipasvir	12 weeks
	2	Sofosbuvir **PLUS** Velpatasvir	12 weeks
	3	Sofosbuvir **PLUS** Velpatasvir	12 weeks
	4	Grazoprevir **PLUS** Elbasvir	12 weeks
	5/6	Sofosbuvir **PLUS** Velpatasvir	12 weeks
Decompensated cirrhosis	1a	Sofosbuvir **PLUS** Ledipasvir **PLUS** Ribavirin	12 weeks
	1b	Sofosbuvir **PLUS** Velpatasvir **PLUS** Ribavirin	12 weeks
	2	Sofosbuvir **PLUS** Velpatasvir **PLUS** Ribavirin	12 weeks
	3	Sofosbuvir **PLUS** Velpatasvir **PLUS** Ribavirin	12 weeks
	4	Grazoprevir **PLUS** Elbasvir **PLUS** Ribavirin	12 weeks

The main drawback to the treatment of HCV is the cost. In the UK, current treatment costs £40,000 per person. However, this is a clinically superior treatment and the cost compares favourably long-term when calculating the current cost of treatment including blood tests, side effect management, hospital visits and long term complications.

Prognosis and Complications
- Hepatitis A – 0.1-0.3% mortality (1.8% if >50 years old)
- Hepatitis B - 10% of acute infections become chronic
- Hepatitis C - 85% of acute infections become chronic, 20% develop cirrhosis, 5% die from liver failure or hepatocellular carcinoma
  - Treatment of HCV with DAA results in 95-99% cure (<1% relapse)
- Hepatitis B with *Hepatitis D Virus* – 20% mortality
- Hepatitis E – similar to hepatitis A, except pregnancy (20% mortality)

Prophylaxis and Prevention
- Vaccination against *Hepatitis A Virus* and *Hepatitis B Virus* (hepatitis B vaccine also protects against *Hepatitis D Virus*)
- No vaccine for hepatitis C or E, CMV or EBV
- Avoid exposure through sexual intercourse or IV drug abuse for hepatitis B, C and D
- Avoid contaminated food and water for hepatitis A and hepatitis E
- See management of needlestick injuries - *Hepatitis B Virus* and *Hepatitis C Virus* (see section – Infection Control, Needlestick Injuries)

Peptic Ulcer Disease

Peptic ulcers can be gastric or duodenal and occur in 10-15% of adults during their life-time. 75% of peptic ulcers in Europe and the USA are caused by *Helicobacter pylori*.

Clinical features
- Can be asymptomatic
- Upper abdominal pain or discomfort (stomach ulcers hurt shortly after eating whereas duodenal ulcers hurt several hours later)
- Haematemesis – vomiting blood
- Melaena – black tarry stool due to partially digested blood

Causes

Peptic ulcer disease	• *Helicobacter pylori*

Investigations
Patients being investigated for *Helicobacter pylori* should be off antibiotics and antacids for 4 weeks prior to testing to reduce the likelihood of false negative tests
- Stool antigen test (SAT)
- Urease breath test (UBT)
- If treatment failure consider endoscopic biopsy for culture and sensitivity

It is likely that there will be a recommendation in the near future to confirm cures with repeat SAT or UBT at 4-6 weeks after treatment as the incidence of treatment failure due to resistance is increasing.

Treatment

1st line	PPI e.g. Lansoprazole 30mg BD **PLUS** Amoxicillin 1g BD **PLUS** Clarithromycin 500mg BD
2nd line (if 1st line contraindicated)	PPI e.g. Lansoprazole 30mg BD **PLUS** Clarithromycin 500mg BD **PLUS** Metronidazole 400mg BD
Alternative treatment regimens	PPI **PLUS TWO** of the following: Tetracycline hydrochloride 500mg QDS Doxycycline 100mg BD Levofloxacin 250mg BD Rifabutin 150mg BD

Total Duration
7 days (10 days if third attempt at treatment)

Dosing
See section – Antibiotics, Empirical Antibiotic Guidelines

Prognosis and complications
First line antibiotic treatment is effective in >85% patients
The main complications of gastritis and peptic ulcer disease:
- Bleeding (5-20%)
- Perforation (5-10%)
- Gastric malignancy – chronic gastritis can predispose to cancer

Other Infections

Infective Endocarditis

Infective endocarditis is an infection of the endocardium of the heart. Diagnosis is based upon Duke's criteria. Infective endocarditis usually implies infection of the heart valves; however infection can also be related to transmural thrombosis and congenital heart defects such as atrioseptal defects and ventriculoseptal defects.

Clinical Features
- Fever
- Emboli e.g. CVA
- Haematuria
- Finger clubbing
- Splenomegaly
- Meningism
- New or changing heart murmur
- Janeway lesions (non-tender red lesions on palms and soles due to micro-emboli)
- Roth's spots (retinal haemorrhages)
- Splinter haemorrhages (due to micro-emboli in the nail bed)
- Pneumonia or pulmonary embolus (if right side of heart affected)
- Osler's nodes (painful red lumps on hands due to immune complex deposition)

Causes

Common	
Native valve (slow onset – weeks to months)	• Alpha-haemolytic *Streptococcus* spp. (also known as "viridans streptococci") • *Enterococcus* spp. • *Streptococcus* spp. • HACEK bacteria (Gram-negative bacilli from oral flora)
Native valve (severe sepsis or fast onset – days to weeks)	• *Staphylococcus aureus*

Variations	
Prosthetic valve	• *Staphylococcus aureus* • Coagulase negative *Staphylococcus* spp. • *Enterococcus* spp.
Intravenous Drug Users (IVDU)	• *Staphylococcus aureus* • *Candida* spp.
Culture Negative	• *Coxiella* spp. • *Brucella* spp. • *Bartonella* spp. • *Mycoplasma* spp. • *Chlamydia* spp. • *Legionella* spp. • *Tropheryma whipplei*

Investigations
- Blood cultures
  - At least 3 sets separated in time over 24 hours (see Hints and Tips)
  - Can take up to 2 weeks to be positive as some bacteria are slow growing
- Urine for haematuria
- Serology for culture negative causes
- Echocardiography
  - Transthoracic (TTE) 60-75% sensitivity
  - Transoesophageal (TOE) 95-97% sensitivity

Hints and Tips
Schedule when to take blood cultures. Take 1 set now, another in 1-2 hours and plan the 3rd set for 12-24 hours later (e.g. next day). That way if the patient deteriorates suddenly after the first hour a 3rd set of blood cultures can be taken and treatment started knowing 3 sets of blood cultures have been taken before starting antibiotics.

Duke's Criteria
Diagnosis of infective endocarditis requires either: 2 major criteria **OR**, 1 major **PLUS** 3 minor criteria, **OR** 5 minor criteria, using Duke's criteria:

Major criteria	Minor criteria
• Typical microorganism from 2 or more sets of blood cultures, ideally more than 12 hours apart • Positive echocardiogram showing vegetation, abscess, dehiscence of prosthetic valve or new valve regurgitation	• Predisposing heart condition **OR** IVDU • Fever >38°C • Vascular phenomena – emboli, mycotic aneurysm, haemorrhages, Janeway lesions • Immunological phenomena – glomerulonephritis, Osler's nodes, Roth's spots, rheumatoid factor • Microbiological evidence – positive blood culture but falls short of major criteria (e.g. 1 set with typical microorganism, 2 or more sets with uncommon microorganism) • Echocardiography findings – consistent with endocarditis but not a major criteria (e.g. thickened valve leaflets, transmural thrombus)

Culture negative endocarditis

Culture negative endocarditis is endocarditis where nothing grows in the cultures. Reasons for culture-negative infective endocarditis include:

- Previous administration of antibiotics
  - Antibiotics given prior to blood cultures reduce positivity by 35-40%
- Non-culturable bacteria
  - e.g. *Coxiella burnetii* (Q fever), *Bartonella* spp., *Tropheryma whipplei*, *Mycoplasma* spp., *Chlamydia* spp. and *Legionella* spp.
  - These bacteria are detected by serology or molecular methods
- Slow growing or fastidious bacteria
  - e.g. *Brucella* spp. and HACEK bacteria
  - These bacteria may require extended culture for 14 days and when positive should be sub-cultured onto more nutritious agar
- Fungi
  - *Candida* spp. grow in blood cultures but *Aspergillus* spp. do not
  - Diagnosis requires serology for galactomannan or (1,3)-Beta-d-glucan or histological examination of the heart valve

Non-infectious causes of endocarditis:

- Antiphospholipid syndrome with antiphospholipid antibodies allowing sterile vegetations to form on heart valves in rheumatological disorders e.g. systemic lupus erythematosus (SLE) as well as malignancies
- Malignancy e.g. atrial myxoma, carcinoid and direct invasion by cancer
- Autoimmune e.g. rheumatic heart disease, SLE, polyarteritis nodosa, Behcet's disease
- Post-valvular surgery e.g. stitches promote sterile clot formation
- Miscellaneous e.g. eosinophilic heart disease, ruptured chordae and myxomatous degeneration, all promote clot formation

Investigation of Culture Negative Endocarditis (CNE)

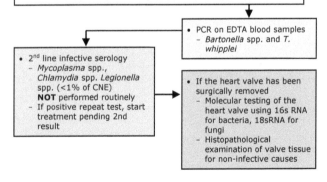

- Repeat 3 sets of blood cultures **OFF** antibiotics (14 days incubation)
- 1st line infective serology
  - *Coxiella burnetii* and *Bartonella* spp. (25-50% of CNE)
  - *Brucella* spp. if risk of exposure e.g. dietary (unpasteurised milk), occupational (veterinarians, dairy farmers, abattoir workers) or travel (Africa, Middle East, Latin America and Caribbean)
- Investigate non-infective serology
  - Rheumatoid factor and antinuclear antibodies

- PCR on EDTA blood samples
  - *Bartonella* spp. and *T. whipplei*

- 2nd line infective serology
  - *Mycoplasma* spp., *Chlamydia* spp. *Legionella* spp. (<1% of CNE) **NOT** performed routinely
  - If positive repeat test, start treatment pending 2nd result

- If the heart valve has been surgically removed
  - Molecular testing of the heart valve using 16s RNA for bacteria, 18sRNA for fungi
  - Histopathological examination of valve tissue for non-infective causes

Non-invasive imaging in infective endocarditis

Non-echocardiographic imaging can help diagnose infective endocarditis:

- Cardiac CT angiography (CTA)
  - CTA is becoming increasingly available and is excellent at showing paravalvular extension of infection e.g. abscesses, fistulas, dehiscence of prosthetic valves and perivalvular leakage and abscesses. It can also help diagnose endocarditis in some patients when echocardiography is unable to visualise a prosthetic heart valve due to artefact or the patient cannot tolerate a TOE.
- Electrocardiogram-gated multidetector CT angiography (MDCTA)
  - MDCTA may have a future role in patients who are unable to tolerate TOE as it is able to identify valve perforations and paravalvular extension.
- 18F-fluorodeoxyglucose positron emission tomography CT (PET CT)
  - PET CT can identify extracardiac foci of infection e.g. abscesses in the lungs, spleen, liver, etc.

At present there is insufficient evidence to recommend the routine use of MDCTA or PET CT, and they are not widely available.

Treatment

Treatment should be discussed with a Microbiologist before antibiotics are given. It is rarely necessary to rush in with antibiotics as most patients are stable enough to delay treatment until a cause is identified. If Gentamicin is contraindicated then omit until able to discuss with a Microbiologist.

If microbiology advice is unavailable **AND** the patient is unwell, treatment may be started after taking a set of blood cultures. It is important to know what is causing the infection as the long-term treatment depends on the identification of a specific bacterium and antibiotic sensitivities. Starting antibiotics before the causative microorganism is known may confuse or delay the diagnosis and make treatment more difficult.

Native Valve		
	(Slow onset)	**(Severe sepsis or fast onset)**
1st Line	IV Amoxicillin **PLUS** IV Gentamicin	IV Vancomycin **PLUS** IV Gentamicin
2nd line (if 1st line contraindicated)	IV Vancomycin **PLUS** IV Gentamicin	IV Daptomycin **PLUS** IV Gentamicin

Prosthetic valve	
1st Line	IV Vancomycin **PLUS** IV Gentamicin **PLUS** PO Rifampicin
2nd line (if 1st line contraindicated)	Discuss with Microbiologist

Adapted from: BSAC Guidelines for the diagnosis and antibiotic treatment of endocarditis in adults

Total Duration
4-6 weeks

Dosing
See section - Antibiotics, Empirical Antibiotic Guidelines.

Prognosis and Complications
Mortality is 100% without treatment. With treatment, mortality depends on the causative bacterium:
- *Staphylococcus aureus* 30-40%
- Alpha-haemolytic *Streptococcus* spp. 2%
- *Candida* spp. >50%

Indications for Referral to Cardiothoracic Surgeons Include:
- Worsening cardiac failure
- Aortic root abscess
- Progressive heart block (monitor PR interval on ECG)
- Recurrent emboli
- Antibiotic resistance
- Fungal infection

Prophylaxis and Prevention
Most hospitals have their own guidelines for antibiotic prophylaxis to prevent endocarditis in at-risk patients undergoing certain procedures. There is a guideline from the National Institute for Health and Care Excellence (NICE) that now suggests considering antibiotic prophylaxis to prevent endocarditis but NICE does not give specific recommendations.

The following is based upon the American Heart Association Guidelines.
REMEMBER endocarditis is rare therefore there is insufficient evidence to draw firm conclusions on prophylaxis. Many Microbiologists and Cardiologists believe absence of evidence does not mean evidence of absence and as endocarditis is a life-threatening infection prevention is more effective than treatment.

At-Risk Patients:
- Previous infective endocarditis
- Prosthetic heart valve
- Acquired valvular heart disease with stenosis or regurgitation
- Cyanotic congenital heart disease

At-Risk Patients who are undergoing the Following Procedures:
- Dento-gingival manipulation or endodontics
- Surgery to the jaw and oral cavity
- Tonsillectomy and adenoidectomy
- Respiratory tract procedures with incision or biopsy of the respiratory mucosa
- Gastrointestinal or urogenital procedures

Antibiotic prophylaxis	
1st Line	PO Amoxicillin 3g **OR** IV Amoxicillin 2g
2nd line (if 1st line contraindicated **OR** recent treatment with Beta-lactam antibiotics)	PO Clindamycin 450mg **OR** IV Clindamycin 600mg

Pyrexia of unknown origin (PUO) is a fever >38°C classified as below:

Classic	A temperature >38°C for >3 weeks **PLUS** >2 visits to hospital **OR** >3 days of investigation in hospital
Nosocomial	A temperature >38°C occurring >48 hours after admission to hospital **PLUS** >3 days of hospital investigation
HIV- related	A temperature >38°C for >3 weeks **PLUS** >2 visits to hospital **OR** >3 days of investigation in hospital **PLUS** a previous diagnosis of HIV infection

Warning
>3 days of investigation in hospital means the patient has undergone investigation e.g. blood cultures, urine, sputum. It is not enough to admit a patient for 3 days, do no investigations, and diagnose PUO.

Causes

Classic (approx.% of patients)	<ul><li>Infection (11-19%)<ul><li>Abscess</li><li>Infective endocarditis</li><li>Tuberculosis</li><li>Urinary tract infection</li></ul></li><li>Malignancy (7-20%)<ul><li>Lymphoma</li></ul></li><li>Connective tissue disorder (22-33%)<ul><li>Still's disease</li><li>Systemic Lupus Erythematosus (SLE)</li><li>Rheumatoid arthritis</li><li>Temporal arteritis</li><li>Polymyalgia rheumatica</li></ul></li><li>Other diagnosis (4-10%)</li><li>Undiagnosed (33-51%)</li></ul>
Nosocomial	<ul><li>Infection<ul><li>Abscess</li><li>Infective endocarditis</li><li>Reactivation of tuberculosis</li><li>Urinary tract infection</li></ul></li><li>IV device</li><li>Surgery</li><li>Drugs</li></ul>
HIV-related	As for classic plus:<ul><li>HIV</li><li>Opportunists<ul><li>*Mycobacteria* spp.</li><li>*Pneumocystis jirovecii* (PCP)</li><li>*Cytomegalovirus*</li><li>*Toxoplasma gondii*</li><li>*Cryptococcus neoformans*</li></ul></li></ul>

The proportion of each cause of PUO is changing over time as improved diagnostic tests are able to identify more causes of PUO. Recent studies from Europe suggest that connective tissue disorders are now the most common cause of PUO.

Investigations

Patients with PUO should not routinely be started on antibiotics unless they are septic (see section – Emergencies, Sepsis). Antibiotics prevent bacteria growing in cultures and make diagnosing infections difficult, including infection with *M. tuberculosis* (see section – Antibiotics, Antimycobacterials).

- Blood cultures on 3 separate occasions off antibiotics
- Serology for HIV, CMV and EBV
- Urine for microscopy, culture and sensitivity
- Sputum culture for *Mycobacteria* spp.
- Early morning urine culture for *Mycobacteria* spp.
- Interferon Gamma Release Assay for *M. tuberculosis* complex
- Radiological investigation such as abdominal ultrasound or PET CT scan
- Non-infection
  - Antinuclear antibody (ANA)
  - Antineutrophil cytoplasmic antibody (ANCA)
  - Rheumatoid factor

1st line investigations (generic infection screen)
- History & examination including localizing symptoms, travel, animal contact
- Drug history (prescribed and not prescribed)
- Blood tests (daily FBC, U&Es, LFTs, CRP +/- ESR)
- Midstream urine (MC&S)
- Blood cultures (3 sets over 24 hours for infective endocarditis)
- Chest X-ray
- If localizing symptoms or signs consider CT chest, abdomen and pelvis +/- biopsy
DO NOT give empirical antibiotics until a diagnosis is made

↓

2nd line investigations if no diagnosis after 3-7 days (diagnosis specific tests)
- Repeat history & examination
- Tuberculosis (sputum, early morning urine, IGRA for latent TB)
- Viral infections (blood for HIV, CMV, EBV, Hepatitis A, B and C if LFTs abnormal)
- Infectious mononucleosis (Monospot or Paul Bunnell in <30 year old)
- Haematological malignancy (LDH, Ferritin)
- Connective tissue disorder (rheumatoid factor, ANA, ANCA, Ferritin)
- Localization of tissue for biopsy (CT chest, abdomen and pelvis)

↓

3rd line investigations if no diagnosis after 2 weeks
- Consider PET CT scan to look for potential diagnostic biopsy target
- Consider echocardiography if infective endocarditis strongly suspected
- If foreign travel or unusual occupational/recreational exposure discuss further investigations with a Microbiologist

The most important aspect in determining the cause of a PUO is the patient's history followed by the clinical examination (see section – Basic Concepts, Diagnosing Infection: History, Examination and Non-Microbiological Investigations)

PET CT is said to help in finding the cause of PUO in up to 50% of cases, therefore if available should be done when routine infection and connective tissue disorder investigations have failed to yield a diagnosis. However, PET CT scans are not yet widely available.

PET CT detects an increased uptake of the chemical 18F-fluorodeoxyglucose into inflammatory cells in infection and connective tissue disorders as well as cancer cells. The increased uptake indicates a site that warrants further investigation, usually by biopsy.

Treatment
Antibiotics are not normally indicated, unless the patient is septic, as they may confuse or delay the diagnosis. If in doubt discuss with a Microbiologist before starting antibiotics.

Septic patient	Follow sepsis guidelines (see section – Emergencies, Sepsis
Neutropaenic or Immunosuppressed septic patient	Follow neutropaenic sepsis guidelines (see section – Emergencies, Neutropaenic Sepsis and Febrile Neutropaenia

Prognosis and Complications
Depends on the cause. If all investigations are normal and the patient is otherwise well mortality <1%

Rash Illness

Many infections cause skin rashes, which makes diagnosis difficult unless a method is used to reduce the possible number of causes before ordering investigations. One method is to use a combination of clinical history and appearance of the skin lesions, as in the tables below:

Rash Illness with Systemic Symptoms

Type of rash	Causes
Multiple purpuric lesions and sepsis	• Meningococcal sepsis • *Capnocytophaga canimorsus* sepsis • Rickettsiae • Gram-negative bacilli e.g. Enterobacteriaceae
Ecthyma gangrenosum or other bullae	• *Pseudomonas aeruginosa* • Gram-negative bacilli e.g. Enterobacteriaceae • *Vibrio vulnificus*
Rose spots	• *Salmonella typhi* (typhoid)
Erythema	• Toxic Shock Syndrome e.g. *Staphylococcus aureus* and Group A Beta-haemolytic *Streptococcus*

Rash Illness Acquired in the UK

Type of rash	Causes
Macules and papules	• *Human Immunodeficiency Virus* (HIV) • Enteroviruses e.g. *Echovirus, Coxsackie Virus* • *Measles Virus* • *Adenovirus* • *Rubella Virus* • Herpes viruses e.g. *Cytomegalovirus* , *Epstein Barr Virus, Human Herpes Virus 6* and *7* • *Parvovirus* B19 • *Chlamydophila psittaci* • *Mycoplasma pneumoniae* • *Staphylococcus aureus* • *Candida* spp.
Vesicles and bullae	• Enteroviruses e.g. *Echovirus, Coxsackie Virus* • *Varicella Zoster Virus* • *Chlamydophila psittaci* • *Candida* spp.
Petechiae and purpura	• Enteroviruses e.g. *Echovirus, Coxsackie Virus* • *Adenovirus* • *Rubella Virus* • *Epstein Barr Virus* • *Neisseria meningitidis*

Rash Illness after Contact with Animals

Type of rash	Causes
Macules and papules	• *Bartonella* spp. • Rat bite fever • Leptospirosis • *Borrelia burgdorferi* (Lyme disease)
Petechiae and purpura	• Rat bite fever • *Capnocytophaga canimorsus*

Type of rash	Causes
Macules and papules	• *Human Immunodeficiency Virus* (HIV) • Dengue • Ehrlichia • Rickettsiae • *Cryptococcus neoformans* • Fungal e.g. *Histoplasma capsulatum, Blastomyces dermatitidis, Coccidioides immitis* • *Salmonella* spp.
Vesicles and bullae	• Rickettsiae • *Vibrio vulnificus*
Petechiae and purpura	• Dengue • Viral Haemorrhagic Fever (VHF) • Yellow fever • Rickettsiae • Malaria

Rash Illness with Risk of Sexually Transmitted Diseases (STDs)

Type of rash	Causes
Macules and papules	• *Human Immunodeficiency Virus* (HIV) • *Hepatitis B Virus* • *Treponema pallidum* (syphilis) • *Neisseria gonorrhoeae*
Vesicles and bullae	• *Herpes Simplex Virus*
Petechiae and purpura	• *Hepatitis B Virus* • *Neisseria gonorrhoeae*

Investigations
• For each cause of rash illness see specific tests (see section – Microbiology, A-Z of Microbiology Tests)
• If systemic symptoms consider taking blood cultures
• If malaria is part of the differential diagnosis, do malaria antigen test and thick and thin films

Treatment
Antibiotics are not normally indicated, unless the patient is septic, as they may confuse or delay the diagnosis. Specific treatment should be targeted to causative microorganisms when they are known. If in doubt, discuss with a Microbiologist before starting antibiotics.

Septic patient	Follow sepsis guidelines (see section – Emergencies, Sepsis
Neutropaenic or Immunosuppressed septic patient	Follow neutropaenic sepsis guidelines (see section – Emergencies, Neutropaenic Sepsis and Febrile Neutropaenia

Lyme Disease

Lyme disease (borreliosis) is an infection caused by the bacterium *Borrelia burgdorferi*. It is transmitted by the bite of an infected tick, normally of the *Ixodes* spp. e.g. *Ixodes ricinus*.

Clinical Features
- **Erythema migrans** – usually at the site of the tick bite, spreading red rash that clears centrally; not painful or itchy.
- **Non-focal illness** - Flu-like illness (fever, sweats, lymphadenopathy and fatigue), joint or muscle pains, memory problems and difficulty concentrating, headache, numbness and tingling
- **Neurological symptoms**
  - Cranial or peripheral nerves e.g. facial palsy (especially in children)
  - Meningitis, encephalitis
  - Neuropsychiatric illness
- **Cardiac symptoms** – arrhythmias, heart block and pericarditis
- **Inflammatory arthritis** – single or multiple joints
- **Acrodermatitis chronica atrophicans** (chronic skin changes culminating in skin atrophy and plaque formation)
- **Eye symptoms** – uveitis or keratitis

Causes

Borreliosis Lyme disease	• *Borrelia burgdorferi*

> **Warning**
> Lyme disease testing should not be performed as a screening test in patients with non-specific symptoms or signs, or following a tick bite in an asymptomatic patient; when the pre-test probability is low the post-test probability of a positive test indicating actual disease is also low. A positive test in this context is likely to be a false positive and may prevent further investigation and result in unnecessary treatment (see section – Microbiology, How to Interpret Microbiology Result - Bacteriology).

Investigations
Lyme disease testing should only be carried out in an accredited laboratory (in the UK this is the United Kingdom Accreditation Service UKAS) that uses validated tests and participates in an external quality assurance scheme.
- Serology
  - ELISA for combined IgM and IgG against C6 antigen
  - Immunoblot for IgM and IgG, as separate tests if ELISA positive
- CSF
  - Immunoblot for IgM and IgG, as separate tests if ELISA positive
  - PCR if acute infection suspected
- Joint fluid or tissue biopsy
  - PCR if acute infection suspected

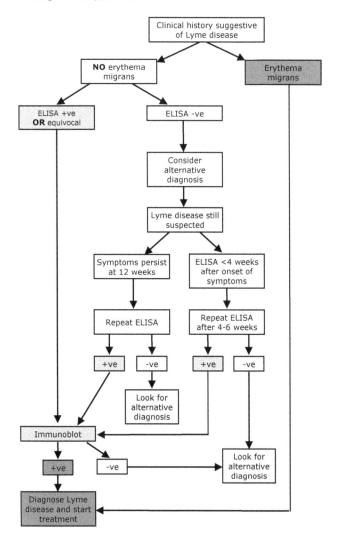

The Lyme disease immunoblot can be confusing to interpret. The test produces a series of lines corresponding to different parts of the test, a bit like a bar code. There are 3 IgM bands and 10 IgG bands. The test is considered positive if 2 of the 3 IgM bands are present or 5 of the 10 IgG bands.

IgM is produced in the first 2-3 weeks of illness and then starts to disappear; IgG is produced after about 4 weeks and persists for many years and even life-long. The presence of IgM on its own is insufficient to diagnose Lyme disease as IgM is prone to false positives (IgM can cross react from other illnesses) and in this case the test should be repeated 4-6 weeks later to look for IgG production. IgG is much more reliable and a negative IgG immunoblot after 4-6 weeks makes a diagnosis of Lyme disease very unlikely even if the IgM is positive.

Treatment
The treatment is based upon clinical features. If symptoms worsen during the first 24 hours of treatment then consider the Jarisch-Herxheimer reaction; dead and dying bacteria release proteins and toxins causing an immunological reaction.

Erythema migrans	
1st Line	PO Doxycycline 100mg BD (or 200mg OD)
2nd line (if 1st line contraindicated)	PO Amoxicillin 1g TDS
Children	PO Amoxicillin 30mg/kg TDS

Non-focal illness	
1st Line	PO Doxycycline 100mg BD (or 200mg OD)
2nd line (if 1st line contraindicated)	PO Amoxicillin 1g TDS
Children	PO Amoxicillin 30mg/kg TDS

Neurological (cranial or peripheral nerves)	
1st Line	PO Doxycycline 100mg BD (or 200mg OD)
2nd line (if 1st line contraindicated)	PO Amoxicillin 1g TDS
Children	PO Amoxicillin 30mg/kg TDS

Neurological (CNS e.g. meningitis, encephalitis)	
1st Line	IV Ceftriaxone 2g BD
2nd line (if 1st line contraindicated)	PO Doxycycline 200mg BD (or 400mg OD)
Children	IV Ceftriaxone 80mg OD

Cardiac	
1st Line	PO Doxycycline 100mg BD (or 200mg OD)
2nd line (if 1st line contraindicated)	IV Ceftriaxone 2g OD
Children	IV Ceftriaxone 80mg OD

Inflammatory arthritis	
1st Line	PO Doxycycline 100mg BD (or 200mg OD)
2nd line (if 1st line contraindicated)	PO Amoxicillin 1g TDS
Children	IV Ceftriaxone 80mg OD

Acrodermatitis chronica atrophicans	
1st Line	PO Doxycycline 100mg BD (or 200mg OD)
2nd line (if 1st line contraindicated)	PO Amoxicillin 1g TDS
Children	PO Amoxicillin 30mg/kg TDS

Adapted from: NICE guideline (NG95) Lyme disease

Uveitis or Keratitis
Treatment should be discussed with an Ophthalmologist

Total Duration
21 days
Inflammatory arthritis: 28 days
Acrodermatitis chronica atrophicans: 28 days

Prognosis and Complications
Mortality from Lyme disease is rare. Up to 5% of those treated for Lyme disease have some form of ongoing symptoms.

Hints and Tips
Symptoms can persist despite antibiotic treatment for serologically confirmed Lyme disease; often known as chronic Lyme disease. This may represent treatment failure or re-infection. A second treatment course with an alternative antibiotic may be indicated. If symptoms still persist after a second course then further antibiotics are not recommended. Consider sending samples from affected sites e.g. CSF, joint aspiration or tissue biopsy or seek an alternative diagnosis.

Symptoms following Lyme disease may persist for months or years due to tissue damage from the initial infection. Prolonged courses of antibiotics make no difference to these symptoms.

Depression, anxiety, chronic pain, sleep disturbance and fatigue may occur after Lyme disease and can require ongoing management.

Prophylaxis and Prevention
There is no role in the UK for prophylactic antibiotics following a tick bite in asymptomatic patients.

<u>**Human Immunodeficiency Virus (HIV and AIDS)**</u>

Human Immunodeficiency Virus (HIV) causes an infection that ultimately leads to a reduced ability to fight disease through the loss of the CD4 subset of lymphocytes. HIV infection can lead to the clinical diagnosis of Acquired Immune Deficiency Syndrome (AIDS). AIDS is defined by a certain group of clinical conditions which only occur when the immune system is profoundly compromised. Patients are not infected with AIDS; they are infected with HIV which can cause AIDS.

Clinical Features
- Acute retroviral syndrome 2-3 weeks after acquisition of HIV
- Fever
- Lymphadenopathy
- Pharyngitis
- Rash
- Myalgia
- Diarrhoea
- Headache
- Nausea and vomiting

Causes

Acquired Immune Deficiency Syndrome (AIDS)	• *Human Immunodeficiency Virus* 1 • *Human Immunodeficiency Virus* 2

Investigations
- HIV test for antigen and antibody to both HIV 1 and HIV 2
  - Test at 4 weeks after exposure; if test negative but high risk exposure then repeat at 8 weeks before excluding HIV infection
- CD4 count
  - Patients with established HIV infection often have a low blood lymphocyte count on presentation

Common Mistake
Some doctors are reluctant to test patients for HIV infection. **This is a mistake.** Patients usually don't mind being asked if they can be tested and almost all will readily consent to testing. After all, it is in their best interest to know if they have the infection because it can be treated even if it cannot currently be cured. In general, patients diagnosed with HIV in the era of modern anti-retroviral drugs are much more likely to die from a non-HIV related cause, including old age, rather than the HIV infection itself or its complications.

Treatment
No treatment guidelines are given here as HIV is a rapidly changing area of medicine; in the last 20 years there have been >25 new anti-retrovirals available for HIV treatment. Treatment of HIV infection should be under the care of a doctor experienced in HIV medicine, usually an Infectious Diseases or Genitourinary Medicine Physician.

Prognosis and Complications

HIV infection is usually progressive following acquisition:

2-3 weeks	Acute retroviral syndrome
2-4 weeks	Seroconversion
4 weeks - 8 years	Asymptomatic carriage
8-11 years	Symptomatic HIV or AIDS
10-11 years	Death if untreated

Complications are usually related to the patient's CD4 count. AIDS defining illnesses* usually occur with CD4 counts ≤200/mm^3

CD4 Count	Complications
CD4 >500/mm^3	• Acute retroviral illness • Candida vaginitis • Lymphadenopathy • Guillain-Barre syndrome • Aseptic meningitis
CD4 200-500/mm^3	• Recurrent pneumonia*, especially pneumococcal pneumonia • Tuberculosis* • Shingles • Oropharyngeal candidiasis* • Kaposi sarcoma* • Oral hairy leukoplakia • Anaemia • Lymphoma*
CD4 <200/mm^3	• Pneumocystis pneumonia (PCP)* • Miliary **OR** extra-pulmonary tuberculosis* • Progressive Multifocal Leukoencephalopathy* (PML) • Dementia* • Cardiomyopathy • Neuropathies
CD4 <100/mm^3	• Disseminated *Herpes Simplex Virus* • *Toxoplasma gondii* • *Cryptococcus neoformans* • Oesophageal candidiasis* • Persistent cryptosporidiosis
CD4 <50/mm^3	• Disseminated *Cytomegalovirus* • *Mycobacterium avium*

If patients with risk factors for HIV infection, or who are known to have HIV infection, develop pneumonia that fails to respond to conventional antibiotic therapy then consider a diagnosis of **Pneumocystis Pneumonia** (PCP).

PCP is a fungal lower respiratory tract infection caused by *Pneumocystis jirovecii*. The fungus is common and widespread in the environment but acquisition does not usually cause serious illness. Most people have been exposed by the age of 5 years old through either inhalation or hand transmission of the fungus.

The clinical features of PCP include fever, progressive shortness of breath, profound hypoxia (particularly on exertion) and ground glass shadowing on a chest X-ray. Bronchoalveolar lavage (BAL) and molecular testing is diagnostic in 95% of patients. The serology test (1,3)-Beta-d-glucan (BDG) detects fungal cell wall; a negative BDG has an NPV of 97% in PCP.

Treatment is usually with IV **OR** PO Co-trimoxazole (Septrin) 30mg/kg QDS **PLUS** PO Prednisolone 40mg BD.

Prophylaxis and Prevention
The risk of transmission of HIV depends on the type of exposure to the virus and the incidence of HIV in the population.

Risk of transmission with known HIV-positive donor	
Blood transfusion	9 in 10 (very high risk)
Needle sharing IVDU	1 in 150
Needlestick injury	1 in 300
Anal sexual intercourse	1 in 200
Vaginal sexual intercourse	1 in 1,000

Risk of transmission with unknown HIV status of donor	
IVDU needlestick injury	1 in 2,000
Low risk patient needlestick injury	1 in 20,000
Mucosal splash blood	1 in 20,000
Mucosal splash other body fluid	1 in 100,000

In order to help patients and healthcare staff understand the risk of HIV acquisition, it often helps to present risk in a non-clinical context for comparison.

Non-clinical context of risk of death	
Car crash	1 in 6,000
Falling over	1 in 20,000
Lightning strike	1 in 100,000

Post-Exposure Prophylaxis Following Sexual Exposure (PEPSE)
Certain patient groups are now being offered prophylaxis against HIV infection.
These should normally be managed by GUM or Infectious Diseases Physicians
and are supported by the British Association of Sexual Health and HIV
(BASHH), British HIV Association (BHIVA) and the National Institute for Health
and Care Excellence (NICE). Whilst they are safe and effective, they do not
prevent all HIV acquisition and therefore they are not a replacement for safe
sexual practice and barrier contraception.

PEPSE	PO Truvada (Tenofovir-emtricitabine) 1 tablet OD **PLUS** Raltegravir 1 tablet BD within 24-72 hours of exposure for 28 days

Recommended for:
- Known HIV-positive exposure on anti-retroviral therapy for <6 months **AND/OR** HIV viral load >200 copies/ml
  - Receptive and insertive anal intercourse
  - Receptive vaginal intercourse
  - Insertive vaginal intercourse if factors present that increase risk of transmission e.g. high viral load, other STDs and genital ulcers
- Unknown HIV status exposure if high HIV prevalence in country or risk-group
  - Receptive and insertive anal intercourse
  - Receptive vaginal intercourse
  - Insertive vaginal intercourse if factors present that increase risk of transmission e.g. high viral load, other STDs and genital ulcers

Pre-Exposure Prophylaxis (PrEP)

PrEP	PO Truvada (Tenofovir-emtricitabine) event-based dosing (on demand) or daily • **Event based dosing** = 2 tablets 2-24 hours before sex followed by 1 tablet 24 and 48 hours after the first dose • **Daily dosing** = 1 tablet OD started 7 days before sex

Note: PrEP takes 2-24 hours to give effective antimicrobial levels in anal and rectal tissue, and 7 days in vaginal tissue

Recommended for:
- **Event-based dosing** in HIV-negative men who have sex with men (MSM) at risk of HIV acquisition through condomless anal sex 3-6 months previously and ongoing, have HIV-positive partners on anti-retroviral therapy for <6 months **AND/OR** have HIV viral loads >200 copies/ml
- **Daily dosing** in HIV-negative male or female heterosexual or transsexual having condomless sex with HIV-positive partners on anti-retroviral therapy for <6 months **AND/OR** have HIV viral loads >200 copies/ml
- Other patients on a cases-by-case basis with close follow up by GUM Physicians
- **NOT** routinely recommended for intravenous drug users (IVDU)

For practical purposes a "returned traveller" is someone who has returned from travel within the last month. This is only a guide as some infections present up to a year after returning. Most infections in returned travellers are not tropical but rather non-travel-related infections which they would normally present with. However, tropical infections do occur and should be considered in the differential diagnosis and the patient should be isolated in a side room until the risk of a potentially transmissible infection has been excluded.

20-70% of travellers to developing countries develop a fever. Of these:
• 1-5% seek medical attention
• 0.1% need medical treatment (tropical and non-tropical)
• Only 0.001% will actually die (i.e. 1 in 100,000)

The most important part of the assessment of fever in a returned traveller is the history.

Clinical Features
Clinical features vary, but the essential components of the history are:
• Where have they been, for how long, and was it rural or urban?
• Have they had any contact with animals and insects?
• Have they been exposed to anyone else ill and how long ago was it?
• How long have they been unwell and when did it start?
• Have they received immunisations including both the primary childhood course and travel related?
• Did they take malaria prophylaxis? What and for how long?

These questions indicate what microorganisms the patient might have been exposed to and what investigations and specimens are required.

Causes

<14 days incubation or Return from travel within 14 days	• Blood-borne – malaria, dengue, rickettsiae, leptospirosis, typhoid, paratyphoid • Gastrointestinal – gastroenteritis, typhoid, paratyphoid • Respiratory – influenza, legionellosis • CNS – meningitis, cerebral malaria, typhoid, typhus, rabies • HIV
>14 days incubation or More than 14 days after return from travel	• Malaria • Typhoid • Hepatitis A, B or E • Parasites • HIV • Tuberculosis

Warning
Clinical information is critical on laboratory request forms to ensure full investigations are done and also to warn the laboratory staff if they are at risk of infection from handling the sample. If unclear what to request then discuss with Infectious Diseases Physician or Microbiologist to ensure the correct samples are sent.

Destinations and Travel-Related Diseases

Diagnosis	Sub-Saharan Africa	North Africa, Middle East & Mediterranean	Eastern Europe & Scandinavia	South & Central Asia	South East Asia	North Australia	Latin America & Caribbean	North America
Malaria	✓			✓	✓		✓	
Enteric fever (Typhoid and Paratyphoid)	✓			✓	✓		✓	
Meningococcal sepsis	✓							
Viral Haemorrhagic Fever (VHF)	✓							
HIV	✓	✓	✓	✓	✓	✓	✓	✓
Rickettsiae (Typhus)	✓					✓		
Amoebic liver abscess	✓							
Brucellosis	✓	✓					✓	
Dengue	✓			✓	✓	✓	✓	
Zika	✓			✓	✓		✓	
MERS-CoV		✓1						
Q Fever		✓				✓		
Lyme Disease			✓					✓
Tick-borne encephalitis			✓					
Chikungunya				✓	✓			
Leptospirosis					✓		✓	
Melliodosis					✓			
Rocky Mountain Spotted Fever								✓
West Nile fever								✓
Antibiotic resistant enterobacteriaceae				✓				✓
Rabies	✓	✓	✓2	✓	✓		✓	
Hepatitis A, B or E	✓	✓	✓	✓	✓	✓	✓	✓
Tuberculosis	✓	✓	✓	✓	✓	✓	✓	✓

1) Middle East ONLY
2) Eastern Europe ONLY

Investigations

- MSU to rule out simple UTI
- Stool for ova, cysts and parasites, as well as culture and sensitivity
  - Serum to save in case first line investigations do not yield the cause
- Biopsy of any skin lesions
- If systemic symptoms, consider taking blood cultures (**label high risk**)
- Serology for *Hepatitis A, B* or *E Viruses*
- Chest X-ray for pneumonia including tuberculosis
- Abdominal ultrasound if suspecting hepatic pathology e.g. abscess

Diagnosis	Investigations
Malaria	Antigen test and thick and thin films on 3 different whole blood (EDTA) samples, taken over a 72 hour period
Enteric fever (Typhoid and Paratyphoid)	Blood and stool cultures labelled as **HIGH RISK**
Meningococcal sepsis	Blood cultures **PLUS** PCR on whole blood (EDTA)
Viral Haemorrhagic Fever (VHF)	PCR on whole blood (EDTA), serum and urine **MUST** discuss with Microbiologist before sending
HIV	Combined antigen and antibody test on serum (red or yellow vacutainer) but may not detect seroconversion illness
Rickettsiae (Typhus)	Antibody test on acute serum (red or yellow vacutainer) and 3-6 week serum looking for seroconversion
Amoebic liver abscess	Antibody test on serum (red or yellow vacutainer) **PLUS** abdominal ultrasound scan
Brucellosis (*Brucella* spp.)	Blood cultures with extended incubation up to 2 weeks labelled as **HIGH RISK, PLUS** antibody test on acute serum (red or yellow vacutainer)
Dengue	Onset of symptoms <4 days – PCR on whole blood (EDTA) sample Onset of symptoms >4 days - antibody test for IgM on serum (red or yellow vacutainer)
Zika	Antibody test for IgM and IgG on serum (red or yellow vacutainer) PCR on whole blood (EDTA) sample, serum (red or yellow vacutainer), urine or semen
MERS-CoV	PCR on nose and throat swab (green viral swab) and sputum if available
Q Fever (*Coxiella* spp.)	Antibody test on serum (red or yellow vacutainer)
Lyme Disease	Antibody test on serum (red or yellow vacutainer)
Tick-borne encephalitis	Antibody test on serum (red or yellow vacutainer) **OR** PCR on CSF
Chikungunya	Antibody test on serum (red or yellow vacutainer) **OR** PCR on whole blood (EDTA)
Leptospirosis	Antibody test on serum (red or yellow vacutainer) **OR** PCR on whole blood (EDTA) or urine

Melliodosis (*Burkholderia pseudomallei*)	Blood or urine culture labelled as **HIGH RISK**
Rocky Mountain Spotted Fever	Antibody test on acute serum (red or yellow vacutainer) and 3-6 week serum looking for seroconversion
West Nile fever	Antibody test on serum (red or yellow vacutainer) **OR** PCR on whole blood (EDTA) or CSF
Antibiotic resistant enterobacteriaceae	Blood or urine culture
Rabies	Seek specialist advice from Infectious Diseases Physician or Microbiologist
Hepatitis A, B or E	See section – Clinical Scenarios, Viral Hepatitis
Tuberculosis (TB)	See section – Clinical Scenarios, Tuberculosis (TB)

Treatment

Malaria is the most common tropical infection that requires treatment (see section – Emergencies, Malaria). For all travel-related diseases discuss with an Infectious Diseases Physician or Microbiologist.

Diagnosis	Treatment
Malaria	See section – Emergencies, Malaria
Enteric fever (Typhoid and Paratyphoid)	IV Ceftriaxone (patients can be converted to PO Ciprofloxacin **OR** PO Azithromycin once antibiotic sensitivities known)
Meningococcal sepsis	See section – Emergencies, Meningococcal sepsis
Viral Haemorrhagic Fever (VHF)	See section – Infection Control, Viral Haemorrhagic Fever (VHF)
HIV	See section – Clinical Scenarios, *Human Immunodeficiency Virus* (HIV and AIDS)
Rickettsiae (Typhus)	PO Doxycycline **OR** IV Tetracyclines
Amoebic liver abscess	IV or PO Metronidazole **THEN** PO Paromomycin **OR** PO Diiodohydroxyquin **OR** PO Diloxanide furoate
Brucellosis	PO Doxycycline **PLUS** PO Rifampicin
Dengue	No specific treatment, **HOWEVER** observe carefully for signs of dengue haemorrhagic fever or dengue shock syndrome, which require critical care support and have a mortality up to 40% • **Dengue haemorrhagic fever** = platelet count <100x10^9/L **PLUS** objective evidence or clinical signs of plasma leakage (>20% increase in packed cell volume, effusions, hypoproteinaemia) • **Dengue shock syndrome** = narrow pulse pressure <20mmHg **OR** systolic blood pressure <90mmHg

Zika	No specific treatment
MERS-CoV	No specific treatment
Q Fever	PO Doxycycline
Lyme Disease	See section – Clinical Scenarios, Lyme Disease
Tick-borne encephalitis	No specific treatment
Chikungunya	No specific treatment
Leptospirosis	IV Benzylpenicillin **OR** PO Doxycycline
Melliodosis	IV Meropenem **PLUS** PO Co-trimoxazole
Rocky Mountain Spotted Fever	PO Doxycycline **OR** IV Tetracyclines
West Nile fever	No specific treatment
Antibiotic resistant enterobacteriaceae	Dependent on antibiotic sensitivities
Rabies	No specific treatment
Hepatitis A, B or E	See section – Clinical Scenarios, Viral Hepatitis
Tuberculosis (TB)	See section – Clinical Scenarios, Tuberculosis (TB)

Warning
Returning travellers who are septic should be started on empirical treatment to cover sepsis, enteric fever and malaria, whilst waiting for laboratory results.

An appropriate empirical antimicrobial regimen is:
IV Ceftriaxone **PLUS** IV Gentamicin **PLUS** IV Artesunate

If antibiotic resistant Gram-negative bacteria are suspected (e.g. travel to South-East Asia) then consider instead:
IV Meropenem **PLUS** IV Gentamicin **PLUS** IV Artesunate

REMEMBER: at least a third of septic returning travellers have the normal causes of sepsis they would have developed had they not travelled, e.g. UTI, pneumonia, and abscesses. However, if they have a life-threatening tropical disease, 77% have falciparum malaria and 18% have enteric fever, hence the empirical treatment above.

Prophylaxis and Prevention
Those intending to travel should be encouraged to seek specialist advice about vaccinations and malaria prophylaxis specific to their destination at least 8 weeks before they travel. Useful sources of advice for travellers online include NaTHNac (https://nathnac.net/) and the Centre for Disease Control (CDC).

Antibiotics

Antimicrobial Stewardship

It is widely acknowledged that 50% of antibiotic prescriptions are inappropriate; meaning that the antibiotic is incorrect for the condition, the dose is wrong or infection is not the actual diagnosis, therefore antibiotics are not the correct management. Global antibiotic resistance is becoming increasingly prevalent and worryingly the world faces a post-antibiotic era where there are no longer antibiotics to treat common infections.

Antimicrobial stewardship is the response to the increasing misuse of antibiotics. It promotes the use of the right antibiotic, at the right dose, route and duration, for the right infection at the right time in order to improve patient care whilst reducing antibiotic resistance. At the forefront of this fight are Antimicrobial Pharmacists; specialist clinical pharmacists who help optimise antibiotic use within hospitals and the community.

Common Mistakes in prescribing antibiotics
- Using antibiotics that do not cover the causes of the infection
- Unnecessary use of broad-spectrum (or narrow-spectrum) antibiotics
- Prescribing antibiotics where there is no evidence of infection
- Unnecessarily long courses of antibiotics
- Incorrect dosing
- Overuse of intravenous antibiotics
- Delaying antibiotics in the critically ill
- Failing to modify antibiotic treatments when microbiology results are available

The Role of the Antimicrobial Pharmacist involves:
- Expert advice regarding antibiotic usage in specific individual patients in conjunction with Microbiologists or Infectious Diseases Physicians
- Participation in Route Cause Analysis (RCA) for cases of Healthcare Associated Infections e.g. *Clostridium difficile* Associated Disease and MRSA bacteraemias
- Educating healthcare staff about prudent antibiotic usage
- Developing evidence-based guidelines for:
  - Empirical antibiotic treatment and surgical prophylaxis
  - Restricted antibiotics which specifically require the approval of a Microbiologist or Infectious Diseases Physician before their use
  - Intravenous to oral switching to reduce the unnecessary use of IV antibiotics
  - Stop and review to reduce unnecessarily long courses of antibiotics
- Providing clinical tools such as antibiotic drug charts to facilitate compliance with guidelines
- Surveillance and audit of antibiotic usage to ensure compliance with guidelines
- Antibiotic formulary decision-making and horizon-scanning for information about new antibiotics
- Representation at Infection Prevention and Control Committees and Antibiotic Steering Groups (sub-committees of Hospital Drug and Therapeutic Committees)

Essentially there are only 5 basic mechanisms of action or sites where the antibiotic works, either in the bacterium's cytoplasm, on its chromosome, at its cell membrane, on its ribosome or its cell wall. The flagella and plasmid have no role in antibiotic mechanisms of action.

1. Cytoplasm
- Nitroimidazoles (e.g. Metronidazole) produce oxygen free radicals which damage proteins and DNA
- Lipopeptides (e.g. Daptomycin) depolarise cell membranes inside the cell

2. Chromosome
- Diaminopyramidines (e.g. Trimethoprim) interfere with folic acid synthesis
- Quinolones (e.g. Ciprofloxacin, Levofloxacin) inhibit DNA coiling
- Rifampicin and Fidaxomicin inhibit RNA polymerase
- Nitrofurantoin's actual mechanism is unknown but it causes direct damage to DNA

3. Cell Membrane
- Polymyxin (e.g. Colistin) binds to phospholipids disrupting the cell membrane

4. Ribosome
- Macrolides and Lincosamides (e.g. Erythromycin, Clarithromycin, Azithromycin, Clindamycin) prevent protein elongation and inhibit ribosome formation
- Aminoglycosides (e.g. Gentamicin, Amikacin, Tobramycin) interfere with translation and protein formation
- Tetracyclines and Glycylcyclines (e.g. Doxycycline, Tigecycline) prevent protein synthesis
- Oxazolidinones (e.g. Linezolid) prevent ribosome formation
- Fusidic Acid blocks elongation factor G, preventing protein formation
- Chloramphenicol inhibits protein synthesis
- Nitrofurantoin's actual mechanism is unknown but it interferes with translation

5. Cell Wall
- Beta-Lactams (e.g. Penicillins, Cephalosporins, Carbapenems) inhibit cell wall formation
- Glycopeptides (Vancomycin, Teicoplanin) prevent peptidoglycan cross-linkage
- Fosfomycin blocks peptidoglycan synthesis

How to Choose an Antibiotic

Before deciding whether to prescribe an antibiotic there are a number of things to consider and questions to ask. Firstly:
- Make sure you know normal flora and the causes of common infections
- Know your speciality's serious and common infections, the microorganisms that cause these and the usual treatments for them
- Use the British National Formulary (BNF) for interactions, cautions and contraindications as well as dosing information
- Discuss patients with your own senior team members and Consultant
- Know your own hospital's empirical antibiotic guidelines for your specialty

Empirical antibiotic guidelines are established by answering many of the questions below. It is essential to understand the relevance of these questions and the effect of the answers. Relying on empirical antibiotic guidelines without knowing why or how these guidelines are produced can be dangerous and is poor practice.

Questions to ask:

Does the patient have an infection?	There are many non-infectious reasons for "signs of infections" • Fever caused by drugs, malignancy, connective tissue disorders • Increased CRP caused by inflammation, malignancy, connective tissue disorders • Chest crackles caused by heart failure, pulmonary fibrosis • Pyuria caused by appendicitis, connective tissue disorders, malignancy
If the patient has an infection what is the likely source?	Urine, respiratory tract, skin, bone, joint, heart, CNS etc....
What are the likely causative microorganisms?	Viruses, bacteria, fungi, parasites
Does the patient need an antibiotic or is the infection self-limiting?	• Viral infections are usually self-limiting • Urethral syndrome and gastroenteritis do not usually require antibiotics
Does the patient need urgent treatment or is there time to make a diagnosis?	There is often time to make a diagnosis before starting treatment **HOWEVER** certain infections require immediate management without waiting for investigations: • Sepsis • Neutropaenic sepsis • Meningitis • Meningococcal sepsis • Encephalitis • Epiglottitis • Spinal epidural abscess • Necrotising fasciitis • Toxic shock syndrome
Is the antibiotic active against the microorganisms?	See section – Antibiotics, Table of Antibiotic Spectrum of Activity

Does the antibiotic get into the site of infection?	See section
	  – Antibiotics, Table of Antibiotic Tissue
	     Penetration

Does the patient need a bactericidal antibiotic or is bacteriostatic adequate?	Immunodeficient patients require bactericidal antibiotics because they are unable to fight infections themselves
What route of administration should be used?	• **DO NOT** use oral antibiotics to treat systemic infections if patients are unable to absorb from the gastrointestinal tract • Antibiotics with good oral bioavailability rarely need to be given intravenously (see section – Antibiotics, for individual antibiotic agents)
How much antibiotic should be prescribed?	• Patients in renal failure may need doses of antibiotics reducing • Patients over 60-70kg may need increased doses of antibiotics as normal doses are calculated for previously normal body size (see section – Antibiotics, Antibiotic Dosing in Obesity)
Are there any contraindications or cautions for prescribing this antibiotic?	• **DO NOT** use any Beta-lactam antibiotics if the patient has a history of severe penicillin allergy • Many antibiotics interact with Methotrexate e.g. Trimethoprim, Ciprofloxacin, Doxycycline • Many antibiotics are contraindicated in myasthenia gravis e.g. macrolides, quinolones, aminoglycosides, Colistin • Always check the BNF for interactions, cautions and contraindications as well as dosing information
What are the side effects of this antibiotic?	See section – Antibiotics, for individual antibiotic agents • Always check the BNF for side effects
When should the patient be reviewed?	• Septic patients should be reviewed within 1 hour of starting treatment • Daily review of **ALL** patients on antibiotics • Don't forget "stop and review" dates as these help prevent over-treatment and CDAD

When can I switch from IV to oral, and how long should I treat the patient for?	See sections
	  – Clinical Scenarios, for individual
	     conditions
	  – Antibiotics, IV to Oral Switching of
	     Antibiotics

Do the results of the microbiology investigations identify a specific causative microorganism?	Once the cause is known, antibiotics should be narrowed down to cover the specific microorganisms identified e.g. CAP caused by *Streptococcus pneumoniae* can be treated with Penicillin rather than Co-amoxiclav and Clarithromycin

Prophylaxis vs. Treatment

Prophylaxis is the use of antibiotics to prevent infection of a previously uninfected site.

Primary Prophylaxis	• Aims to prevent initial infection e.g. surgical prophylaxis • Duration – prophylactic antibiotics usually required for <24 hours • Only required whilst ongoing entry of bacteria into sterile body sites e.g. at the time of surgery
Secondary Prophylaxis	• Aims to prevent recurrent episodes of infection • Duration – usually long courses of antibiotics at reduced doses e.g. post-splenectomy, rheumatic fever, recurrent UTIs in children

Treatment is the use of antibiotics to eliminate infection from an already infected site. Treatment and duration of treatment varies between clinical conditions (see section – Clinical Scenarios, individual conditions).

How to Prescribe an Antibiotic

- Name of Antibiotic
  - This should be the generic name, not a specific product name
- Indication
  - In order to know if the stop date is correct, you need to know why the antibiotic has been prescribed
- Start Date
  - This is the date the antibiotic was first prescribed **NOT** the date the prescription was re-written
- Frequency of Dosing
  - Antibiotics need to be spaced out evenly in order to maintain therapeutic levels in a patient
- Stop or Review Date
  - Should be set at the time of prescribing based on the original diagnosis, e.g. CAP is diagnosed and treated for up to 7 days
- Name and signature
- GMC number

> **Warning**
> The information forgotten when prescribing is usually the **indication** and the **stop or review dates**. These are important to document because they allow other healthcare staff to know when the antibiotic should be stopped. This ensures patients do not get unnecessarily long courses of antibiotics which would increase the risk of side effects, antibiotic resistance and CDAD.
>
> **REMEMBER** check the indication against the stop date. The indication might not match the current diagnosis as the diagnosis may have changed e.g. patient with crackles in the chest treated for CAP with Co-amoxiclav and Clarithromycin prescribed for 7 days actually has a UTI, which only needs treating for 3 days with Co-amoxiclav.

The Daily Review of Antibiotic Therapy

Patients on antibiotics should be reviewed every day to ensure they are responding to treatment and that they are not getting any side effects.

Questions to ask:

Is the patient getting better?	• Are they improving subjectively i.e. feeling better? • Are they improving objectively i.e. blood test results such as white blood cell count, CRP improving? • Is the diagnosis still correct? • If the patient is not feeling better follow the method for failing to respond to antibiotics (see section – Antibiotics, Reasons for Failing Antibiotic Therapy)
Can the patient be converted from IV to oral antibiotics?	See section – Antibiotics, Intravenous to Oral Switching of Antibiotics
Can the antibiotics be narrowed down to a specific treatment?	• Review the microbiology results • Empirical antibiotics cover all common causes of a particular type of infection, they are not specific • Narrowing down antibiotics reduces side effects and risks of complications such as CDAD
Are antibiotic levels required?	• Have levels been taken? • Are they within acceptable ranges (see section – Antibiotics, Therapeutic Drug Monitoring)
Is the patient's renal and liver function stable?	• If not, then dosage of antibiotic may require adjusting (see section – Antibiotics, Antibiotic Dosing in Adult Renal Impairment)
Is the patient experiencing side effects?	• If side effects are severe the antibiotic may require changing (see section – Antibiotics, for individual antibiotic agents) • Consult the BNF • Do not forget to ask about symptoms of CDAD for patients on Cephalosporins, Ciprofloxacin, Clindamycin and Co-amoxiclav
Have any other drugs been started that might interact with the antibiotics?	See section – Antibiotics, for individual antibiotic agents • Consult the BNF
Can the antibiotics be stopped?	• Is there an indication? • Is there a stop date? • Has the patient received the correct duration of antibiotics for the infection? • Is the patient better? Not necessarily the same as back to normal, which may take longer

Reasons for Failing Antibiotic Therapy

There are many reasons why patients might fail to respond to empirical treatment regimens. The following is a method for exploring these by **answering each question in turn**.

Questions to ask:

1. Has the antibiotic been given for long enough to assess for failed response?	• Few infections respond in <24-48 hours
2. Is the diagnosis correct?	• Review the clinical history and investigations • If diagnosis incorrect initiate treatment for correct diagnosis
3. Is the antibiotic choice correct for the diagnosis and common causative microorganisms?	• If incorrect antibiotic choice prescribe correct treatment
4. Does the patient have a new problem or secondary infection?	• Examples: cannula site infections, bacterial infections following viral chest infections, CDAD • If patient has new problem then commence new treatment
5. Is the patient compliant with treatment?	• Review the drug chart for missing doses • If patient refusing antibiotics then educate patient or prescribe more acceptable treatment
6. Is the patient actually being given the antibiotic?	• Review the drug chart for missing doses • If the patient is not being given the antibiotic then correct the reasons why e.g. IV antibiotics are not being given due to lack of IV access. Therefore gain IV access
7. If patient on oral antibiotics is the patient able to swallow and absorb oral medication?	• If patient unable to take oral antibiotics, or absorb from the gastrointestinal tract, consider converting to IV
8. Is the dose of antibiotic appropriate for the patient?	• Does the patient weigh more than 70kg? If patient overweight, dose of antibiotic may need increasing (see section – Antibiotics, Antibiotic Dosing in Obesity)
9. Is the patient on any drugs that might interact with the antibiotics e.g. folic acid and Trimethoprim?	• If uncertain then check with the BNF or discuss with the ward pharmacist • Consider stopping drug that is interacting or change antibiotic

10. Does the patient have prosthetic material that needs to be removed before the antibiotics will be effective? e.g. IV lines in cannula site infections	• Remove prosthetic material and continue current treatment
11. Does the patient have an infection with a microorganism resistant to antibiotics e.g. MRSA, GRE, ESBL or AmpC producer, *Pseudomonas* spp.	• Prescribe an antibiotic with activity against the resistant bacteria

If still unable to ascertain why the patient is not responding to treatment then discuss with a Microbiologist (see section – Microbiology, Considerations When Contacting a Microbiologist for Advice).

<u>Intravenous to Oral Switching of Antibiotics</u>

The majority of patients with severe infections, who are started on IV antibiotics and are able to absorb orally, can be safely switched to oral antibiotics within 48 hours. It is not usually necessary for patients to need more than 48 hours of IV antibiotics. **In general patients should be switched to the oral version of the IV antibiotic they have been receiving.**

The benefits of switching from IV to oral antibiotics include:
• Reduced risk of IV device related infection
• Improved adherence to correct dosing intervals of antibiotics
• Reduced staff time for antibiotic administration
• Reduced length of stay in hospital
• Reduced cost of healthcare

Criteria for Safe IV to Oral Switch

If YES to ALL consider changing to oral	If YES to ANY continue IV
Is the patient able to swallow and tolerate oral fluids?	Is the patient's swallow unsafe?
Is the patient's temperature settling and <38°C for 24-48 hours?	Does the patient have continuing sepsis?
Has the patient's heart rate been <100 bpm for 12 hours?	Does the patient have an infection that specifically indicates the need for IV antibiotics, because there is no oral treatment? • Meningitis • Infective endocarditis • Encephalitis • Osteomyelitis • Febrile neutropaenia
Is the patient's peripheral white blood cell count 4-12 x10^9/L?	
Is the patient's blood pressure stable?	
Is the patient's respiratory rate <20bpm?	
Is the patient's CRP falling?	
Are oral antibiotic formulations available?	

Therapeutic Drug Monitoring (TDM)

The majority of systemic antibiotics do not need to have their levels monitored. However, for others it is essential:

- Aminoglycosides - Gentamicin, Tobramycin, Amikacin
- Glycopeptides – Vancomycin, Teicoplanin (doses in excess of 400mg)
- Daptomycin (doses in excess of 6mg/kg or renal failure)
- Chloramphenicol (children under 4 years old, the elderly and those with hepatic impairment)
- Antifungals – Itraconazole, Posaconazole, Voriconazole, Isavuconazole

Antibiotic assays should be taken at the correct times, usually:

- **Peak** - 1 hour after administration
- **Trough** - immediately before administration of the next dose

Serum samples should be sent at the time of the 3rd or 4th dose, approximately 2-4mls of blood = 1-2mls of serum, in red or yellow topped vacutainers. Subsequent levels should be checked twice weekly if renal function is stable or more frequently if renal function changes.

Hints and Tips

Best practice is to give the dose, take the peak as appropriate, **THEN** take the trough immediately before the next dose is given. For convenience the trough and peak levels are often taken around the same dose i.e. the trough is taken, the dose given, then the peak taken. Although adequate when the patient is on an established dose of antibiotic and their renal function is stable, this is not best practice.

It should be remembered that a trough level is related to the previous dose, (which may have been given many hours or days before) and shows how effectively the drug has been cleared by the patient's metabolism. If a patient's renal function has deteriorated since the last dose, clearance will be worse leading to an accumulation of the drug. Likewise an improving renal function would result in faster than expected clearance leading to under treatment.

Timing of Samples and Target Levels

Antibiotic	Timing of Sample	Target Level
Gentamicin BD or TDS	Peak (1hr after administration) Trough (immediately pre-dose)	Peak 5-10mg/L Trough <2mg/L
Gentamicin in Infective Endocarditis	Peak (1hr after administration) Trough (immediately pre-dose)	Peak 3-5mg/L Trough <1mg/L
Gentamicin OD	Trough (immediately pre-dose) **OR** 8 hours post-dose **OR** Follow locally agreed nomogram	Trough <1mg/L 8 hours 1.5-6mg/L **Note:** no peak level necessary
Tobramycin BD or TDS	Peak (1hr after administration) Trough (immediately pre-dose)	Peak 5-10mg/L Trough <2mg/L
Tobramycin OD	Trough (immediately pre-dose)	Trough <1mg/L

Antibiotic	Timing of Sample	Target Level
Amikacin BD or TDS	Peak (1hr after administration) Trough (immediately pre-dose)	Peak 20-30mg/L Trough <10mg/L
Amikacin OD	Trough (immediately pre-dose)	Trough <5mg/L
Vancomycin	Trough (immediately pre-dose)	Trough 10-20mg/L
Teicoplanin	Trough (immediately pre-dose) • Skin & soft tissue infection or pneumonia • Osteomyelitis or septic arthritis • Infective endocarditis	Trough 15-60mg/L Trough 20-60mg/L Trough 30-60mg/L
Daptomycin >6mg/kg or renal failure	Trough (immediately pre-dose) • Sepsis	Trough 5-20mg/L Trough 10-20mg/L
Chloramphenicol QDS	Peak (2hr after administration) Trough (immediately pre-dose)	Peak 10-25mg/L Trough <15mg/L
Itraconazole	Trough (immediately pre-dose) after 7 days • Prophylaxis • Invasive disease	Trough 0.5-1mg/L Trough 1-2mg/L
Posaconazole	Trough (immediately pre-dose) after 5 days • Prophylaxis • Invasive disease	Trough 0.7-1.5mg/L Trough 1-3.75mg/L
Voriconazole	Trough (immediately pre-dose) after 3-5 days	Trough 1-6mg/L
Isavuconazole	Trough (immediately pre-dose) after 3-5 days	Trough 1-4.5mg/L

Interpretation of TDM

Gentamicin, Tobramycin and Amikacin
- Peak level (post-dose) generally assesses whether a therapeutic level has been achieved, therefore levels not required for once daily dosing
    - If peak too low: dose inadequate therefore increase dose by approximately 10% (Graph A, Diagrammatic Interpretation of TDM)
    - If peak too high: dose too high therefore reduce dose by approximately 10% (Graph B, Diagrammatic Interpretation of TDM)
- Trough level (pre-dose) generally assesses whether toxic levels are accumulating
    - If trough too high: patient is unable to eliminate the antibiotic quickly enough therefore increase the time between doses, usually in 12 or 24 hour blocks of time (Graph C, Diagrammatic Interpretation of TDM)
    - In severe renal failure check levels daily and redose when target level achieved

Vancomycin

In order to interpret Vancomycin TDM, the dosing regimen must be followed accurately otherwise the result cannot be interpreted.

Dosing Regimen Step 1: Give a Loading Dose
This is based on Actual Body Weight

Actual Body Weight (kg)	Dose (mg)	Volume of 0.9% sodium chloride (ml)*	Duration of infusion
<40	750	250	90minutes
40-59	1000	250	2 hours
60-90	1500	500	3 hours
>90	2000	500	4 hours

Note: *5% Glucose may be used in patients with sodium restriction

Dosing Regimen Step 2: Give the Maintenance Dose
The dose and frequency is based on the Cockcroft Gault equation (see below) for Calculated Creatinine Clearance (CrCl). Dose Intervals are either 12, 24 or 48 hours after the Loading Dose.

$$CrCl\ (ml/min) = \frac{F \times (140\text{-age}) \times \text{weight in kg}}{\text{Creatinine in micromol/L}}$$

$F =$
1.23 (Male)
1.04 (Female)

The CrCl **MUST** be used not the creatinine value as the creatinine value does not give an accurate reflection of renal function on its own.

CrCl (ml/min)	Dose (mg)	Volume of 0.9% sodium chloride (ml)*	Duration of infusion (hours)	Dose Interval (hours)
<20	500	250	1	48
20-29	500	250	1	24
30-39	750	250	1.5	24
40-54	500	250	1	12
55-74	750	250	1.5	12
75-89	1000	250	2	12
90-110	1250	250	2.5	12
>110	1500	500	3	12

Note: *5% Glucose may be used in patients with sodium restriction

Dosing Regimen Step 3: Measure the Trough Level
A trough level should be taken within 48 hours of starting treatment (e.g. just before the 4th maintenance dose if on 12 hourly dose interval or just before the 1st maintenance dose if on 48 hourly dose interval), **THEN** at least every 3 days if stable renal function, to reach the target 10-20mg/L (15-20mg/L in severe or deep-seated infections).

REMEMBER in changing renal function take trough levels more frequently (i.e. just before every dose).

Trough concentration (mg/L)		Action: Suggested dose change
Too Low	<10	• Reduce dose interval by 12 hours (i.e. 48 hourly to 36 hourly **OR** 24 hourly to 12 hourly) • If dose interval **ALREADY 12 HOURLY** then increase dose by 50%
Target 10-20mg/L	10-15	• If patient responding to treatment then continue • If seriously ill, reduce dose interval **OR** increase dose (as per <10mg/L above) to achieve trough level of 15-20mg/L
	15-20	• Maintain dosing regime
Too High	>20	• **STOP** Vancomycin until trough <20mg/L • **THEN** restart at increased dose intervals **Note:** How long did the patient's levels take to reduce below 20mg/L? e.g. if patient took 72 hours to reduce to 20mg/L **THEN** give dose every 72 hours and recheck trough level • Seek specialist advice, Microbiologist or Infectious Diseases Physician

Teicoplanin
• Levels are not normally required unless patient is on high doses (>400mg)
  - If trough too low: patient is eliminating antibiotic too quickly therefore reduce time between doses in 12 or 24 hour blocks of time (Graph D and/or E, Diagrammatic Interpretation of TDM)
  - If trough too high: patient is unable to eliminate antibiotic quickly enough therefore increase the time between doses usually in 12 or 24 hour blocks of time (Graph C and/or F, Diagrammatic Interpretation of TDM)
  - In severe renal failure check levels daily and redose when target level achieved
• Occasionally it is necessary to reduce the dose in order to avoid too frequent dosing but this should be discussed with a Microbiologist beforehand

Daptomycin
• Trough level (pre-dose) generally assesses whether toxic levels are accumulating, but also indicates if Daptomycin is therapeutic
  - If trough too low: patient is eliminating antibiotic too quickly therefore reduce time between doses in 6 or 12 hour blocks of time (Graph D and/or E, Diagrammatic Interpretation of TDM)
  - If trough too high: patient is unable to eliminate antibiotic quickly enough therefore increase the time between doses usually to alternate daily dosing (Graph C, Diagrammatic Interpretation of TDM)

Chloramphenicol

- Peak level (post-dose) generally assesses whether a therapeutic level has been achieved
  - If peak too low: dose inadequate therefore increase dose by approximately 10% (Graph A, Diagrammatic Interpretation of TDM)
  - If peak too high: dose too high therefore reduce dose by approximately 10% (Graph B, Diagrammatic Interpretation of TDM)
- Trough level (pre-dose) generally assesses whether toxic levels are accumulating
  - If trough too high: patient is unable to eliminate antibiotic quickly enough therefore increase the time between doses usually to TDS then BD (Graph C, Diagrammatic Interpretation of TDM)

Itraconazole, Posaconazole, Voriconazole and Isavuconazole

- Trough level (pre-dose) assesses whether both therapeutic levels are achieved or toxic levels are accumulating; usual practice is to adjust the dose before adjusting the frequency of dosing for antifungals as these are usually once a day dosing regimens and giving as fractions of days is problematic
  - If trough too low: dose is usually too low therefore increase dose by approximately 10% (Graph A, Diagrammatic Interpretation of TDM)
  - If trough too high: dose is usually too high therefore reduce dose by approximately 10% (Graph B, Diagrammatic Interpretation of TDM)

Diagrammatic Interpretation of TDM

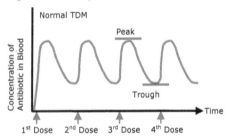

Incorrect TDM Dosing:

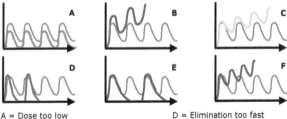

A = Dose too low
B = Dose too high
C = Elimination too slow

D = Elimination too fast
E = Too infrequent dosing
F = Too frequent dosing Time

230

Antibiotic Dosing in Adult Renal Impairment

Many antibiotics require dose reduction in patients with renal impairment. Doses should be based upon the patient's creatinine clearance (CrCl) using the Cockcroft-Gault equation below.

$$CrCl\ (ml/min) = \frac{F \times (140\text{-age}) \times \text{weight in kg}}{\text{Creatinine in micromol/L}}$$

$F =$
1.23 (Male)
1.04 (Female)

Level of Impairment	CrCl (ml/min)
Mild	50-20ml/min
Moderate	20-10ml/min
Severe	<10ml/min

REMEMBER if the patient is anuric, morbidly obese **OR** in acute renal failure the Cockcroft-Gault equation **WILL NOT** give a true reflection of creatinine clearance.

For those who are:
- Morbidly obese (Body Mass Index >40) use ideal body weight (IBW) instead of actual body weight in the calculation
  - Male IBW = 50 + (2.3 x height in inches above 60 inches)
  - Female IBW = 45 + (2.3 x height in inches above 60 inches)
- Anuric or oliguric (<500ml urine per day) patients should be assumed to have a CrCl <10ml/min i.e. severe renal impairment
- In acute renal failure monitor the creatinine frequently as it may change rapidly. Be prepared to adjust doses accordingly

> **Warning**
> **DO NOT** use an estimated glomerular filtration rate (eGFR) to calculate drug doses. The eGFR is a tool used to detect trends in renal function but does not take body habitus into account. It can therefore be significantly different from a calculated CrCl, especially in the elderly or those with little body mass.

Adjustment of Antibiotic Doses in Adult Renal Impairment

Antibiotic	Creatinine Clearance		
	(50-20ml/min)	**(20-10ml/min)**	**(<10ml/min)**
Gentamicin - Conventional Dosing	80mg BD (60mg BD if <60kg)	80mg OD (60mg OD if <60kg)	80mg 48 hourly (60mg 48 hourly if <60kg)

Antibiotic	Creatinine Clearance	
	40-10ml/min	**<10ml/min**
Gentamicin – Once Daily Dosing	3mg/kg (max 300mg) check level at 24 hour intervals and redose when levels <1mg/L	2mg/kg (max 200mg) check level at 24 hour intervals and redose when levels <1mg/L

Normal = normal dose and frequency for specified antibiotic

Antibiotic	Creatinine Clearance		
	(50-20ml/min)	**(20-10ml/min)**	**(<10ml/min)**
Amikacin	5-6mg/kg BD	3-4mg/kg OD	2mg/kg 24-48 hourly
Amoxicillin PO	Normal	Normal	250mg TDS
Amoxicillin IV	Normal	Normal	250mg-1g TDS (Max 6g/day in infective endocarditis)
Lipid based Amphotericin B	Normal	Normal	Normal
Benzylpenicillin	Normal	600mg-2.4g QDS	600mg-1.2g QDS
Caspofungin	Normal	Normal	Normal
Cefradine	Normal	Normal	250-500mg QDS
Ceftazidime	1g BD	1g OD	500mg-1g OD
Ceftriaxone	Normal	Normal	Normal (max 2g/day)
Cefuroxime IV	Normal	750mg-1.5g BD	750mg-1.5g OD
Chloramphenicol PO	Normal	Normal	Normal
Chloramphenicol IV	Normal	Normal	Normal
Clindamycin PO	Normal	Normal	Normal
Clindamycin IV	Normal	Normal	Normal
Doxycycline	Normal	Normal	Normal
Erythromycin PO	Normal	Normal	Normal
Ethambutol	Normal	7.5-15mg/kg OD	5-7.5mg/kg OD
Flucloxacillin PO	Normal	Normal	Normal (Max 4g/day)
Flucloxacillin IV	Normal	Normal	Normal (max 4g/day)
Fluconazole PO	Normal	Normal	50% dose (min 50mg)
Fluconazole IV	Normal	Normal	50% dose
Fosfomycin PO	Normal	Normal	3g PO lasts 7-10 days
Fosfomycin IV	Normal	Normal	**DO NOT USE**
Fusidic Acid	Normal	Normal	Normal
Isoniazid	Normal	Normal	200-300mg OD
Levofloxacin	500mg stat **THEN** 250mg BD	500mg stat **THEN** 125mg BD	500mg stat **THEN** 125mg OD
Linezolid	Normal	Normal	Normal
Meropenem	500mg-2g BD	500mg-1g BD	500mg-1g OD
Metronidazole	Normal	Normal	Normal

Antibiotic	Creatinine Clearance		
	(50-20ml/min)	(20-10ml/min)	(<10ml/min)
Phenoxymethyl-penicillin (Penicillin V)	Normal	Normal	Normal
Pivmecillinam Hydrochloride	Normal	Normal	Normal
Pyrazinamide	Normal	Normal	50-100% dose
Rifampicin	Normal	Normal	50-100% dose
Tigecycline	Normal	Normal	Normal
Trimethoprim	Normal	Normal for 3 days **THEN** 50% dose 12 hourly	**DO NOT USE**
Vancomycin PO	Normal	Normal	Normal
Vancomycin IV	See section - Antibiotics, Therapeutic Drug Monitoring		
Voriconazole	Normal	Normal	Normal

Antibiotic	Creatinine Clearance		
	50-30ml/min	30-10ml/min	<10ml/min
Ciprofloxacin PO or IV	Normal	50-100% dose	50% dose
Clarithromycin PO or IV	Normal	250-500mg BD	250-500mg BD
Co-amoxiclav PO	Normal	Normal	Normal
Co-amoxiclav IV	Normal	1.2g BD	1.2g BD
Ertapenem	Normal	50-100% dose	50% dose

Antibiotic	Creatinine Clearance		
	50-40ml/min	40-20ml/min	<20 ml/min
Piptazobactam	Normal	4.5g TDS	4.5g BD

Antibiotic	Creatinine Clearance		
	50-30ml/min	30-15ml/min	<15 ml/min
Ceftaroline IV	400mg BD	300mg BD	200mg BD
Co-trimoxazole – PCP (PO or IV)	Normal	60mg/kg BD 3 days **THEN** 30mg/kg BD	30mg/kg BD (only if haemodialysis available)
Co-trimoxazole - Other (PO or IV)	Normal	50% dose	50% dose
Daptomycin	Normal	6mg/kg 48 hourly	

Normal = normal dose and frequency for specified antibiotic

Antibiotic	Creatinine Clearance		
	50-25ml/min	25-10ml/min	<10ml/min
Aciclovir PO	Normal	HSV 200mg QDS VZV 800mg TDS	HSV 200mg BD VZV 800mg BD
Aciclovir IV	Normal dose BD	Normal dose OD	50% dose OD

Antibiotic	Creatinine Clearance		
	60-30ml/min	30-10ml/min	<10ml/min
Oseltamivir	30mgBD	30mg OD	30mg stat
Temocillin	1g BD	1g OD	1g 48 hourly **OR** 500mg OD

Antibiotic	Creatinine Clearance		
	>25/min	25-15ml/min	<15ml/min
Trimethoprim	Normal	Normal	50-100% dose

Antibiotic	Creatinine Clearance			
	50-31ml/min	30-16ml/min	15-6ml/min	<5ml/min
Ceftazidime	1-2g BD	1-2g OD	500mg-1g OD	500mg-1g 48 hourly
Ceftazidime + Avibactam	1.25g TDS	940mg BD	940mg OD	940mg 48 hourly
Ceftolozane + Tazobactam	750mg TDS	375mg TDS	750mg stat **THEN** 150mg TDS	

Antibiotic	Creatinine Clearance	
	60-40ml/min	<40ml/min
Nitrofurantoin	Normal dose – use with caution risk of treatment failure and toxicity	**DO NOT USE**

Antibiotic	Creatinine Clearance	
	80-30ml/min	<30ml/min
Teicoplanin	Normal dose for 4 days **THEN** 48 hourly	Normal dose for 4 days **THEN** 72 hourly

Antibiotic	Creatinine Clearance			
	90-60ml/min	60-30ml/min	30-15ml/min	<15ml/min
Imipenem	500mg QDS	500mg TDS	500mg BD	Use Meropenem

Adapted from: The Renal Drug Handbook (2018)

Morbidly obese patients (BMI >40) are often treated with inadequate doses of antibiotics. Most antibiotic dosing has been evaluated for patients of average weights of 60-70kg; there is currently little data available to help doctors prescribe correct doses for obese patients. For average height patients the following weights correspond to a BMI >40:

Gender	Average Height (m)	Weight (kg) for BMI >40
Male	1.76 m	125 kg
Female	1.62 m	105 kg

Body Mass Index Calculation (BMI)

$$BMI = \frac{Weight\ (kg)}{Height\ (m)^2}$$

Height Conversion Table

Ft & In	Metres	Ft & In	Metres	Ft & In	Metres
5.0	1.52	5.8	1.73	6.4	1.93
5.1	1.55	5.9	1.75	6.5	1.96
5.2	1.57	5.10	1.78	6.6	1.98
5.3	1.60	5.11	1.80	6.7	2.01
5.4	1.63	6.0	1.83	6.8	2.03
5.5	1.65	6.1	1.85	6.9	2.06
5.6	1.68	6.2	1.88	6.10	2.08
5.7	1.70	6.3	1.91	6.11	2.11

Dosing in obesity is based on ideal body weight (IBW), actual body weight (Actual) or adjusted body weight (ABW) and varies for each drug. The table below gives doses for where there is some evidence about dosing in obesity; if in doubt check doses with a pharmacist.

Antibiotic Dosing

Antibiotic	Weight	Dose
IV Aciclovir	IBW	10mg/kg TDS
IV AmBisome	Actual	3-5mg/kg OD
IV Amikacin	ABW	7.5mg/kg TDS
IV Benzylpenicillin	-	2.4g 4 hourly
IV Ceftriaxone	-	2g BD
IV Ciprofloxacin	-	600mg BD
IV Clindamycin	-	1.2g QDS
IV Daptomycin	Actual	4-6mg/kg OD
IV Gentamicin	ABW	5mg/kg OD
IV Meropenem	-	2g TDS
IV Metronidazole	-	500mg QDS
IV Piptazobactam	-	4.5g QDS
IV Teicoplanin	Actual	6mg/kg BD for 3 doses **THEN** OD
IV Vancomycin	Actual	15mg/kg BD

To Calculate IBW or ABW use the following:

Ideal Body Weight (IBW)

Male IBW   = 50 + (2.3 x height in inches above 60 inches)

Female IBW   = 45 + (2.3 x height in inches above 60 inches)

Adjusted Body Weight (ABW)

ABW   = 0.4 x (Actual Body Weight − IBW) + IBW

Treatment of Common Clinical Scenarios in Obesity

Doses and drugs can be different when considering obesity; the 3 most common clinical scenarios in obese patients are cellulitis, hospital acquired pneumonia and pyelonephritis:

Cellulitis in obesity	
1st line	IV Teicoplanin 6mg/kg BD for 3 doses **THEN** OD (actual body weight) **OR** IV Vancomycin 15mg/kg BD (actual body weight)
2nd line (if 1st line contraindicated)	IV Clindamycin 1.2g QDS

Hospital Acquired Pneumonia in obesity	
1st line	IV Piptazobactam 4.5g QDS
2nd line (if 1st line contraindicated)	IV Meropenem 2g TDS **OR** IV Teicoplanin 6mg/kg BD for 3 doses **THEN** OD (actual body weight) **PLUS** IV Ciprofloxacin 600mg BD

Pyelonephritis in obesity	
1st line	IV Gentamicin 5mg/kg OD (adjusted body weight)
2nd line (if 1st line contraindicated)	IV Ciprofloxacin 600mg BD

<u>What is Antibiotic Resistance?</u>

Antibiotic resistance is the term used to indicate that a microorganism will not respond to treatment with a particular antibiotic. The resistance is related to the microorganism not the patient. All microorganisms have the potential to be resistant to antibiotics. Resistance can be:

Relative resistance occurs when a microorganism in a particular body site of a patient with normal physiology and body size will not respond to standard doses of antibiotic. It can sometimes be overcome by using higher doses of antibiotic. Most antibiotic resistance is relative.

Absolute resistance cannot be overcome whatever concentration of antibiotic is used. Examples of absolute resistance:

Microorganism	Absolute Resistance
Staphylococcus spp.	<ul><li>Ceftazidime</li><li>Temocillin</li><li>Aztreonam</li><li>Colistin</li></ul>
Streptococcus spp.	<ul><li>Fusidic acid</li><li>Ceftazidime</li><li>Gentamicin, Tobramycin, Amikacin</li><li>Temocillin</li><li>Aztreonam</li><li>Colistin</li></ul>
MRSA	As for *Staphylococcus* spp. plus:<ul><li>Beta-lactams</li></ul>
Enterococcus spp.	As for *Streptococcus* spp. plus:<ul><li>Cefuroxime, Cefotaxime, Ceftriaxone, Ceftazidime</li><li>Ciprofloxacin</li><li>Erythromycin, Clarithromycin, Azithromycin, Clindamycin</li></ul>
Listeria monocytogenes	<ul><li>Cefuroxime, Cefotaxime, Ceftriaxone, Ceftazidime</li><li>Chloramphenicol</li></ul>
Gram-negative bacteria	<ul><li>Fusidic acid</li><li>Teicoplanin, Vancomycin</li><li>Linezolid</li><li>Daptomycin</li></ul>
Pseudomonas spp.	As for Gram-negative bacteria plus:<ul><li>Ampicillin, Amoxicillin</li><li>Cefuroxime, Cefotaxime, Ceftriaxone</li><li>Ertapenem</li><li>Trimethoprim</li><li>Tetracycline, Doxycycline</li><li>Tigecycline</li><li>Chloramphenicol</li><li>Neomycin</li></ul>
Klebsiella spp.	As for Gram-negative bacteria plus:<ul><li>Ampicillin, Amoxicillin</li></ul>

Proteus spp. and *Morganella morganii*	As for Gram-negative bacteria plus: • Nitrofurantoin • Tetracycline, Doxycycline • Tigecycline • Colistin
AmpC producing bacteria e.g. *Enterobacter cloacae*, *Citrobacter freundii*, *Serratia marcescens*	As for Gram-negative bacteria plus: • Ampicillin, Amoxicillin • Co-amoxiclav • Cefuroxime, Cefotaxime, Ceftriaxone, Ceftazidime
Non-Culturable bacteria e.g. *Mycoplasma* spp. and *Chlamydia* spp.	• Beta-lactams • Teicoplanin, Vancomycin
Aerobes	• Metronidazole

The naming of antibiotic resistance genes is confusing and does not really follow any standard pattern. Some are named after the person they were first isolated from, others after the antibiotic to which they cause resistance and still others after the place where they were discovered. There can even be a mixture within each class of resistance. Do not try and find a logical method for learning them; there isn't one.

Types of Beta-lactamase	
TEM	Named after the first patient from whom this type of enzyme was isolated, Temoniera
SHV	Named after part of the enzyme structure; sulfhydryl variable
CTX-M	Named after the antibiotic to which this causes resistance, CTX is the abbreviation for Cefotaxime. The M stands for Munich; the place where it was first isolated
NDM	Named after the place which first described this enzyme, New Delhi Metallo-Beta-lactamase

Bacteria develop mechanisms of resistance in 4 ways; these are the bacterium's survival response to the antibiotics trying to kill it. Knowledge of individual classes of antibiotics can all be fitted into these groups.

1. Production of a Protein (▲) that Interferes Before the Action of Antibiotic
- **Enzymes**
  - Beta-lactams (e.g. ESBLs, AmpC)
  - Macrolides and Lincosamides
  - Aminoglycosides (e.g. aminoglycoside modifying enzymes)
  - Nitroimidazoles (e.g. Catalase)
  - Tetracyclines and Chloramphenicol (e.g. Acetyl transferases)
- **Inhibitors**
  - Tetracyclines (proteins knock Tetracyclines off ribosome)
  - Nitrofurantoin (inhibition of activating enzyme)
  - Fosfomycin (prevents binding to active site)

2. Mutation or Change in Active Site Prevents Binding of the Antibiotic
- **At the Ribosome**
  - Macrolides, Lincosamides, Aminoglycosides, Oxazolidinones, Fusidic Acid and Chloramphenicol
- **At the Cell Wall**
  - Beta-lactams and Glycopeptides
- **At the Chromosome**
  - Diaminopyramidines, Quinolones, Rifampicin and Fidaxomicin
- **Excessive Target Site**
  - Diaminopyramidines and Glycopeptides
- **No Target Site**
  - Colistin in Gram-positive bacteria
- **At Cell Membrane**
  - Daptomycin and Colistin

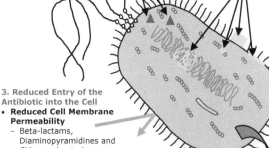

3. Reduced Entry of the Antibiotic into the Cell
- **Reduced Cell Membrane Permeability**
  - Beta-lactams, Diaminopyramidines and Chloramphenicol
- **Gram-negative Cell Membrane Blocks Entry**
  - Macrolides, Lincosamides, Glycopeptides and Lipopeptides
- **Loss of Porin**
  - Quinolones
- **Loss of Active Transport Mechanism**
  - Aminoglycosides and Fosfomycin

4. Efflux Pumps Remove the Antibiotic from the Bacterium Before its Action
- Beta-lactams, Diaminopyramidines, Macrolides, Lincosamides, Aminoglycosides, Quinolones and Tetracyclines

How is Antibiotic Resistance Spread?

Antibiotic resistance can be spread between bacteria and bacterial species by mobile genetic elements. There are two principal mobile genetic elements which carry resistance genes:

Plasmid – a circular piece of self-replicating DNA (○) located outside of the bacterial chromosome (∿). They can carry multiple resistance mechanisms e.g. ESBL, and transfer them via a pilus. A pilus is an appendage that allows bacteria to adhere to each other and transfer genetic material.

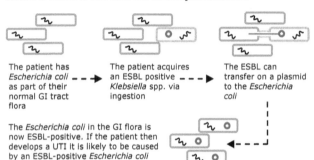

The patient has *Escherichia coli* as part of their normal GI tract flora

The patient acquires an ESBL positive *Klebsiella* spp. via ingestion

The ESBL can transfer on a plasmid to the *Escherichia coli*

The *Escherichia coli* in the GI flora is now ESBL-positive. If the patient then develops a UTI it is likely to be caused by an ESBL-positive *Escherichia coli*

Transposon – a mobile gene or group of genes which cannot self-replicate. They need to be inserted into a chromosome (∿) or a plasmid in order to be expressed e.g. vanA gene in GRE can transfer on its transposon (↝) via a pilus to MRSA.

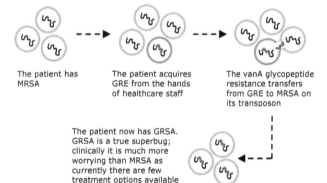

The patient has MRSA

The patient acquires GRE from the hands of healthcare staff

The vanA glycopeptide resistance transfers from GRE to MRSA on its transposon

The patient now has GRSA. GRSA is a true superbug; clinically it is much more worrying than MRSA as currently there are few treatment options available

How is Antibiotic Resistance Detected in the Laboratory?

Antibiotic resistance is determined using four methods in the laboratory:
- Implication of resistance from bacterial species identification
- Disc diffusion using, for example, the European Committee on Antimicrobial Susceptibility Testing (EUCAST) method
- Measurement of the minimum inhibitory concentration (MIC)
- Measurement of the minimum bactericidal concentration (MBC)

Bacterial Species Identification
Each bacterium has a different pattern of sensitivity and resistance to the array of antibiotics available. Once bacteria have been identified (Gram stain, ZN stain etc.) resistance patterns can be implied as certain bacteria are known to be consistently resistant to certain antibiotics (see section – Antibiotics, What is Antibiotic Resistance?)

Disc Diffusion
Antibiotic-impregnated filter paper discs are placed on specific agar plates, which have been inoculated with the bacteria to be tested. If the bacteria are sensitive to the antibiotic they will not be able to grow in a zone around the antibiotic, called the zone of inhibition. Resistant bacteria will be able to grow close to the disc. Because resistance is usually relative it is necessary to measure the zone diameter to see if it is large enough to correspond to physiologically achievable concentrations of antibiotic. EUCAST publish regular updates to their method including the zone sizes for bacteria and antibiotic combinations. This method takes 24-48 hours.

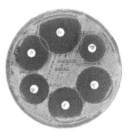

Disc diffusion testing of antibiotic sensitivity

Minimum Inhibitory Concentration (MIC)

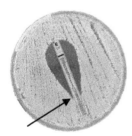

Etest for determining MIC

The MIC is the least amount of antibiotic required to prevent a bacterium from multiplying. The bacterium may still be alive. It is only usually performed in specific clinical scenarios under the instruction of a Microbiologist, e.g. infective endocarditis. The most common method employed in most UK laboratories is the Etest method whereby a strip impregnated with an antibiotic gradient is placed on an inoculated agar plate. The MIC is determined by how far up the strip the bacterium can grow. Low concentrations (bottom of strip) allow growth whereas higher concentrations (top of strip) inhibit the growth. The MIC is the point at which the growth meets the strip. This method takes 24-48 hours.

Minimum Bactericidal Concentration (MBC)

The MBC is the least amount of antibiotic required to kill a bacterium. It is very rarely performed. It is difficult to do and labour intensive. Different dilutions of antibiotic are prepared in liquid culture media from low concentration to high concentration. After 24-48 hours the tubes where the bacterium is growing become cloudy (green tubes in the diagram below); some tubes show no bacterial growth (clear tubes in the diagram below).

This test allows the laboratory to initially determine the MIC (the lowest concentration of antibiotic required to prevent a bacterium from multiplying). The first clear tube shows inhibition of growth and corresponds to the MIC.

The MBC is determined by plating out the liquid cultures to agar. The first cloudy tube is known to have the bacterium growing and is used as a positive control, while the clear tubes have either inhibited or killed bacteria in them. The agar does not contain antibiotic therefore any living bacteria will now not be inhibited and start to grow (e.g. tube A). Tube B is the MBC; the bacterium in the tube has not grown on the agar because it has been killed by the concentration of antibiotic that was in tube B.

Calculation of Minimum Bactericidal Concentration (MBC)

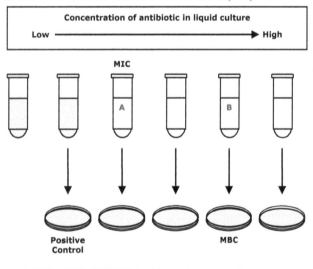

In certain circumstances it is possible to use a combination of a bacterium's name and an antimicrobial sensitivity result to infer its sensitivity to other antibiotics. If the report states that the bacterium is sensitive to the first antibiotic (column 2) in the table, then the bacterium is also sensitive to the antibiotics listed in column 3.

Bacterium	Reported sensitive	Inferred sensitivity
Staphylococcus aureus	Flucloxacillin	• Co-amoxiclav • Cephalosporins • Piptazobactam • Carbapenems
	Erythromycin	• Clarithromycin • Azithromycin • Clindamycin
Streptococcus spp.	Penicillin	• Amoxicillin • Co-amoxiclav • Cephalosporins • Piptazobactam • Carbapenems
	Erythromycin	• Clarithromycin • Azithromycin • Clindamycin
Enterococcus spp.	Amoxicillin	• Co-amoxiclav • Piptazobactam • Carbapenems
Enterobacteriaceae	Amoxicillin	• Co-amoxiclav • Cephalosporins • Piptazobactam • Carbapenems • Pivmecillinam Hydrochloride
	Cephalosporins	• Ceftriaxone • Cefotaxime • Ceftazidime • Carbapenems
Haemophilus influenzae	Amoxicillin	• Co-amoxiclav • Cephalosporins • Piptazobactam • Carbapenems
Neisseria meningitidis	Penicillin	• Ceftriaxone • Cefotaxime • Carbapenems
Neisseria gonorrhoea	Penicillin	• Ceftriaxone

Table of Antibiotic Spectrum of Activity

✓ = Usually sensitive   − = usually resistant **OR** inappropriate therapy

Antibiotic	Gram-positive Bacteria								Anaero-	
	Staphylococcus aureus (MSSA)	Staphylococcus aureus (MRSA)	Coagulase Negative Staphylococcus	Beta-haemolytic Streptococcus (A, B, C, G)	Enterococcus faecalis	Enterococcus faecium	Streptococcus pneumoniae	Listeria monocytogenes	Clostridium perfringens	Clostridium difficile
Penicillins										
Benzylpenicillin	−	−	−	✓	✓	−	✓	✓	✓	−
Amoxicillin / Ampicillin	−	−	−	✓	✓	−	✓	✓	✓	−
Co-amoxiclav	✓	−	−	✓	✓	−	✓	−	✓	−
Flucloxacillin	✓	−	?	✓	−	−	✓	−	−	−
Temocillin	−	−	−	−	−	−	−	−	−	−
Pivmecillinam Hydrochloride	−	−	−	−	−	−	−	−	−	−
Piptazobactam	✓	−	−	✓	✓	−	✓	−	✓	−
Cephalosporins										
Cefradine	✓	−	?	✓	−	−	✓	−	−	−
Cefalexin	✓	−	?	✓	−	−	✓	−	−	−
Cefuroxime	✓	−	?	✓	−	−	✓	−	−	−
Ceftriaxone / Cefotaxime	✓	−	−	✓	−	−	✓	−	−	−
Ceftazidime	−	−	−	−	−	−	−	−	−	−
Ceftazidime + Avibactam	−	−	−	−	−	−	−	−	−	−
Ceftolozane + Tazobactam	−	−	−	−	−	−	−	−	−	−
Ceftaroline	✓	✓	✓	✓	−	−	✓	−	✓	−
Carbapenems										
Ertapenem	✓	−	−	✓	✓	−	✓	−	✓	−
Meropenem	✓	−	−	✓	✓	−	✓	✓	✓	−
Diaminopyramidines										
Trimethoprim	?	?	−	−	−	−	−	−	−	−
Macrolides and Lincosamides										
Erythromycin	✓	?	−	✓	−	−	✓	−	−	−
Clarithromycin	✓	?	−	✓	−	−	✓	−	−	−
Azithromycin	✓	−	−	✓	−	−	✓	−	−	−
Clindamycin	✓	?	−	✓	−	−	✓	−	✓	−

Gram-negative Bacteria									Non-Culturable		
bes											
Bacteroides fragilis	Neisseria meningitidis	Neisseria gonorrhoeae	Haemophilus influenzae	Escherichia coli	ESBL-positive Escherichia coli	Enterobacteriaceae	Pseudomonas aeruginosa	Moraxella catarrhalis	Legionella pneumophila	Mycoplasma pneumoniae	Chlamydia spp.
–	✓	?	–	–	–	–	–	–	–	–	–
–	✓	?	?	?	–	–	–	–	–	–	–
✓	–	?	✓	✓	–	?1	–	✓	–	–	–
–	–	–	–	–	–	–	–	–	–	–	–
–	–	–	✓	✓	✓	✓	–	✓	–	–	–
–	–	–	–	✓	✓	✓	–	–	–	–	–
✓	–	–	✓	✓	–	✓1	✓	✓	–	–	–
–	–	–	–	✓	–	–	–	–	–	–	–
–	–	–	–	✓	–	–	–	–	–	–	–
–	–	–	✓	✓	–	?	–	✓	–	–	–
–	✓	✓	✓	✓	–	✓2	–	✓	–	–	–
–	–	–	✓	✓	–	✓2	✓	✓	–	–	–
–	–	–	✓	✓6	✓6	✓6	✓6	✓	–	–	–
–	–	–	✓	✓	✓	–	✓	✓	–	–	–
–	–	–	✓	✓	–	✓2	–	✓	–	–	–
✓	–	–	✓	✓	✓	✓	–	✓	–	–	–
✓	✓	–	✓	✓	✓	✓	✓	✓	–	–	–
–	–	–	?	✓	–	✓	–	–	–	–	–
–	–	–	–	–	–	–	–	✓	✓	✓	✓
–	–	–	–	–	–	–	–	✓	✓	✓	✓
–	–	–	–	–	–	–	–	✓	✓	✓	✓
✓	–	–	–	–	–	–	–	✓	–	–	–

✓ = Usually sensitive   – = usually resistant **OR** inappropriate therapy

Antibiotic	Gram-positive Bacteria								Anaero-	
	Staphylococcus aureus (MSSA)	Staphylococcus aureus (MRSA)	Coagulase Negative Staphylococcus	Beta-haemolytic Streptococcus (A, B, C, G)	Enterococcus faecalis	Enterococcus faecium	Streptococcus pneumoniae	Listeria monocytogenes	Clostridium perfringens	Clostridium difficile
Aminoglycosides										
Gentamicin	✓	✓	–	–	–	–	–	–	–	–
Amikacin	✓	✓	–	–	–	–	–	–	–	–
Quinolones										
Ciprofloxacin	✓	–	–	–	–	–	–	–	–	–
Levofloxacin	✓	–	–	✓	–	–	✓	–	–	–
Glycopeptides and Lipopeptides										
Vancomycin IV	✓	✓	✓	✓	✓	✓	✓	✓	✓	–
Vancomycin PO	–	–	–	–	–	–	–	–	–	✓
Teicoplanin	✓	✓	✓	✓	✓	✓	✓	✓	✓	–
Daptomycin	✓	✓	✓	✓	✓	✓	✓	–	✓	–
Nitroimidazoles										
Metronidazole	–	–	–	–	–	–	–	–	✓	✓
Tetracyclines and Glycylcyclines										
Doxycycline	✓	✓	–	?	–	–	✓	–	–	–
Tigecycline	✓	✓	✓	✓	✓	✓	✓	–	–	–
Oxazolidinones										
Linezolid	✓	✓	✓	✓	✓	✓	✓	✓	✓	–
Other										
Co-trimoxazole	✓	✓	?	✓	–	–	✓	✓	–	–
Rifampicin	✓5	✓5	✓5	✓5	–	–	✓5	–	–	–
Fusidic Acid	✓5	✓5	✓5	–	–	–	–	–	–	–
Colistin	–	–	–	–	–	–	–	–	–	–
Chloramphenicol	?	?	?	?	–	–	✓	–	–	–
Fidaxomicin	–	–	–	–	–	–	–	–	–	✓
Fosfomycin	✓	✓	✓	?	✓	✓	✓	–	✓	–

1. May not be active against bacteria producing AmpC e.g. *Enterobacter cloacae*, *Serratia marcescens*, *Citrobacter freundii*, *Morganella* spp.
2. Not active against bacteria producing AmpC e.g. *Enterobacter cloacae*, *Serratia marcescens*, *Citrobacter freundii*, *Morganella* spp.
3. Most ESBL-positive *Escherichia coli* clones are resistant to Gentamicin and Ciprofloxacin, but this is unpredictable

? = Variable sensitivity   **P** = Prophylaxis only

Bacteroides fragilis	Neisseria meningitidis	Neisseria gonorrhoeae	Haemophilus influenzae	Escherichia coli	ESBL-positive Escherichia coli	Enterobacteriaceae	Pseudomonas aeruginosa	Moraxella catarrhalis	Legionella pneumophila	Mycoplasma pneumoniae	Chlamydia spp.
Gram-negative Bacteria											
bes									**Non-Culturable**		
–	–	–	–	✓	? 3	✓	✓	–	–	—	—
–	–	–	–	✓	✓	✓	✓	–	–	—	—
–	P	?	✓	✓	? 3	✓	✓	✓	✓	✓	✓
–	–	–	✓	✓	?3	✓	✓	✓	✓	✓	✓
–	–	–	–	–	–	–	–	–	–	—	—
–	–	–	–	–	–	–	–	–	–	—	—
–	–	–	–	–	–	–	–	–	–	—	—
–	–	–	–	–	–	–	–	–	–	—	—
✓	–	–	–	–	–	–	–	–	–	—	—
–	–	?	✓	–	–	–	–	✓	✓	✓	✓
–	–	–	✓	✓4	✓4	? 4	–	✓	–	—	—
–	–	–	–	–	–	–	–	–	–	—	—
–	–	–	✓	?	?	?	–	✓	–	—	—
–	P	–	✓	–	–	–	–	–	–	—	—
–	–	–	–	–	–	–	–	–	–	—	—
✓	–	–	–	✓	✓	✓?	✓	-	–	—	—
–	✓	–	✓	?	?	?	–	?	–	—	—
–	–	–	–	–	–	–	–	–	–	—	—
–	–	–	✓	✓	✓	✓	✓	✓	–	—	—

4. Not active in the urinary tract or against Proteus spp.
5. Should not be used as single therapy, should only be used as adjuncts to other antibiotics
6. Including most CPE positive bacteria except NDM

Table of Antibiotic Tissue Penetration

✓ Good penetration	− Poor penetration OR no activity OR no data						? Variable penetration		
Antibiotic	CSF	Urine	Prostate	Lung	Pleural fluid	Liver & biliary tract	GI tract	Bone	Synovial fluid	Abscess
Penicillins										
Benzylpenicillin	✓1	-	-	✓	✓	✓	-	✓	✓	✓
Amoxicillin	✓1	✓	-	✓	✓	✓	-	✓	✓	✓
Ampicillin	✓1	✓	-	✓	✓	✓	-	✓	✓	✓
Co-amoxiclav	-	✓	-	✓	✓	✓	-	✓	✓	✓
Flucloxacillin	-	✓	-	✓	✓	✓	-	✓	✓	✓
Temocillin	-	✓	✓	✓	✓	✓	-	-	✓	✓
Pivmecillinam Hydrochloride	-	✓	-	-	-	✓	-	-	-	-
Piptazobactam	-	✓	✓	✓	✓	✓	-	✓	✓	✓
Cephalosporins										
Cefradine	-	-	-	✓	-	-	-	✓	-	-
Cefalexin	-	-	-	✓	-	-	-	-	-	-
Cefuroxime	-	✓	-	✓	✓	✓	-	✓	✓	✓
Cefotaxime	✓	✓	✓	✓	✓	✓	-	✓	✓	✓
Ceftriaxone	✓	✓	✓	✓	✓	✓	-	✓	✓	✓
Ceftazidime	-	✓	✓	✓	✓	✓	-	✓	✓	✓
Ceftazidime + Avibactam	-	✓	✓	✓	✓	✓	-	✓	✓	✓
Ceftolozane + Tazobactam	-	✓	-	✓	✓	✓	-	✓	✓	✓
Ceftaroline	-	✓	-	✓	✓	✓	-	✓	✓	✓
Carbapenems										
Ertapenem	-	✓	✓	✓	✓	✓	-	✓	✓	✓
Meropenem	✓	✓	✓	✓	✓	✓	-	✓	✓	✓
Macrolides and Lincosamides										
Erythromycin	-	-	✓	✓	✓	-	-	-	-	-
Clarithromycin	-	-	✓	✓	✓	-	-	-	-	-
Azithromycin	-	-	✓	✓	✓	-	-	-	-	-
Clindamycin	-	-	✓	✓	✓	✓	-	✓	✓	✓
Aminoglycosides										
Gentamicin	-1	✓	-	-2	-	✓	-	-	-	-
Amikacin	-	✓	-	-2	-	✓	-	-	-	-

Table of Antibiotic Tissue Penetration Cont.

✓ Good penetration		− Poor penetration OR no activity OR no data						? Variable penetration		
Antibiotic	CSF	Urine	Prostate	Lung	Pleural fluid	Liver & biliary tract	GI tract	Bone	Synovial fluid	Abscess
Diaminopyramidines										
Trimethoprim	-	✓	✓	-	-	-	-	-	-	-
Quinolones										
Ciprofloxacin	-	✓	✓	✓	✓	✓	-	✓	✓	✓
Levofloxacin	-	✓	✓	✓	✓	✓	-	✓	✓	✓
Glycopeptides and Lipopeptides										
Vancomycin IV	✓1	✓	-	✓	✓	✓	-	✓	✓	✓
Vancomycin PO	-	-	-	-	-	-	✓	-	-	-
Teicoplanin	-	✓	-	✓	✓	✓	-	✓	✓	✓
Daptomycin	-	✓	-	-	-	-	-	✓	✓	✓
Nitroimidazoles										
Metronidazole	✓	-	-	✓	✓	✓	✓	-	-	✓
Tetracyclines and Glycylcyclines										
Doxycycline	?4	✓	✓	✓	✓	✓	-	-	-	✓
Tigecycline	-	-	-	✓	✓	✓	-	✓	✓	✓
Oxazolidinones										
Linezolid	?3	-	-	✓	✓	✓	-	✓	✓	✓
Other										
Co-trimoxazole	✓	✓	✓	✓	✓	✓		✓	✓	✓
Rifampicin	✓5	✓6	-	✓5	✓5	-	-	✓	✓	✓
Fusidic Acid	-	-	-	-	-	-	-	✓	✓	✓
Colistin	-	✓	-	✓	-	-	-	-	-	✓
Chloramphenicol	✓	-	-	✓	✓	-	-	✓	✓	✓
Fidaxomicin	-	-	-	-	-	-	✓	-	-	-
Fosfomycin	-	✓	✓	✓	✓	✓	-	✓	✓	✓

1. If meninges inflamed penetration increases
2. Unless used at very high doses such as in cystic fibrosis patients
3. Depends on MIC of microorganism as drug has narrow therapeutic window
4. Can be used to treat Lyme disease
5. Usually used as part of treatment for tuberculosis
6. Colours urine orange/red

Collectively penicillins, cephalosporins, carbapenems and Aztreonam are known as Beta-lactams. Strictly speaking Aztreonam is a monobactam.

Penicillins	• Benzylpenicillin (Penicillin G) • Phenoxymethylpenicillin (Penicillin V) • Amoxicillin • Ampicillin • Temocillin • Pivmecillinam Hydrochloride • Piperacillin • Flucloxacillin
Beta-lactam-Beta-lactamase inhibitor combinations	• Co-amoxiclav = (Amoxicillin + Clavulanic Acid) = Augmentin® • Piptazobactam = (Piperacillin + Tazobactam) = Tazocin® • Ceftazidime + Avibactam • Ceftolozane + Tazobactam
Cephalosporins	• Cefalexin • Cefradine • Cefaclor • Cefuroxime • Cefotaxime • Ceftriaxone • Ceftazidime • Ceftaroline
Carbapenems	• Ertapenem • Imipenem • Meropenem
Monobactams	• Aztreonam

Mechanism of Action
- Bactericidal
- Bind to penicillin binding proteins (PBP) in the cell wall or cell cytoplasm, thereby inhibiting cell wall formation
- Ceftaroline has a high affinity for PBP2a as well as PBPs 1-4 which means it is the only currently available beta-lactam in the UK active against Meticillin resistant *Staphylococcus aureus* (MRSA)
- Beta-lactamase inhibitors (e.g. Clavulanic Acid, Tazobactam and Avibactam) are molecules within the antibiotic that irreversibly bind to beta-lactamase enzymes (resistance mechanism) and prevent the enzyme breaking down the antibiotic
- May trigger cell enzymes causing the bacteria to undergo cell death
- Different antibiotics have different affinities for different PBPs leading to different spectrums of activity

Mechanisms of Resistance
- Mutation of active site preventing binding, such as decreased affinity of PBPs for the antibiotic. MRSA has a mutated PBP called PBP2a (encoded by the *mecA* gene), which leads to resistance to all commonly used Beta-lactams
- Reduced antibiotic entry into bacteria due to inability to penetrate the bacterial cell membrane
- Antibiotic is removed from the bacteria by a multi-efflux pump before it is able to act

- Production of Beta-lactamase enzymes such as AmpC, ESBL or CPE which break down the antibiotic before it can reach its active site
  - AmpC usually chromosomally mediated (non-transferable between bacterial species) in *Enterobacter cloacae*, *Citrobacter freundii*, *Serratia marcescens*, *Morganella morganii*
  - ESBL usually plasmid mediated (transferable between bacterial species) in *Escherichia coli* and *Klebsiella* spp.
  - CPE usually plasmid mediated (transferable between bacterial species) in enterobacteriaceae and *Pseudomonas* spp.
- Combinations of resistance mechanisms can lead to antibiotic resistance, even if each mechanism on its own would not give resistance e.g. reduced entry (loss of porin) into the cell **PLUS** AmpC gives carbapenem resistance in enterobacteriaceae

Pharmacology and Pharmacodynamics
- Variable oral absorption
  - Phenoxymethylpenicillin 60%
  - Amoxicillin 75-90%
  - Flucloxacillin 60%
  - Pivmecillinam Hydrochloride 60-70%
  - Meropenem 0%
- Renal excretion - dose reduction in renal failure is often necessary
- Good distribution into body tissues (see section – Antibiotics, Table of Antibiotic Tissue Penetration)

Spectrum of Activity of Beta-lactams

Antibiotic	Bacteria active against
Benzylpenicillin and Phenoxymethylpenicillin (Penicillin V)	• *Streptococcus* spp. • *Neisseria meningitidis* • *Clostridium perfringens*
Amoxicillin and Ampicillin	As for Benzylpenicillin and Penicillin V plus: • *Escherichia coli* • *Enterococcus faecalis* • *Listeria monocytogenes*
Flucloxacillin	• Meticillin sensitive *Staphylococcus aureus* (MSSA) • Beta-haemolytic *Streptococcus* (Groups A, C, G)
Co-amoxiclav	As for Amoxicillin and Ampicillin plus: • Meticillin sensitive *Staphylococcus aureus* (MSSA) • *Klebsiella* spp. • *Proteus* spp. • Anaerobes
Temocillin	No Gram-positive activity • Enterobacteriaceae including AmpC and ESBL producers • *Burkholderia cenocepacia*
Piptazobactam	As for Co-amoxiclav plus: • *Pseudomonas* spp.

1st Generation Cephalosporins e.g. Cefalexin and Cefradine	Less Gram-negative activity • *Streptococcus* spp. • Meticillin sensitive *Staphylococcus aureus* (MSSA) • *Escherichia coli* • *Klebsiella* spp. • *Proteus* spp.
2nd Generation Cephalosporins e.g. Cefaclor and Cefuroxime	Some Gram-positive and Gram-negative activity • *Streptococcus* spp. • Meticillin sensitive *Staphylococcus aureus* (MSSA) • *Escherichia coli* • *Klebsiella* spp. • *Proteus* spp. • *Haemophilus* spp. • *Moraxella catarrhalis*
3rd Generation Cephalosporins e.g. Cefotaxime and Ceftriaxone	Less Gram-positive activity • *Streptococcus* spp. • Meticillin sensitive *Staphylococcus aureus* (MSSA) • *Escherichia coli* • *Klebsiella* spp. • *Proteus* spp. • *Haemophilus* spp. • *Neisseria meningitidis* • *Neisseria gonorrhoeae* • *Borrelia burgdorferi*
3rd Generation Cephalosporins e.g. Ceftazidime	No Gram-positive activity • *Escherichia coli* • *Klebsiella* spp. • *Proteus* spp. • *Pseudomonas* spp.
5th Generation Cephalosporins (unique) e.g. Ceftaroline	• *Staphylococcus aureus* including MRSA, glycopeptide resistant *S. aureus* (GRSA) • Coagulase negative *Staphylococcus* spp. • *Streptococcus* spp. (including *S. pneumoniae* resistant to Ceftriaxone and Cefotaxime) • *Haemophilus influenzae* • *Moraxella catarrhalis* • *Escherichia coli* • *Klebsiella* spp. • *Proteus* spp. • Anaerobes
Ertapenem	• *Streptococcus* spp. • Meticillin sensitive *Staphylococcus aureus* (MSSA) • *Haemophilus* spp. • *Enterococcus faecalis* • Enterobacteriaceae including AmpC and ESBL producers • Anaerobes

Meropenem and Imipenem	As for Ertapenem plus: • *Moraxella catarrhalis* • *Neisseria meningitidis* • *Listeria monocytogenes* • *Pseudomonas aeruginosa* • *Acinetobacter* spp.
Aztreonam	• *Escherichia coli* • *Klebsiella* spp. • *Proteus* spp. • *Pseudomonas* spp.

Common Misunderstanding

Doctors find the classification of cephalosporins confusing for good reason. There is no easy way to remember the differences. However, getting the 3rd generation confused can have the biggest impact on patient care. The 3rd generation of cephalosporins are all based on a similar modification to the original cephalosporin. However, they can be split into two on the basis of their spectrum of activity. Some have good Gram-positive activity but no anti-pseudomonal activity (e.g. Cefotaxime and Ceftriaxone) whereas others have no Gram-positive activity but good anti-pseudomonal activity (e.g. Ceftazidime).

If you can remember nothing else, REMEMBER this:

Ceftazidime has no Gram-positive activity but is the only commonly used cephalosporin with good anti-pseudomonal activity.

Cautions and Contraindications

• See BNF for full details
• History of severe Beta-lactam allergy (see section – Antibiotics, Allergy to Beta-lactam Antibiotics)
• Renal failure (reduce dose in severe renal failure)
• Epilepsy (reduced seizure threshold can occur with any Beta-lactam but more common with Imipenem)
• Drugs
  - Carbapenems reduce Valproate levels in epileptics
  - Reduced excretion of Methotrexate with penicillins

Side Effects

• Significant predisposition to *Clostridium difficile* with cephalosporins and Co-amoxiclav
• Gastrointestinal disturbance (diarrhoea)
• Neutropaenia and thrombocytopaenia (1-4% of patients given Beta-lactams)
• Cholestasis
• Fever (usually only after 10 days of administration)
• Hepatitis (particularly with Flucloxacillin, up to 2 months after stopping antibiotic)
• Encephalopathy
• Rash (Amoxicillin can cause a rash in patients with acute EBV infection)

Monitoring

• Warn patients about risk of *Clostridium difficile* and check daily for symptoms
• Weekly full blood count and liver function tests

Allergy to Beta-Lactam Antibiotics

Side effects from antibiotics are common (e.g. diarrhoea and vomiting) and do not usually represent allergy. If patients are unclear about the nature of any drug reaction it is important to seek clarification from their relatives, carers or general practitioner.

Up to 20% of patients say they are allergic to penicillin; the actual rate is only 5%. On closer questioning what patients are describing are either side effects or a symptom unrelated to the antibiotic. It is important to distinguish true allergy from side effects and to explain to patients that restricting choices of antibiotics, due to incorrect reporting of penicillin allergy, can cause unnecessary risks to patient safety through less effective or more toxic treatments. For example, a patient with an ESBL-positive *Escherichia coli* UTI and a history of severe Beta-lactam allergy may require treatment with Colistin and Amikacin, which predisposes to a high risk of renal failure.

Side effects do not necessarily prevent the use of antibiotics in future episodes of infection.

Allergic Reactions to Beta-Lactams		
Mild	1 in 20 (5% of the population)	• Rash • Fever
Severe	1 in 2,000 (0.05% of the population)	• Anaphylaxis • Angioedema and facial swelling • Breathing difficulties • Stevens-Johnson Reaction

Relative Risks of Severe Allergic Reactions to Beta-Lactams		
Mild reaction to penicillin	Severe cross-reaction to cephalosporin	1 in 40,000
	Severe cross-reaction to carbapenem	1 in 400,000
Severe reaction to penicillin	Severe cross-reaction to cephalosporin	1 in 20
	Severe cross-reaction to carbapenem	1 in 200

Warning
If a patient has a history of severe allergic reaction to penicillin **DO NOT GIVE OTHER BETA-LACTAMS** including penicillins, Beta-lactam-Beta-lactamase inhibitor combinations, cephalosporins and carbapenems.

If there is a history of a mild reaction to penicillin then there is a low risk of cross-reaction to other classes of Beta-lactams, such as cephalosporins and carbapenems. Therefore it is usually safe to give these antibiotics.

There is no 100% safe method for excluding penicillin allergy but the risks can be reduced with careful history taking regarding the reported reaction to the penicillin.

Taking a penicillin allergy history

1. **What was the name of the antibiotic that caused the reaction?**
   - If necessary suggest examples e.g. Amoxicillin, Augmentin, Cephalexin
2. **Why was the antibiotic given?**
   - Amoxicillin can cause a rash if given in glandular fever due to an autoimmune reaction, this is not an allergy
3. **Did the reaction happen immediately or within 60 minutes?**
   - IgE mediated reactions occur quickly and include anaphylaxis, rashes and urticaria (hives, weals, welts); these reactions are a contraindication to beta-lactams
4. **What was the reaction; rash, shortness of breath, facial swelling, shock, diarrhoea, vomiting?**
   - Reactions occurring after 60 minutes are usually mediated by cytokines from T cells and include maculopapular or urticarial rashes, as well as the less common but more severe Stevens-Johnson syndrome, toxic epidermal necrolysis and DRESS syndrome (in these conditions the skin reaction is severe and life-threatening with extensive sloughing of the skin appearing like a burn); these severe reactions are a contraindication to beta-lactams
5. **How long ago was this reaction? How old where they?**
   - If a patient hasn't been given a penicillin for more than 15 years their body will almost certainly have "forgotten" the allergy and they will no longer be allergic (including severe) **BUT** if it is essential to give a penicillin, try one of the Beta-lactams but do so with care e.g. in an HDU
6. **Have they been given an antibiotic whose name began with "Ceph"? What happened?**
   - Cross reactivity between penicillins and cephalosporins occurs in about 5% of patients but if a patient has been given cephalosporins safely in the past then it is usually safe for them to be given them again
7. **Where they admitted to hospital with the allergic reaction?**
   - This helps describe the severity of the reaction as patients with severe reactions are likely to be admitted to hospital, if they weren't it wasn't a severe reaction

Trimethoprim and Co-Trimoxazole (Septrin®)

Trimethoprim is a diaminopyramidine antibiotic. It is sometimes used in combination with the sulphonamide antibiotic, Sulfamethoxazole, as Co-trimoxazole (Septrin®). Sulfamethoxazole is only available as part of Co-trimoxazole.

- Trimethoprim is usually only used to treat urinary tract infections and prostatitis
- Co-trimoxazole is usually only used to treat PCP and infections with the bacterium *Stenotrophomonas maltophilia*

Mechanism of Action of Trimethoprim
- Bactericidal
- Interferes with folic acid synthesis by inhibiting dihydrofolate reductase thereby preventing DNA synthesis

Mechanism of Action of Sulfamethoxazole
- Bacteriostatic
- Interferes with folic acid synthesis by competitively inhibiting the use of Para-amino benzoic acid (PABA)

Mechanisms of Resistance
- Bacteria increase production of dihydrofolate reductase to levels that Trimethoprim is unable to overcome
- Mutation of active site therefore the antibiotic does not bind
- Reduced entry of the antibiotic into bacteria due to alteration of cell membrane permeability
- Antibiotic is removed from the bacteria by an efflux pump before it is able to act
- *Enterococcus* spp. are inherently resistant to Trimethoprim because they are able to scavenge and use thymidine from other sources to bypass dihydrofolate reductase, even if they are sensitive on laboratory testing

Pharmacology and Pharmacodynamics
- Trimethoprim is only available orally
- Co-trimoxazole is available both orally and intravenously
- 60-80% renally excreted
- Good penetration into tissue (see section – Antibiotics, Table of Antibiotic Tissue Penetration)

Spectrum of Activity of Trimethoprim

Gram-positive	• *Staphylococcus aureus* (but rarely used)
Gram-negative	• Enterobacteriaceae e.g. *Escherichia coli*, *Klebsiella* spp., *Enterobacter* spp, *Salmonella* spp.

Spectrum of Activity of Co-Trimoxazole (Septrin)

Gram-positive	• *Staphylococcus aureus* (but rarely used)
Gram-negative	• Enterobacteriaceae e.g. *Escherichia coli*, *Klebsiella* spp., *Enterobacter* spp., *Salmonella* spp. • *Stenotrophomonas maltophilia*
Fungi	• *Pneumocystis jirovecii* (PCP)

Cautions and Contraindications
- See BNF for full details
- Renal failure (reduce dose in renal failure although if severe, Trimethoprim and Co-trimoxazole are unlikely to be therapeutic in UTI)
- Use with caution if preceding blood disorder
- Pregnancy (avoid particularly in the first trimester as risk of neural tube defects)
- Drugs
    - Risk of hyperkalaemia when used in combination with ACE inhibitors or diuretics
    - Causes bone marrow suppression, which is worsened with other bone marrow suppressing agents, such as Methotrexate
    - Increases Phenytoin levels

Side Effects
- Gastrointestinal disturbance (nausea and vomiting)
- Allergic reaction
- Hyperkalaemia
- Bone marrow toxicity (Trimethoprim has the same mechanism of action as the chemotherapeutic Methotrexate)

Monitoring
- Baseline and weekly full blood count and urea and electrolytes required for treatment doses. However, prophylactic doses require at least monthly full blood count and urea and electrolytes

Erythromycin, Clarithromycin, Azithromycin and Clindamycin

Erythromycin, Clarithromycin and Azithromycin are macrolide antibiotics. Clindamycin is in the related group of antibiotics, called the lincosamides.

Mechanism of Action
- Bactericidal at high concentration
- Binds to ribosome preventing protein elongation and also inhibits ribosome formation
- The theoretical antitoxin effect of Clindamycin, through the inhibition of protein synthesis, is used in the treatment of severe toxin-mediated diseases e.g. Group A Beta-haemolytic *Streptococcus* and Panton-Valentine Leukocidin (PVL) positive *Staphylococcus aureus* infections

Mechanisms of Resistance
- Reduced entry of antibiotic through Gram-negative cell membrane therefore not usually active against Gram-negative bacilli (exceptions are *Bordetella pertussis* and *Campylobacter* spp.)
- Mutation of active site therefore antibiotic does not bind
- Production of enzymes that inactivate antibiotic before binding
- Antibiotic is removed from the bacteria by an efflux pump before it is able to act

Pharmacology and Pharmacodynamics
- Available as oral and intravenous preparations
- Good oral bioavailability, between 50-100%, therefore intravenous administration is rarely necessary
- Excreted in urine and bile
- Good penetration into most body tissues (see section – Antibiotics, Table of Antibiotic Tissue Penetration)

Spectrum of Activity of Erythromycin, Clarithromycin, Azithromycin

Gram-positive	• *Staphylococcus aureus* • *Streptococcus* spp.
Gram-negative	• *Bordetella pertussis* • *Campylobacter* spp.
Non-Culturable	• *Legionella* spp. • *Mycoplasma pneumoniae* • *Chlamydia* spp.

Spectrum of Activity of Clindamycin

Bacteria	• *Staphylococcus aureus* • *Streptococcus* spp. • Anaerobes
Other	• Parasites e.g. *Toxoplasma gondii*, malaria • *Pneumocystis jirovecii* (PCP)

Cautions and Contraindications
- See BNF for full details
- Renal failure (reduce dose in severe renal failure)
- Liver failure (contraindicated in severe liver failure)
- Myasthenia gravis (macrolides and lincosamides are contraindicated in myasthenia gravis as they can precipitate a myasthenic crisis)
- Prolonged QT interval on ECG (risk of arrhythmia in patients with prolonged QT interval)
- Drugs
  - Risk of myopathy when given with statins e.g. Simvastatin
  - Increased levels when given with proton pump inhibitor e.g. Omeprazole
  - Increases Warfarin effect
  - Increases Phenytoin levels
  - Arrhythmias with other drugs that affect QT interval on ECG e.g. antidepressants, Beta-blockers, antipsychotics

Side Effects
- Significant predisposition to *Clostridium difficile* associated diarrhoea especially with Clindamycin
- Gastrointestinal disturbance (nausea and vomiting)
- Hepatotoxicity
- Neutropaenia and thrombocytopaenia
- Localised thrombophlebitis with intravenous administration
- Allergic reaction
- Fever
- Rash
- Prolonged QT interval

Monitoring
- Warn patients about risk of *Clostridium difficile* and check daily for symptoms
- If prescribing for more than 10 days monitor full blood count, urea and electrolytes and liver function tests at least weekly

Gentamicin, Amikacin and Tobramycin

Gentamicin, Amikacin and Tobramycin are aminoglycoside antibiotics.

Mechanism of Action
- Bactericidal
- Antibiotic binds to the ribosome causing a shape change that interferes with mRNA translation thereby preventing protein synthesis
- Aminoglycosides are taken up into bacterial cells by an energy-dependent mechanism (not concentration-dependent) which results in very high intracellular levels. This is responsible for the "post-antibiotic effect" seen with these drugs (continued potent antibacterial activity despite sub-therapeutic levels in blood), because the level in the bacteria remains therapeutic

Mechanisms of Resistance
- Reduced entry of antibiotic into anaerobic bacteria because these lack an energy-dependent transport mechanism
- Mutation of the active site therefore antibiotic does not bind
- Production of aminoglycoside modifying enzymes which break down the antibiotic before it reaches the active site. This is usually specific to each individual antibiotic so other aminoglycosides often remain active
- Antibiotic is removed from the bacteria by an efflux pump before it is able to act, often leading to resistance to all aminoglycosides

Hints and Tips
Complete antibiotic class resistance is very unusual in aminoglycosides. It is common for bacteria to be resistant to Gentamicin but sensitive to Amikacin. In this situation Amikacin is a good antibiotic to use instead of Gentamicin for septic patients when there is concern about potential antibiotic resistance e.g. previous courses of Gentamicin or known colonisation with a Gentamicin-resistant Enterobacteriaceae.

Pharmacology and Pharmacodynamics
- Intravenous and topical only
- Aminoglycosides display concentration-dependent killing, i.e. more bacteria are killed at higher peak concentrations. Once daily dosing gives higher peak concentrations and is therefore preferable to conventional TDS dosing
- 99% excreted unchanged in urine
- Bile level achieves 30% of serum levels
- Aminoglycosides are often used in combination with cell wall active agents (e.g. Beta-lactams) as this leads to synergy, i.e. the combination of the antibiotics is more effective than the sum of both agents used alone

Spectrum of Activity of Gentamicin, Amikacin and Tobramycin

Gram-positive	• *Staphylococcus aureus* (including MRSA)
Gram-negative	• Enterobacteriaceae e.g. *Escherichia coli*, *Klebsiella* spp., *Enterobacter* spp., *Salmonella* spp. • *Pseudomonas* spp.
Mycobacteria	• *Mycobacterium tuberculosis* (including MDR)

- See BNF for full details
- Renal failure (reduce dose in severe renal failure or **DO NOT** use)
- Pregnancy (avoid unless benefit outweighs risk)
- Myasthenia gravis (aminoglycosides are contraindicated in myasthenia gravis as they can precipitate a myasthenic crisis)
- Drugs
  - Increased ototoxicity when used in conjunction with Furosemide
  - Increased renal toxicity if used with other nephrotoxic agents e.g. Colistin, Vancomycin, Ciclosporin, Tacrolimus

Common Mistake
Some doctors withhold Gentamicin in septic patients with renal failure because of concern it will make the renal failure worse. **This is a mistake.** Gentamicin is an essential part of sepsis treatment in many empirical guidelines. Withholding it means patients may die from sepsis due to worries about the potential for worsening renal failure.

If in doubt give a stat dose of Gentamicin and review.

Side Effects
- Nephrotoxic
- Ototoxic
- Side effects tend to be related to concentration in blood therefore doses should be calculated for ideal body weight in renal failure (**NOT** actual body weight) and serum levels must be monitored.

Ideal body weight (IBW) calculation:
- Male IBW = 50 + (2.3 x height in inches above 60 inches)
- Female IBW = 45 + (2.3 x height in inches above 60 inches)

Monitoring
- Monitor serum levels on the 3rd - 4th dose, then weekly or more frequently if renal function changes
- For peak and trough levels (see section – Antibiotics, Therapeutic Drug Monitoring)
- Warn patients to report hearing and balance disturbances, and review daily for symptoms
- At least twice weekly monitoring of urea and electrolytes

Hints and Tips
Renal failure with Gentamicin occurs in 10% of patients but is rarely severe and usually recovers in <21 days of stopping Gentamicin.

Gentamicin induced renal failure is more common in:
- Prolonged courses of Gentamicin (≥7 days)
- Comorbidities (old age, diabetes mellitus, leukaemia)
- Reduced intravascular volume
- Drug interactions (e.g. Furosemide, non-steroidal anti-inflammatory drugs NSAIDS, Ciclosporin, Vancomycin)
- High serum Gentamicin concentrations

The risk of renal failure with Gentamicin can be reduced by:
- Using the correct dose for the individual patient
- Correcting fluid and electrolyte disturbances
- Limiting treatment to <7 days
- Avoiding co-administration with other nephrotoxic drugs

Ciprofloxacin and Levofloxacin

Ciprofloxacin and Levofloxacin are fluoroquinolone antibiotics. Other antibiotics in the class include Gatifloxacin, Moxifloxacin and Ofloxacin.

Mechanism of Action
- Bactericidal
- Inhibit topoisomerase and DNA gyrase which are enzymes involved in the coiling of bacterial DNA

Mechanisms of Resistance
Fluoroquinolone resistance is normally encoded by genes on the bacterial chromosome, therefore not usually transferable to other bacteria. It is often associated with resistance to other antibiotics by other mechanisms e.g. ESBL production via a plasmid.
- Mutation of active site therefore antibiotic does not bind
- Reduced entry of antibiotic into bacteria via loss of a porin
- Antibiotic is removed from the bacteria by a multi-efflux pump before it is able to act

Pharmacology and Pharmacodynamics
- Available as oral and intravenous preparations
- Very good oral bioavailability, between 50-100%, therefore intravenous administration is rarely necessary
- Oral absorption is reduced with concurrent use of antacids
- Renally excreted but effective levels also achieved in bile
- Good penetration into prostate, lung and bone (see section – Antibiotics, Table of Antibiotic Tissue Penetration)
- Fluoroquinolones are the only oral anti-pseudomonal antibiotics

Spectrum of Activity of Ciprofloxacin and Levofloxacin

Gram-positive	<ul><li>*Staphylococcus aureus* but usually **NOT ACTIVE** against MRSA</li><li>*Streptococcus pneumoniae*</li></ul>
Gram-negative	<ul><li>Enterobacteriaceae e.g. *Escherichia coli, Klebsiella* spp., *Enterobacter* spp.,</li><li>*Salmonella* spp.</li><li>*Pseudomonas* spp.</li><li>*Campylobacter* spp.</li><li>*Neisseria* spp.</li></ul>
Non-Culturable	<ul><li>*Legionella pneumophila*</li><li>*Mycoplasma pneumoniae*</li><li>*Chlamydia* spp.</li></ul>
Mycobacteria	<ul><li>*Mycobacterium tuberculosis* (including MDR)</li></ul>

Hints and Tips
Ciprofloxacin and Levofloxacin are the **ONLY** oral antibiotics with activity against *Pseudomonas* spp. requiring a high dose:
- PO Ciprofloxacin 750mg BD
- PO Levofloxacin 500mg BD

Cautions and Contraindications

- See BNF for full details
- Renal failure (reduce dose in severe renal failure)
- Epilepsy (reduced seizure threshold can occur with fluoroquinolones)
- G6PD deficiency (fluoroquinolones can precipitate haemolysis)
- Myasthenia gravis (fluoroquinolones are contraindicated in myasthenia gravis as they can precipitate a myasthenic crisis)
- Prolonged QT interval on ECG (risk of arrhythmia in patients with prolonged QT interval)
- Drugs
  - Ciprofloxacin increases Methotrexate levels
  - Increases Warfarin effect
  - Increases or decreases Phenytoin levels
  - Arrhythmias with other drugs that effect QT interval on ECG e.g. antidepressants, Beta-blockers, antipsychotics

Side Effects

- Significant predisposition to CDAD, MRSA and ESBL-positive *Escherichia coli*
- Gastrointestinal disturbance (nausea and vomiting)
- CNS (altered mood, headache, hallucinations, convulsions)
- Allergic reaction
- Prolonged QT interval
- Arthropathy and tendon rupture (fluoroquinolones are not recommended in children or adults with a risk of tendon rupture unless benefit outweighs the risk)
- Aortic dissection

Monitoring

- Warn patients about risk of *Clostridium difficile* and check daily for symptoms

Vancomycin and Teicoplanin are glycopeptide antibiotics.

Mechanism of Action
- Bactericidal
- Bind to the *d-ala-d-ala* tail of peptidoglycan and block cross linkage of the peptidoglycans, preventing bacterial cell wall formation

Mechanisms of Resistance
- Antibiotics are unable to penetrate the cell membrane of Gram-negative bacteria therefore cannot reach the active site on the cell wall
- Mutation of active site therefore antibiotic does not bind. This is the main resistance mechanism in Glycopeptide Resistant *Enterococcus* (GRE) of which there are three common types:
  - VanA causes high level resistance to both Vancomycin and Teicoplanin, transferable on transposon between bacterial species including MRSA creating Glycopeptide Resistant *Staphylococcus aureus* (GRSA)
  - VanB causes high level resistance to Vancomycin which induces the genes giving resistance, and low level resistance to Teicoplanin which does not induce the genes giving resistance, rarely transferable. Can become Teicoplanin resistant during treatment due to further changes in the regulatory genes so that resistance becomes constitutive
  - VanC causes low level resistance to Vancomycin and Teicoplanin, non-transferable and is inherent in *Enterococcus casseliflavus* and *Enterococcus gallinarum*
- Production of thicker bacterial cell wall preventing antibiotic penetration to the active site, seen in Glycopeptide Intermediate-Resistant *Staphylococcus aureus* (GISA) (gives co-resistance to Daptomycin)

Pharmacology and Pharmacodynamics
- Intravenous, do not transfer from the systemic circulation into the GI tract
- Renally excreted therefore may need dose reduction in renal failure
- Oral Vancomycin is only used for CDAD. It stays in the GI tract and is not absorbed and therefore cannot be used for any other infections

Spectrum of Activity of Vancomycin and Teicoplanin

Gram-positive	• *Staphylococcus aureus* • Coagulase negative *Staphylococcus* spp. • *Streptococcus* spp. • *Enterococcus* spp. • Coryneform bacteria ("Diphtheroids") • *Clostridium* spp. • **NOT ACTIVE** against Glycopeptide Resistant *Enterococcus* (GRE), *Leuconostoc* spp., *Lactococcus* spp., *Lactobacillus* spp., *Erysipelothrix rhusiopathiae*
Gram-negative	• *Acinetobacter* spp. (only used under specialist supervision for MDR *Acinetobacter* spp.)

Cautions and Contraindications
- See BNF for full details
- Renal failure (increase dosing interval to allow excretion)
- Drugs
  - Increased risk of renal failure if Vancomycin given with Colistin, aminoglycosides, Ciclosporin or Tacrolimus

Side Effects
- Nephrotoxicity
- Red man syndrome if Vancomycin infused too quickly
- Neutropaenia
- Thrombocytopaenia
- Fever
- Allergy

Monitoring
- Vancomycin levels required routinely to ensure therapeutic without being toxic
  - Monitor serum levels on the 3rd - 4th dose, then weekly or more frequently if renal function changes
- For trough levels (see section – Antibiotics, Therapeutic Drug Monitoring)
- Full blood count and urea and electrolytes initially daily, then at least weekly once regimen established

Daptomycin

Daptomycin is a lipopeptide antibiotic.

Mechanism of Action
- Bactericidal
- Depolarises cell membranes preventing protein, DNA and RNA synthesis

Mechanisms of Resistance
- Resistance is rare in Gram-positive bacteria
- Increased +ve charge of cell membrane repels Daptomycin preventing binding to active site (*Staphylococcus aureus, Enterococcus faecium*)
- Cell membrane mutation causes inefficient binding (*Enterococcus faecalis*)
- Production of thicker bacterial cell wall prevents antibiotic penetration to the active site (gives co-resistance to glycopeptides)
- Daptomycin is unable to penetrate the cell membrane of Gram-negative bacteria, therefore cannot reach its active site

Pharmacology and Pharmacodynamics
- Intravenous only
- Renally excreted therefore may need dose reduction in renal failure
- Inactivated by surfactant in the lungs therefore not used to treat pneumonia

Spectrum of Activity of Daptomycin

Gram-positive	- *Staphylococcus aureus* (including MRSA) - Coagulase negative *Staphylococcus* spp. - *Streptococcus* spp. (including Penicillin-resistant *Streptococcus pneumoniae*) - *Enterococcus* spp. (including GRE) - Gram-positive anaerobes

Cautions and Contraindications
- See BNF for full details
- Interferes with measurement of prothrombin time and INR
- Renal failure (increase dosing interval to allow excretion)
- Increased risk of myopathy when given with Ciclosporin and lipid regulating drugs e.g. statins

Side Effects
- Myalgia, muscle weakness, myositis, rhabdomyolysis
- Gastrointestinal disturbance (nausea and vomiting)
- Headache, anxiety, insomnia
- Rash
- Eosinophilic pneumonia 2-4 weeks after starting treatment
- Peripheral neuropathy
- Eosinophilia, thrombocythaemia and electrolyte disturbances

Monitoring
- Baseline full blood count, urea and electrolytes and creatine kinase tests then repeat at least weekly
- If muscle pain and raised creatine kinase (x5 higher than baseline) then consider stopping Daptomycin
- If using doses >6mg/kg or in renal failure monitor Daptomycin levels to ensure therapeutic without being toxic
  - Monitor serum levels on the 3rd - 4th dose, then weekly or more frequently if renal function changes
- For trough levels (see section – Antibiotics, Therapeutic Drug Monitoring)

Metronidazole

Metronidazole is a nitroimidazole antibiotic.

Mechanism of Action
- Bactericidal to anaerobes, no activity against aerobes
- Forms oxygen free radicals after activation inside the bacteria, which interact with nucleic acid and proteins causing cell death

Mechanisms of Resistance
- Acquired Metronidazole resistance in anaerobes is very rare.
- Aerobic bacteria have enzymes which deactivate oxygen free radicals e.g. catalase

Pharmacology and Pharmacodynamics
- Available as oral, intravenous, topical and per rectal (PR) preparations
- Very good oral bioavailability therefore intravenous administration is rarely necessary
- Hepatically metabolised but renally excreted
- Good penetration into tissues as well as abscesses (see section – Antibiotics, Table of Antibiotic Tissue Penetration)

Spectrum of Activity of Metronidazole

Gram-positive	• Anaerobic bacteria only e.g. *Clostridium* spp.
Gram-negative	• Anaerobic bacteria only e.g. *Bacteroides* spp.
Parasites	• *Giardia lamblia* • Amoebae

Cautions and Contraindications
- See BNF for full details
- Hepatic failure (reduce dose in severe hepatic failure)
- Do not take with alcohol; risk of Disulfiram-like reaction which can be fatal (including nausea, vomiting, flushing, hypotension and psychosis)
- Drugs
  - Increases Lithium levels
  - Increases Warfarin effect
  - Increases or decreases Phenytoin levels

Side Effects
- Gastrointestinal disturbance (nausea and vomiting)
- Allergic reaction
- Taste disturbance
- Prolonged treatment can result in peripheral neuropathy
- Neutropaenia
- Fever
- Hepatitis

Monitoring
- Baseline and weekly full blood count and liver function tests

Doxycycline, Tigecycline and Tetracycline

Doxycycline is a tetracycline antibiotic. Tigecycline is a glycylcycline antibiotic, derived from a related tetracycline called Minocycline.

Mechanism of Action
- Bacteriostatic
- Reversibly bind to the ribosome thereby preventing protein synthesis
- In parasites Doxycycline inhibits mitochondrial protein synthesis

Mechanisms of Resistance
- Production of proteins which knock Doxycycline off the ribosome, reversing its action
- Production of acetyl transferase enzymes that inactivate the antibiotic. This often results in cross-resistance with Chloramphenicol despite this antibiotic being in a different class
- Antibiotic is removed from the bacteria by an efflux pump before it is able to act
- There is less resistance to Tigecycline because it is normally unaffected by the mechanisms that prevent the tetracyclines working

Pharmacology and Pharmacodynamics
- Doxycycline is normally only available orally; IV Doxycycline has to be especially imported into the UK.
- Oral absorption is reduced by milk and antacids
- Tigecycline is only available intravenously
- Good tissue penetration (see section – Antibiotics, Table of Antibiotic Tissue Penetration)
- Primarily excreted in bile
- Tigecycline only enters the renal tract after being metabolised in the liver to a water-soluble inactive form. It cannot be used to treat UTIs

Spectrum of Activity of Doxycycline

Gram-positive	• *Staphylococcus aureus* (including MRSA) • *Streptococcus* spp.
Gram-negative	• *Haemophilus influenzae* • *Rickettsia* spp. • *Coxiella burnetii* (Q fever)
Non-Culturable	• *Legionella pneumophila* • *Mycoplasma* spp. • *Chlamydia* spp.
Spirochaetes	• *Borrelia burgdorferi* (Lyme disease)
Parasites	• Malaria

Spectrum of Activity of Tigecycline

Gram-positive	• *Staphylococcus aureus* (including MRSA) • *Streptococcus* spp. (including Penicillin-resistant *Streptococcus pneumoniae*) • *Enterococcus* spp. (including GRE)
Gram-negative	• *Haemophilus influenzae* • Enterobacteriaceae including AmpC and ESBL producers but **NOT ACTIVE** against *Proteus* spp. and *Morganella morganii*

Cautions and Contraindications

- See BNF for full details
- Contraindicated in children <12 years old, pregnancy and breast feeding as tetracyclines are deposited in growing teeth and bones causing staining and hypoplasia
  - Doxycycline is however **NOT** contraindicated in pregnancy and children for the treatment of infections with *Rickettsia* spp. which have a high mortality
- Renal failure (only use Doxycycline or Tigecycline in renal failure, not other tetracyclines)
- Liver failure (use with caution in liver failure)
- Myasthenia gravis (tetracyclines should be used with caution in myasthenia gravis as they may increase muscle weakness)
- Drugs
  - Doxycycline increases Methotrexate levels

Side Effects

- Gastrointestinal disturbance (nausea and vomiting)
- Photosensitivity reactions (patients should be advised to avoid intense sunlight)
- Hepatotoxicity
- Benign intracranial hypertension
- Allergy

Monitoring

- At least weekly liver function tests

Linezolid is an oxazolidinone antibiotic.

Mechanism of Action
- Predominantly bacteriostatic
- Prevents formation of the ribosome thereby preventing protein synthesis
- The theoretical antitoxin effect of Linezolid, through the inhibition of protein synthesis, is used in the treatment of severe toxin-mediated diseases e.g. Group A Beta-haemolytic *Streptococcus* and Panton-Valentine Leukocidin (PVL) positive *Staphylococcus aureus* infections

Mechanisms of Resistance
- Linezolid resistance is uncommon and usually occurs after prolonged administration
- Mutation of active site therefore antibiotic does not bind

Pharmacology and Pharmacodynamics
- Available as oral and intravenous preparations
- Very good oral bioavailability, approximately 90%, therefore intravenous administration is rarely necessary
- Renally excreted after metabolism in the liver. Does not require dose reduction in renal failure
- Good tissue penetration (see section – Antibiotics, Table of Antibiotic Tissue Penetration)

Spectrum of Activity of Linezolid

Gram-positive	• *Staphylococcus aureus* (including MRSA) • *Streptococcus* spp. (including Penicillin-resistant *Streptococcus pneumoniae*) • *Enterococcus* spp. (including GRE)

Cautions and Contraindications
- See BNF for full details
- Use with caution in patients with a history of seizures, hypertension and pre-existing myelosuppression
- Drugs
  - Use with caution with other drugs that cause bone marrow suppression
  - Linezolid is a monoamine oxidase inhibitor (MAOI) therefore do not give with other MAOIs or within 2 weeks of stopping other MAOIs

Side Effects
Rarely used for more than 2 weeks duration as risk of severe side effects.
- Gastrointestinal disturbance (nausea and vomiting)
- MAOI (avoid tyramine rich foods such as cheese and red wine)
- Myelosuppression after 10-14 days
- Optic neuropathy after 28 days

Monitoring
- Question patient about any visual disturbance daily and assess vision if concerns raised
- Baseline full blood count and liver function tests then repeat at least weekly

<u>**Rifampicin**</u>

Rifampicin is a rifamycin antibiotic.

Mechanism of Action
- Bactericidal
- Inhibits bacterial RNA polymerase

Mechanisms of Resistance
- Mutation of active site via the rpoB gene therefore antibiotic does not bind
- Resistance occurs rapidly with single agent use therefore Rifampicin should never be used alone

Pharmacology and Pharmacodynamics
- Available as oral and intravenous preparations
- Very good oral bioavailability, up to 90%, therefore intravenous administration is rarely necessary
- Good penetration into tissues, but not into CSF unless meninges inflamed (see section – Antibiotics, Table of Antibiotic Tissue Penetration)

Spectrum of Activity of Rifampicin

Gram-positive	• *Staphylococcus aureus* • *Streptococcus pneumoniae*
Gram-negative	• *Haemophilus influenzae* • *Neisseria* spp.
Mycobacteria	• *Mycobacterium tuberculosis* complex • Other Mycobacteria species e.g. *Mycobacterium avium, Mycobacterium abscessus*

Cautions and Contraindications
- See BNF for full details
- Renal failure (reduce dose in severe renal failure)
- Hepatic failure (contraindicated if jaundiced)
- Drugs
  - Decreased effectiveness of oral contraceptives therefore patients should be warned to use other methods of contraception

Side Effects
- Gastrointestinal disturbance (nausea and vomiting)
- Allergic reaction
- Hepatitis
- Thrombocytopaenia
- Orange discolouration of body fluids including tears
  - Can be used to monitor compliance by inspecting a urine sample
  - Will damage contact lenses

Monitoring
- Warn patients about symptoms of liver failure e.g. jaundice
- Baseline and weekly full blood count and liver function tests

Fusidic Acid

Fusidic acid is in a class of its own. It is also available as Sodium Fusidate.

Mechanism of Action
- Bacteriostatic
- Blocks elongation factor G involved in protein chain formation, thereby inhibiting protein synthesis

Mechanisms of Resistance
- Chromosomal mutation in the gene which encodes elongation factor G prevents it being blocked by the antibiotic

> **Warning**
> Resistance occurs rapidly, within 24-48 hours, therefore Fusidic Acid should never be used alone; this is particularly common with topical Fusidic Acid.

Pharmacology and Pharmacodynamics
- Available as oral, intravenous and topical preparations
- Topical preparations rapidly lead to resistance and should be avoided
- Very good oral bioavailability, close to 100%, therefore intravenous administration is rarely necessary
- Biliary excretion
- Good penetration into tissue, especially bone and synovial fluid (see section – Antibiotics, Table of Antibiotic Tissue Penetration)

Spectrum of Activity of Fusidic Acid

Gram-positive	• *Staphylococcus aureus*

Cautions and Contraindications
- See BNF for full details
- Hepatic failure
- Drugs
  - Myopathy and rhabdomyolysis can occur when given with statins therefore avoid use at the same time or within 7 days of stopping the statin

Side Effects
- Gastrointestinal disturbance (nausea and vomiting)
- CNS (altered mood, headache, hallucinations, convulsions)
- Jaundice: more common with intravenous (17% of patients) than oral (6% of patients)
- Thrombocytopaenia

Monitoring
- Baseline and weekly full blood count and liver function tests

Colistin

Colistin is a polymyxin antibiotic; it is also known as Polymyxin E. A related compound is Polymyxin B, which is available for topical use only.

Mechanism of Action
- Bactericidal
- Colistin acts like a detergent by interacting with phospholipids in the bacterial cell membrane leading to disruption of the membrane and cell death

Mechanisms of Resistance
- Gram-positive bacteria do not have a cell membrane and so are inherently resistant to Colistin. Colistin cannot be used to treat infections caused by Gram-positive bacteria
- Normally sensitive Gram-negative bacteria very rarely become resistant to Colistin. However, *Proteus* spp., *Morganella morgani* and *Serratia marcescens* are inherently resistant
- Mutation of the cell membrane by an enzyme preventing Colistin binding (MCR-1)

Pharmacology and Pharmacodynamics
- Available as intravenous, nebulised and topical preparations only
- No oral absorption
- Renally excreted therefore dose reduction required in renal failure
- Does not penetrate into CSF, bile, pleural fluid, bone or synovial fluid (see section – Antibiotics, Table of Antibiotic Tissue Penetration)

Spectrum of Activity of Colistin

Gram-negative	• *Pseudomonas* spp. • Enterobacteriaceae e.g. *Escherichia coli*, *Klebsiella* spp., *Enterobacter* spp., *Salmonella* spp. but **NOT ACTIVE** against *Proteus* spp., *Morganella morgani* and *Serratia marcescens*

Cautions and Contraindications
- See BNF for full details
- Renal failure (reduce dose in severe renal failure)
- Myasthenia gravis (Colistin is contraindicated in myasthenia gravis as it can worsen muscle weakness)
- Drugs
  - Ototoxicity when prescribed with loop diuretics e.g. Furosemide and Bumetanide
  - Increased nephrotoxicity with aminoglycosides, Vancomycin, Ciclosporin and Amphotericin

Side Effects
- Nephrotoxic
- Neurotoxic, especially at high doses (causing apnoea, paresthesia, vertigo, headaches, muscle weakness and cough)
- Nebulised Colistin can cause cough, sore throat, bronchospasm

Monitoring
- Baseline and weekly urea and electrolytes

Chloramphenicol

Chloramphenicol is in a class of its own; there are no related antibiotics.

Mechanism of Action
- Bactericidal against *Streptococcus pneumoniae*, *Neisseria meningitidis* and *Haemophilus influenzae*
- Bacteriostatic against most other bacteria
- Binds to the ribosome preventing attachment of tRNA thereby inhibiting protein synthesis

Mechanisms of Resistance
Resistance to Chloramphenicol does occur in specific bacterial clones therefore sensitivity testing is essential.
- Mutation of active site therefore antibiotic does not bind
- Reduced entry of antibiotic into the bacteria due to changes in membrane permeability
- Production of acetyl transferase enzymes that inactivate the antibiotic. This often results in cross-resistance with tetracyclines despite these antibiotics being in a different class

Pharmacology and Pharmacodynamics
- Available as oral, intravenous, intramuscular and topical preparations
- 90% excreted by the liver after being metabolised to an inactive form
- Good penetration into tissues including CSF (see section – Antibiotics, Table of Antibiotic Tissue Penetration)

Spectrum of Activity of Chloramphenicol

Gram-positive	<ul><li>*Staphylococcus aureus*</li><li>*Streptococcus pneumoniae*</li><li>Anaerobes</li></ul>
Gram-negative	<ul><li>Enterobacteriaceae e.g. *Escherichia coli*, *Klebsiella* spp., *Enterobacter* spp.,</li><li>*Salmonella* spp.</li><li>*Neisseria* spp.</li><li>*Rickettsia* spp.</li><li>Anaerobes</li></ul>
Non-Culturable	<ul><li>*Mycoplasma pneumoniae*</li><li>*Chlamydia* spp.</li></ul>

Cautions and Contraindications
- See BNF for full details
- Hepatic failure
- Pregnancy (avoid unless benefit outweighs risk, **DO NOT** use in third trimester)
- Drugs
  - Chloramphenicol metabolism is increased by Rifampicin
  - Increases Warfarin effect
  - Increases Phenytoin levels
  - Increases Ciclosporin and Tacrolimus levels

Side Effects

- Bone marrow suppression (dose related and reversible)
- Aplastic anaemia (rare, idiosyncratic, but often fatal, occurring in 1 in 25,000 patients)
- Grey baby syndrome (rare but some babies are unable to metabolise Chloramphenicol leading to toxicity, vomiting, cyanosis, circulatory collapse and death)

Monitoring

- Monitor serum levels on the 3rd - 4th dose, then weekly
- For peak and trough levels (see section – Antibiotics, Therapeutic Drug Monitoring)
- Baseline and twice weekly full blood count

<u>Nitrofurantoin</u>

Nitrofurantoin is a nitrofuran antibiotic and the only drug in this class available in the UK.

Mechanism of Action
The mechanism of activity is not completely known.
- Bactericidal
- Requires activation by an enzymatic reaction (nitrofuran reductase) in the bacterial cell in order to be active
- Nitrofurantoin binds to the ribosome to interfere with translation as well as causing direct damage to DNA

Mechanisms of Resistance
- Resistance is caused by inhibition of the enzyme (nitrofuran reductase) within the bacterial cell, some bacteria are inherently resistant as they do not have nitrofuran reductase e.g. *Proteus* spp., *Pseudomonas* spp.
- Resistance can be chromosomal or plasmid mediated

Pharmacology and Pharmacodynamics
- Nitrofurantoin is only available orally
- Predominantly renally excreted with little concentration in serum therefore only used to treat UTIs

Spectrum of Activity of Nitrofurantoin

Gram-positive	• *Staphylococcus saprophyticus* • *Enterococcus* spp. (including GRE)
Gram-negative	• Enterobacteriaceae e.g. *Escherichia coli*, *Klebsiella* spp. but **NOT ACTIVE** against *Proteus* spp., *Morganella morganii*, *Serratia* spp., *Acinetobacter* spp.

Cautions and Contraindications
- See BNF for full details
- Renal failure (inadequate urine concentration and toxicity when GFR <45ml/min)
- G6PD deficiency
- Infants <3 months old (may induce haemolysis)
- Pregnancy (avoid towards term as may induce neonatal haemolysis)
- Drugs
  - Absorption of Nitrofurantoin reduced by antacids
  - Reduced excretion of Nitrofurantoin when used with gout medications such as Probenicid or Sulfinpyrazone leading to toxicity

Side Effects
- Gastrointestinal disturbance (nausea, vomiting and diarrhoea)
- Pulmonary fibrosis (especially with prolonged use)
- Peripheral neuropathy
- Allergic reaction
- Cholestatic jaundice and hepatitis
- Blood disorders

Monitoring
- Baseline and weekly full blood count, urea and electrolytes and liver function tests

Fidaxomicin

Fidaxomicin is a macrocyclic antibiotic and is the only drug in this class available in the UK.

Mechanism of Action
- Bactericidal against *Clostridium difficile*
- Inhibits bacterial RNA polymerase preventing RNA synthesis
- May also inhibit spore formation by *Clostridium difficile*

Mechanisms of Resistance
- Mutation of active site therefore antibiotic does not bind

Pharmacology and Pharmacodynamics
- Fidaxomicin is only available orally and is used for CDAD. It stays in the GI tract and is not absorbed and therefore cannot be used for any other infections
- No dose reduction required in renal or hepatic failure as not absorbed

Spectrum of Activity of Fidaxomicin

Gram-positive	• *Clostridium difficile*

Cautions and Contraindications
- See BNF for full details
- Use with caution in severe CDAD as insufficient data available regarding effectiveness
- History of previous hypersensitivity reaction or allergy to macrolide antibiotics
- Renal and hepatic failure (use with caution as no data available)
- Pregnancy and breast feeding (avoid unless benefit outweighs risk)
- Drugs
  - Increased Fidaxomicin activity when given with Ciclosporin, Verapamil, macrolides and antiarrhythmics

Side Effects
- Gastrointestinal disturbance (nausea and vomiting)
- Hypersensitivity reaction
- Rash

Monitoring
- Check daily for worsening of CDAD

Fosfomycin

Fosfomycin is a derivative of phosphonic acid and is the only drug in this class available in the UK.

Mechanism of Action
- Bactericidal
- Actively transported into the bacterial cell then prevents formation of the bacterial cell wall by blocking peptidoglycan synthesis
- Synergistic effect when given in combination with Beta-lactams, fluoroquinolones and Linezolid

Mechanisms of Resistance
- Fosfomycin resistance can be chromosomal, plasmid or transposon mediated
- Chromosomal mediated resistance is caused by alteration of the active transport mechanisms reducing concentration inside the bacterial cell
- Plasmid or transposon mediated resistance via production of an inhibitor molecule preventing binding to target site or production of an enzyme that breaks down Fosfomycin before it can have any effect

Pharmacology and Pharmacodynamics
- Available as oral and intravenous preparations
- Up to 40% oral bioavailability, reduced when taken with food
- Renally excreted as active compound without being metabolised first
- Good penetration into bone, muscle, eyes, lungs and bile (see section – Antibiotics, Table of Antibiotic Tissue Penetration)

Spectrum of Activity of Fosfomycin

Gram-positive	• *Staphylococcus aureus* including MRSA • Coagulase negative *Staphylococcus* spp. • *Streptococcus* spp. • *Enterococcus* spp. (including GRE) • Gram-positive anaerobes
Gram-negative	• Enterobacteriaceae e.g. *Escherichia coli, Klebsiella* spp. **NOT ACTIVE** against *Morganella morganii* • *Pseudomonas* spp. • Gram-negative anaerobes **NOT ACTIVE** against *Bacteroides* spp.

Cautions and Contraindications
- See BNF for full details
- History of previous hypersensitivity reaction
- Renal failure (reduce dose in renal failure)
- Contains high amounts of sodium therefore use with caution in hypernatraemia, cardiac insufficiency, hypertension, pulmonary oedema and hyperaldosteronism
- Pregnancy and breast feeding (avoid unless benefit outweighs risk)
- No drug interactions

Side Effects

- Gastrointestinal disturbance (nausea and vomiting)
- Hypersensitivity reaction
- Bone marrow suppression including aplastic anaemia
- Rash
- Hepatitis
- Phlebitis at site of intravenous injection
- Vertigo
- Dyspnoea
- Rarely *Clostridium difficile* Associated Disease (CDAD)

Monitoring

- Baseline and weekly full blood count, urea and electrolytes and liver function tests

Antimycobacterials

Antimycobacterials are used to treat a separate group of bacteria called Mycobacteria (acid fast bacilli) which have mycolic acid in their cell wall (see section – Microbiology, Basic Bacterial Identification by Microscopy).

The antimycobacterials are mainly used to treat tuberculosis. The most common are Isoniazid, Rifampicin (see section – Antibiotics, Rifampicin), Pyrazinamide and Ethambutol. In the era of MDR and XDR tuberculosis there have been new agents developed including Bedaquiline, Delamanid and Clofazimine; strictly speaking Clofazimine is an old drug with a new purpose.

Mechanism of Action
- **Isoniazid**
  - Bactericidal
  - Isoniazid inhibits mycolic acid synthesis thereby preventing mycobacterial cell wall formation

- **Pyrazinamide**
  - Bactericidal
  - Unknown mechanism of action

- **Ethambutol**
  - Bactericidal
  - Ethambutol inhibits arabinosyltransferase enzyme thereby interfering with mycobacterial cell wall formation

- **Bedaquiline**
  - Predominantly bacteriostatic (may exhibit delayed bactericidal effects)
  - Bedaquiline inhibits the bacterial electron transport chain depleting the bacterium of energy in the form of adenosine triphosphate (ATP)

- **Delamanid**
  - Bactericidal
  - Pro-drug activated by F_{420}-dependent nitroreductase enzyme
  - Inhibits mycolic acid synthesis used in the cell wall of *Mycobacterium* spp.

- **Clofazimine**
  - Bacteriostatic
  - Clofazimine produces reactive oxygen species e.g. superoxide and hydrogen peroxide inside the bacterial cell, as well as bacterial cell membrane disruption

Mechanisms of Resistance
- **Isoniazid**
  - Mutation at active site

- **Pyrazinamide**
  - Mutation in pyrazinamidase gene

- **Ethambutol**
  - Mutation in arabinosyltransferase gene

- **Bedaquiline**
  - Mutation at active site
  - Very rare, antibiotic is removed from the bacterium by an efflux pump before it is able to act (giving co-resistance to Clofazimine)

- **Delamanid**
  - Mutation of F_{420}-dependent nitroreductase gene leading to pro-drug not being activated

- **Clofazimine**
  - Very rare, antibiotic is removed from the bacterium by an efflux pump before it is able to act (giving co-resistance to Bedaquiline)

Pharmacology and Pharmacodynamics
- **Isoniazid**
  - >95% oral bioavailability
  - Good penetration into tissue including CSF (see section – Antibiotics, Table of Antibiotic Tissue Penetration)
  - Renally excreted therefore dose reduction required in renal failure

- **Pyrazinamide**
  - >90% oral bioavailability
  - Good penetration into tissue including CSF (see section – Antibiotics, Table of Antibiotic Tissue Penetration)
  - Hepatic metabolism, renal excretion (no dose reduction required in renal failure)

- **Ethambutol**
  - 75-80% oral bioavailability
  - Good penetration into tissue including 20-40% in CSF (see section – Antibiotics, Table of Antibiotic Tissue Penetration)
  - Hepatic metabolism
  - Renally excreted therefore dose reduction required in renal failure

- **Bedaquiline**
  - Excellent oral bioavailability
  - High levels in macrophage-rich tissues e.g. lung
  - Low serum levels and does not enter the CSF
  - Hepatic metabolism
  - Synergistic in combination with other antimycobacterials such as Rifampicin, Ethambutol, Linezolid and Clofazimine

- **Delamanid**
  - 25-47% oral bioavailability
  - Highly protein bound
  - Metabolised in blood by albumin
  - Faecal excretion

- **Clofazimine**
  - 45-60% oral bioavailability
  - Highly lipid bound therefore low serum levels
  - Good penetration into lungs and spleen
  - Faecal excretion
  - Synergistic in combination with other antimycobacterials such as Ethambutol, Pyrazinamide, Amikacin, Moxifloxacin, Bedaquiline, Linezolid and Clarithromycin

Spectrum of Activity of Antimycobacterials

Isoniazid	• *Mycobacterium tuberculosis*
Pyrazinamide	• *M. tuberculosis*
Ethambutol	• *M. tuberculosis* • *Mycobacterium kansasii* • *Mycobacterium xenopi* • *Mycobacterium malmoense*
Bedaquiline	• *M. tuberculosis* • *Mycobacterium avium-intracellulare* complex • *Mycobacterium leprae*
Delamanid	• *M. tuberculosis* • *Mycobacterium abscessus* • *Mycobacterium avium-intracellulare* complex
Clofazimine	• *M. tuberculosis* • *Mycobacterium abscessus* • *Mycobacterium fortuitum* • *Mycobacterium avium-intracellulare* complex • *Mycobacterium leprae*

Hints and Tips

A number of more traditional antibiotics have activity against *Mycobacterium* spp. including:

Mycobacterium tuberculosis	Non-tuberculosis mycobacteria
• Fluoroquinolones e.g. Levofloxacin, Moxifloxacin • Aminoglycosides e.g. Gentamicin, Amikacin • Beta-lactams e.g. Co-amoxiclav, Meropenem • Linezolid	• Imipenem • Clarithromycin • Amikacin • Minocycline • Tigecycline • Co-trimoxazole • Linezolid

These antibiotics are sometimes used to treat mycobacterial infections however they can also be responsible for negative mycobacterial cultures if being used to treat other infections.

Cautions and Contraindications

- See BNF for full details
- Renal failure - Reduce dose in renal failure (Isoniazid and Ethambutol)

- **Isoniazid**
  - Risk factors for peripheral neuropathy (diabetes, alcoholism, chronic renal failure, pregnancy, malnutrition, HIV)
  - Increases anti-epileptic drug levels

- **Pyrazinamide**
  - Use with caution in liver disease

- **Ethambutol**
  - Use with caution in the elderly
  - Contraindicated in patients with optic neuritis

- **Bedaquiline**
  - Prolonged QT interval on ECG (risk of arrhythmia in patients with prolonged QT interval)
  - Drugs
    - Arrhythmia with other drugs that affect QT interval on ECG e.g. Delamanid, Clofazimine, antidepressants, Beta-blockers, antipsychotics
    - Reduced levels of Bedaquiline when given with Rifampicin

- **Delamanid**
  - Moderate to severe liver failure
  - Serum albumin <28g/L
  - Prolonged QT interval on ECG (risk of arrhythmia in patients with prolonged QT interval)
  - Drugs
    - Arrhythmia with other drugs that affect QT interval on ECG e.g. Bedaquiline, Delamanid, Clofazimine, antidepressants, Beta-blockers, antipsychotics
    - Increased QT interval with some antiretrovirals (Lopinavir and Ritonavir) and fluoroquinolones e.g. Ciprofloxacin, Levofloxacin and Moxifloxacin

- **Clofazimine**
  - Use with caution in liver disease
  - Possible prolonged QT interval on ECG (risk of arrhythmia in patients with prolonged QT interval)
  - Drugs
    - Arrhythmia with other drugs that affect QT interval on ECG e.g. Bedaquiline, Delamanid, antidepressants, Beta-blockers, antipsychotics

Side Effects
- **Isoniazid**
  - Peripheral neuropathy
  - Hepatitis

- **Pyrazinamide**
  - Liver failure
  - Hepatitis

- **Ethambutol**
  - Visual disturbance (loss of acuity, colour blindness, decreased visual fields)

- **Bedaquiline**
  - Prolonged QT interval on ECG
  - Gastrointestinal disturbance
  - Joint pains
  - Headache
  - Chest pain
  - Haemoptysis
  - Increased aspartate transaminase (AST) and alanine transaminase (ALT)

- **Delamanid**
  - Prolonged QT interval on ECG
  - Gastrointestinal disturbance
  - Headache
  - Insomnia
  - Dizziness
  - Tinnitus
  - Hypokalaemia

- **Clofazimine**
  - Skin pigmentation in 75-100%
  - Rash including photosensitivity
  - Dry skin
  - Gastrointestinal disturbance
  - Hyperglycaemia
  - Discolouration of urine, faeces and other body fluids

Monitoring
- Baseline and weekly liver function tests and urea and electrolytes
- Baseline and monthly ECG (Bedaquiline and Delamanid)
- Baseline visual acuity and warn patients to stop Ethambutol immediately if visual disturbance occurs

Antifungals are antibiotics active against yeasts (e.g. *Candida* spp.) and moulds (e.g. *Aspergillus* spp., *Fusarium* spp. and *Mucor* spp. or Zygomycetes).

Classification of commonly used systemic antifungals:
- **Triazoles** – Fluconazole, Itraconazole, Voriconazole, Posaconazole and Isavuconazole
- **Echinocandins** – Caspofungin, Anidulafungin and Micafungin
- **Polyenes** - Amphotericin B

Mechanism of Action
- **Triazoles**
  - Fungistatic
  - Triazoles inhibit cytochrome P450 14-alpha-demethylase thereby inhibiting ergosterol synthesis for the fungal cell wall
  - Isavuconazole has a higher affinity for cytochrome P450 therefore resistance less common than other azoles

- **Echinocandins**
  - Fungicidal
  - Echinocandins prevent cell wall synthesis by blocking (1,3)-Beta-d-glucan formation

- **Polyenes**
  - Fungicidal
  - Polyenes increase cell membrane permeability by binding to ergosterol within the fungal cell membrane

Mechanisms of Resistance
- **Triazoles**
  - Mutation of 14-alpha-demethylase preventing binding
  - Antibiotic removed from fungi before it is able to act, by an efflux pump
  - *Candida krusei* and 10-15% of *Candida glabrata* are resistant to most azoles
  - Most moulds are resistant to Fluconazole
  - *Mucor* spp. (Zygomycetes) are resistant to voriconazole
  - Resistance to Posaconazole and Isavuconazole is rare

- **Echinocandins**
  - Mutation in (1,3)-Beta-d-glucan synthase preventing antibiotic activity
  - *Candida parapsilosis* is resistant to the echinocandins
  - *Mucor* spp. (Zygomycetes) are resistant to Caspofungin

- **Polyenes**
  - Synthesis of alternative sterols to ergosterol which prevent Amphotericin B from binding
  - Resistance is intrinsic in *Aspergillus terreus*, *Fusarium* spp. and some *Mucor* spp. (Zygomycetes)
  - Resistance is intrinsic and develops on treatment with Amphotericin B in *Candida lusitaniae*

Pharmacology and Pharmacodynamics
- **Triazoles**
  - Fluconazole, Itraconazole, Voriconazole and Isavuconazole are available as both oral and intravenous preparations
  - Posaconazole is only available orally
  - Isavuconazole is metabolised and inactivated in the liver however elimination unknown (possibly faecal)

- Renally excreted therefore dose reduction required in renal failure; Isavuconazole is not excreted by kidneys therefore **NOT** active in urine

- **Echinocandins**
  - Only available as an intravenous preparation
  - Excellent activity in fungal biofilms therefore treatment of choice for infections of prosthetic material with *Candida* spp.
  - Hepatic metabolism followed by biliary and renal excretion

- **Polyenes**
  - Amphotericin B only available as an intravenous preparation
  - Different formulations are available with different dosing regimens:
    - Conventional formulation – Fungizone
    - Lipid formulations – AmBisome, Abelcet, Amphocil

Spectrum of Activity of Antifungals

Fluconazole	• *Candida* spp. but **NOT ACTIVE** against *Candida krusei* and *Candida glabrata* as presumed resistant unless specifically tests sensitive
Itraconazole	*As for* Fluconazole plus: • *Aspergillus* spp.
Voriconazole	*As for* Fluconazole plus: • *Aspergillus* spp.
Posaconazole	*As for* Fluconazole plus: • *Aspergillus* spp. • *Mucor* spp. (Zygomycetes)
Isavuconazole	• *Candida* spp. but **NOT ACTIVE** against all *C. glabrata* as presumed resistant unless specifically tests sensitive • *Aspergillus* spp. • *Mucor* spp. (Zygomycetes)
Caspofungin	• *Candida* spp. but **NOT ACTIVE** against *Candida parapsilosis* as presumed resistant unless specifically tests sensitive • *Aspergillus* spp.
Amphotericin B	• *Candida* spp. but **NOT ACTIVE** against *Candida lusitaniae* which is resistant • *Aspergillus* spp. but **NOT ACTIVE** against *Aspergillus terreus* which is resistant • *Mucor* spp. (Zygomycetes)

Warning
Candida auris is an emerging pathogen associated with resistance to many antifungals:
- Azoles – 86% (although usually remains sensitive to the new azole Isavuconazole)
- Amphotericin B – 43%

C. auris usually remains sensitive to the echinocandins (1% resistance). Treatment of infections with *C. auris* should be based on antifungal sensitivity testing and guided by a Microbiologist or Infectious Diseases Physician

- See BNF for full details

- **Triazoles**
  - Renal failure (reduce dose of Fluconazole in renal failure; Posaconazole, Voriconazole and Isavuconazole are **NOT** dose reduced in renal failure)
  - Hepatic failure
  - Cardiomyopathy
  - Prolonged QT interval
  - Isavuconazole should be avoided in pregnancy and breast feeding
  - Drugs
    - Risk of myopathy when given with statins
    - Reduced concentration when given with proton pump inhibitors
    - Increases concentration of painkillers e.g. NSAIDs
    - Increases Warfarin effect
    - Increases Phenytoin, Ciclosporin and Tacrolimus levels

- **Echinocandins**
  - Hepatic failure

- **Polyenes**
  - Increased renal failure with other nephrotoxic drugs e.g. Ciclosporin, Tacrolimus, aminoglycosides, Colistin, Vancomycin

Side Effects
- **Triazoles**
  - Abnormal liver function tests
  - Voriconazole (visual disturbance)
  - Posaconazole (gastrointestinal disturbance including nausea, vomiting and diarrhoea)
  - Isavuconazole (nausea, vomiting and diarrhoea, headache, rash and shortened QT interval on ECG)

- **Echinocandins**
  - Gastrointestinal disturbance (nausea, vomiting and diarrhoea)
  - Abnormal liver function tests

- **Polyenes**
  - Nephrotoxicity
  - Infusion reactions, e.g. anaphylaxis, therefore give test dose first
  - Gastrointestinal disturbance (nausea, vomiting and diarrhoea)
  - Blood disorders

Monitoring
- **Triazoles**
  - Baseline and at least weekly liver function tests
  - Warn patients about visual disturbance and ask about symptoms daily if on Voriconazole
  - Azole levels required routinely to ensure therapeutic without being toxic
    - Monitor serum levels weekly, more frequently if renal function changes
  - For peak and trough levels (see section – Antibiotics, Therapeutic Drug Monitoring)

- **Echinocandins**
  - Baseline and at least weekly liver function tests

- **Polyenes**
  - Baseline and at least weekly liver function tests, full blood count and urea and electrolytes

Antivirals

Antivirals are antibiotics that are active against viruses.

Classification of commonly used systemic antivirals:
- **Nucleoside analogues** – Aciclovir, Ganciclovir and Ribavirin
- **Neuraminidase inhibitors** – Oseltamivir and Zanamivir

Mechanism of Action
Whilst antivirals can be described as either virucidal or virustatic these terms are not commonly used and are not used in this book.

- **Aciclovir**
  - Nucleoside analogue activated by VZV and HSV specific thymidine kinase thereby interfering with viral DNA polymerase

- **Ganciclovir**
  - Nucleoside analogue activated by CMV protein kinase thereby interfering with viral DNA polymerase

- **Ribavirin**
  - Nucleoside analogue interfering with DNA and RNA synthesis as well as production of viral mRNA

- **Oseltamivir and Zanamivir**
  - Inhibition of neuraminidase preventing release of new viral particles from infected cells

Mechanisms of Resistance
- **Aciclovir**
  - Mutation in VZV and HSV specific thymidine kinase reducing Aciclovir activation

- **Ganciclovir**
  - Mutation in CMV protein kinase reducing Ganciclovir activation
  - Mutation in DNA polymerase preventing nucleoside analogue binding

- **Ribavirin**
  - Resistance to Ribavirin is very rare

- **Oseltamivir and Zanamivir**
  - Mutation in neuraminidase preventing binding of Oseltamivir
  - Resistance to Zanamivir is very rare

Pharmacology and Pharmacodynamics
- **Aciclovir**
  - Available as oral, intravenous and topical preparations
  - Only 15-20% bioavailability orally therefore use intravenously for serious illness
  - Renally excreted therefore dose reduction required in renal failure

- **Ganciclovir**
  - Available as oral and intravenous preparations
  - Only 5-10% bioavailability therefore only used intravenously for serious illness
  - Renally excreted therefore dose reduction required in renal failure

- **Ribavirin**
  - Available as nebulised, oral and intravenous preparations
  - Metabolism and excretion is variable between individuals

- **Oseltamivir and Zanamivir**
  - Oseltamivir only available as an oral preparation
  - Zanamivir is usually only available as an inhaled preparation
    - IV and nebulised preparations are currently unlicensed in the UK but available on a compassionate use named patient basis for those in whom inhaled Zanamivir cannot be given
  - Oseltamivir renally excreted therefore dose reduction required in renal failure

Spectrum of Activity of Antivirals

Aciclovir	• *Herpes Simplex Virus* (HSV) • *Varicella Zoster Virus* (VZV)
Ganciclovir	• *Cytomegalovirus* (CMV)
Ribavirin	• *Respiratory Syncytial Virus* (RSV) • Occasionally used for other viruses e.g. *Hepatitis C Virus*
Oseltamivir and Zanamivir	• *Influenza A Virus* and *Influenza B Virus*

Cautions and Contraindications
- See BNF for full details

- **Aciclovir**
  - Renal failure (reduce dose in severe renal failure)
  - Increased nephrotoxicity with Ciclosporin and Tacrolimus
  - Increases Methotrexate levels

- **Ganciclovir**
  - Bone marrow suppression, especially when prescribed with other bone marrow suppressing agents e.g. chemotherapeutics

- **Ribavirin**
  - Pregnancy (teratogenic)
  - Contraception should be advised after treatment for 4 months in women and 7 months in men

- **Oseltamivir and Zanamivir**
  - Renal failure (reduce dose of Oseltamivir in severe renal failure)
  - Risk of bronchospasm in patients with asthma or COPD with Zanamivir

Side Effects
- **Aciclovir**
  - Nausea
  - Rash
  - Neurotoxicity (1-4% of patients) especially in the elderly
  - Nephrotoxicity

- **Ganciclovir**
  - Bone marrow suppression
  - Headache, confusion, convulsions
  - Nephrotoxicity
  - Hepatotoxicity
  - Fever
  - Myalgia

- **Ribavirin**
  - Bronchospasm
  - Bone marrow suppression

- **Oseltamivir and Zanamivir**
  - Gastrointestinal disturbance with Oseltamivir (nausea, vomiting and diarrhoea)

Monitoring
- **Aciclovir**
  - Baseline and at least weekly urea and electrolytes

- **Ganciclovir**
  - Baseline and at least weekly urea and electrolytes, full blood count and liver function tests

- **Ribavirin**
  - Baseline and at least weekly urea and electrolytes and full blood count

- **Oseltamivir and Zanamivir**
  - Baseline and at least weekly urea and electrolytes with Oseltamivir
  - No monitoring required with inhaled Zanamivir

Antibiotic Guidelines

Antibiotic Guidelines

Finding and accessing the latest guidelines can be difficult. There is no single place where international, national or specialist guidelines are collated and made easily available. Nor do you know if there is a more up-to-date guideline than the one you are using or that the hospital you are currently working in has different guidance to the one you just left!

To make matters worse:
- In order to look at a guideline you have to know that the guideline exists in the first place
- Not all experts agree so guidelines on the same subject can vary
- NICE guidelines do not cover all clinical scenarios
- Some professional bodies only publish their guidelines in medical journals that are not open access
- It can be difficult to know who has written a guideline or what professional authority they hold

For example, a Cardiologist may look for an endocarditis guideline in the British Journal of Cardiology as this is their professional journal. However they may be unaware that BSAC has published guidelines in the Journal of Antimicrobial Chemotherapy and that NICE have also published guidance. On top of these there are new guidelines from Europe and America! These 5 guidelines all differ to some degree. So, which guideline should the Cardiologist follow and which is medically and legally the best?

There is a list of current guidelines relating to infection in section – Numbers & Notes, Sources of Information, Guidelines and Further Reading. The website www.microbiologynutsandbolts.co.uk will endeavour to keep this list up-to-date.

On the Horizon
Microbiologists and Infectious Diseases Physicians are questioning the old adage **"you must finish a course of antibiotics"**. Over recent years courses of antibiotics have become shorter e.g. treatment of pyelonephritis was 4 weeks, now it is 7 days. Soon it may be "here's 7 days, stop them when you feel better".

It used to be thought that inadequate courses caused antibiotic resistance and infections would relapse. **This looks increasingly untrue.** Antibiotic resistance is actually driven by low doses of antibiotics, not short courses of high doses, and once a patient feels better it is unlikely their infection will relapse. Antibiotic courses are likely to continue to get shorter and be tailored to the individual patient's response rather than specific durations.

<u>**Post-Splenectomy Antibiotic Guidelines**</u>

Patients who have no spleen are particularly at risk of infection from capsulated bacteria such as *Streptococcus pneumoniae*, *Neisseria meningitidis* and *Haemophilus influenzae*.

These patients should ideally be immunised against these bacteria before they have their spleen removed or 2 weeks after their spleen has been removed. They should be given a post-splenectomy warning card which includes the dates on which they were immunised.

Post-splenectomy Immunisations	• Pneumovax II (PPV23) stat and 5 yearly • Menitorix (Hib/MenC) stat • Bexsero (MenB) stat and at 1 month • Nimenrix (MenA, C, W135, Y) at 1 month • Influenza vaccination yearly

Antibiotic Prophylaxis
Post-splenectomy patients should be given antibiotic prophylaxis which reduces the incidence of infection by 50% and the risk of death by 90%.

Antibiotic prophylaxis	1st Line PO Penicillin V 250-500mg BD 2nd Line PO Erythromycin 250-500mg OD

Total Duration
2 years
Children should receive prophylaxis until they are 16 years old or for 2 years whichever is longer.

Lifelong prophylaxis for specific post-splenectomy patients
• Inadequate serological response to pneumococcal immunisation
• History of invasive *S. pneumoniae* infection
• Haematological malignancy, especially if on-going immunosuppression

Early Treatment of Infection
Post-splenectomy patients should be given a dose of antibiotic to self-administer if they develop symptoms or signs of infection e.g. fever, sore throat, cough, shortness of breath. **ALL** patients without a functioning spleen should seek urgent medical help if they develop signs of infection, whether they have taken an initial dose of antibiotic or not.

Patient NOT on antibiotic prophylaxis	
1st Line	PO Amoxicillin 500mg stat
2nd line (if 1st line contraindicated)	PO Clarithromycin 500mg stat

Patient ON splenectomy antibiotic prophylaxis	
1st Line	PO Co-amoxiclav 625mg stat
2nd line (if 1st line contraindicated)	PO Levofloxacin 500mg stat

Respiratory Infections	1st Line Antibiotic
Community Acquired Pneumonia (CAP) (CURB-65 score 0-2)	PO Amoxicillin 500mg-1g TDS **PLUS** PO Clarithromycin 500mg BD (If Nil By Mouth use IV)
Community Acquired Pneumonia (CAP) (CURB-65 score 3-5)	IV Co-amoxiclav 1.2g TDS **PLUS** IV Clarithromycin 500mg BD If MRSA **ADD** IV Teicoplanin 400mg BD for 3 doses **THEN** OD (or 6mg/kg if >70kg)
Community Acquired Aspiration Pneumonia	IV Co-amoxiclav 1.2g TDS If MRSA **ADD** IV Teicoplanin 400mg BD for 3 doses **THEN** OD (or 6mg/kg if >70kg)
Hospital Acquired Pneumonia (HAP) (Onset 2-4 days after admission)	IV Co-amoxiclav 1.2g TDS If MRSA **ADD** IV Teicoplanin 400mg BD for 3 doses **THEN** OD (or 6mg/kg if >70kg)
Hospital Acquired Pneumonia (HAP) (Onset ≥4 days after admission)	IV Piptazobactam 4.5g TDS If MRSA **ADD** IV Teicoplanin 400mg BD for 3 doses **THEN** OD (or 6mg/kg if >70kg)
Hospital Acquired Aspiration Pneumonia	IV Piptazobactam 4.5g TDS If MRSA **ADD** IV Teicoplanin 400mg BD for 3 doses **THEN** OD (or 6mg/kg if >70kg)
Ventilator Associated Pneumonia (VAP)	IV Piptazobactam 4.5g TDS If MRSA **ADD** IV Teicoplanin 400mg BD for 3 doses **THEN** OD (or 6mg/kg if >70kg)

2nd line Antibiotic (if 1st line contraindicated)	Oral Treatment (when appropriate)	Duration
PO Doxycycline 200mg stat **THEN** 100mg OD **OR** PO Levofloxacin 500mg BD (If Nil By Mouth use IV)	As for 1st and 2nd line	5-7 days
IV Teicoplanin 400mg BD for 3 doses **THEN** OD (or 6mg/kg if >70kg) **PLUS** PO Levofloxacin 500mg BD (If Nil By Mouth use IV)	PO Co-amoxiclav 625mg TDS **PLUS** PO Clarithromycin 500mg BD **OR** PO Levofloxacin 500mg BD	7 days
IV Teicoplanin 400mg BD for 3 doses **THEN** OD (or 6mg/kg if >70kg) **PLUS** IV Ciprofloxacin 400mg BD-TDS **AND** IV Metronidazole 500mg TDS	PO Co-amoxiclav 625mg TDS	5-7 days
IV Teicoplanin 400mg BD for 3 doses **THEN** OD (or 6mg/kg if >70kg) **PLUS** PO Levofloxacin 500mg BD	PO Co-amoxiclav 625mg TDS	5-7 days
IV Teicoplanin 400mg BD for 3 doses **THEN** OD (or 6mg/kg if >70kg) **PLUS** IV Ciprofloxacin 400mg BD-TDS	PO Co-amoxiclav 625mg TDS depending on culture results	5-7 days
IV Teicoplanin 400mg BD for 3 doses **THEN** OD (or 6mg/kg if >70kg) **PLUS** IV Ciprofloxacin 400mg BD-TDS **AND** IV Metronidazole 500mg TDS	PO Co-amoxiclav 625mg TDS depending on culture results	5-7 days
IV Teicoplanin 400mg BD for 3 doses **THEN** OD (or 6mg/kg if >70kg) **PLUS** IV Ciprofloxacin 400mg BD-TDS	No oral treatment	5-7 days

Respiratory Infections Cont.	1st Line Antibiotic
Infective Exacerbation of COPD	PO Amoxicillin 500mg TDS
Acute Bronchitis	PO Amoxicillin 500mg TDS
Influenza	PO Oseltamivir 75mg BD

Head and Neck Infections	1st Line Antibiotic
Acute Otitis Media	PO Amoxicillin 500mg-1g TDS
Otitis Externa	TOP 2% Acetic Acid TDS
Orbital Cellulitis	IV Cefotaxime 2g QDS **OR** IV Ceftriaxone 2g BD **PLUS** IV Metronidazole 500mg TDS If MRSA **ADD** IV Teicoplanin 400mg BD for 3 doses **THEN** OD (or 6mg/kg if >70kg)
Acute Sinusitis	PO Amoxicillin 500mg-1g TDS

2nd line Antibiotic (if 1st line contraindicated)	Oral Treatment (when appropriate)	Duration
PO Clarithromycin 500mg BD **OR** PO Doxycycline 200mg stat **THEN** 100mg OD	PO Amoxicillin 500mg TDS **OR** PO Clarithromycin 500mg BD **OR** PO Doxycycline 200mg stat **THEN** 100mg OD	5-7 days
PO Clarithromycin 500mg BD **OR** PO Doxycycline 200mg stat **THEN** 100mg OD	PO Amoxicillin 500mg TDS **OR** PO Clarithromycin 500mg BD **OR** PO Doxycycline 200mg stat **THEN** 100mg OD	5-7 days
Inhaled Zanamivir 10mg BD	As for 1st and 2nd line	5 days

2nd line Antibiotic (if 1st line contraindicated)	Oral Treatment (when appropriate)	Duration
PO Clarithromycin 500mg BD	As for 1st and 2nd line	5 days
TOP Neomycin Sulphate + Corticosteroid TDS	No oral treatment	7-10 days
IV Meropenem 500mg-1g TDS If MRSA **ADD** IV Teicoplanin 400mg BD for 3 doses **THEN** OD (or 6mg/kg if >70kg)	Guided by culture results	10-14 days
PO Clarithromycin 500mg BD	As for 1st and 2nd line	7 days

Urogenital Infections	1st Line Antibiotic
Urinary Tract Infection (UTI) Uncomplicated	PO Trimethoprim 200mg BD
Catheter Related UTI	IV Gentamicin as per renal function
UTI in Pregnancy	PO Cefalexin 500mg TDS
Pyelonephritis	IV Gentamicin as per renal function
Pyelonephritis in Pregnancy	IV Cefuroxime 750mg-1.5g TDS
Prostatitis	PO Ciprofloxacin 500mg BD
Pelvic Inflammatory Disease (PID) (Mild)	IM Ceftriaxone 250mg stat **PLUS** PO Doxycycline 100mg BD **PLUS** PO Metronidazole 400mg TDS
Pelvic Inflammatory Disease (PID) (Severe)	IV Ceftriaxone 2g OD for 48 hours **PLUS** PO Doxycycline 100mg BD **PLUS** PO Metronidazole 400mg TDS

2nd line Antibiotic (if 1st line contraindicated)	Oral Treatment (when appropriate)	Duration
PO Nitrofurantoin 50-100mg QDS **OR** PO Pivmecillinam Hydrochloride 400mg TDS **OR** PO Fosfomycin 3g stat (repeat day 3 if required)	As for 1st and 2nd line	Female: 3 days Male: 7 days
IV Piptazobactam 4.5g TDS If MRSA **ADD** IV Teicoplanin 400mg BD for 3 doses **THEN** OD (or 6mg/kg if >70kg)	Guided by culture results	3-5 days
PO Nitrofurantoin 50-100mg QDS	Guided by culture results	5 days
IV Ciprofloxacin 400mg BD or TDS	PO Co-amoxiclav 625mg TDS depending on culture results **OR** PO Ciprofloxacin 500mg BD	7 days
Microbiology advice required	Guided by culture results	14 days
PO Trimethoprim 200mg BD	As for 1st and 2nd line	28 days
PO Ofloxacin 400mg BD **PLUS** PO Metronidazole 400mg TDS	As for 1st and 2nd line	Doxycycline: 14 days Ofloxacin: 14 days Metronidazole: 5 days
IV Clindamycin 600mg QDS for 48 hours **PLUS** IV Gentamicin 7mg/kg OD for 48 hours **THEN** PO Doxycycline 100mg BD **PLUS** PO Metronidazole 400mg TDS	As for 1st and 2nd line	Doxycycline: 14 days Metronidazole: 5 days

Skin, Soft Tissue, Bone and Joint Infections	1st Line Antibiotic
Cellulitis	IV Flucloxacillin 1-2g QDS (or 2g 4 hourly if >85kg)
Cellulitis (if MRSA positive)	IV Teicoplanin 400mg BD for 3 doses **THEN** OD (or 6mg/kg if >70kg)
Cellulitis in Diabetes	IV Flucloxacillin 1-2g QDS (or 2g 4 hourly if >85kg) **PLUS** IV Metronidazole 500mg TDS
Cellulitis in Diabetes (if MRSA positive)	IV Teicoplanin 400mg BD for 3 doses **THEN** OD (or 6mg/kg if >70kg) **PLUS** IV Metronidazole 500mg TDS
Bites	PO Co-amoxiclav 625mg TDS
Infected Burns, Skin Grafts and Post-Operative Wounds	IV Flucloxacillin 1-2g QDS (or 2g 4 hourly if >85kg) **PLUS** IV Gentamicin as per renal function
Infected Burns, Skin Grafts and Post-Operative Wounds (if MRSA positive)	IV Teicoplanin 400mg BD for 3 doses **THEN** OD (or 6mg/kg if >70kg) **PLUS** IV Gentamicin as per renal function
Intravenous Device Associated Infection	IV Teicoplanin 400mg BD for 3 doses **THEN** OD (or 6mg/kg if >70kg)
Osteomyelitis or Septic Arthritis	IV Flucloxacillin 1-2g QDS (or 2g 4 hourly if >85kg) **PLUS** PO Fusidic Acid 500mg TDS
Osteomyelitis* or Septic Arthritis* (*if MRSA positive)	IV Teicoplanin 12mg/kg BD for 5 doses **THEN** OD **PLUS** PO Fusidic Acid 500mg TDS

2nd line Antibiotic (if 1st line contraindicated)	Oral Treatment (when appropriate)	Duration
IV Clindamycin 600mg QDS	PO Flucloxacillin 500mg-1g QDS **OR** PO Clindamycin 150-450mg QDS	10-14 days
IV Daptomycin 6mg/kg OD	PO Doxycycline 100mg BD	10-14 days
IV Clindamycin 600mg QDS	PO Flucloxacillin 500mg-1g QDS **PLUS** PO Metronidazole 400mg TDS	10-14 days
IV Daptomycin 6mg/kg OD **PLUS** IV Metronidazole 500mg TDS	PO Doxycycline 100mg BD **PLUS** PO Metronidazole 400mg TDS	10-14 days
PO Doxycycline 100mg BD **PLUS** PO Metronidazole 400mg TDS	As for 1st and 2nd line	7 days
IV Teicoplanin 400mg BD for 3 doses **THEN** OD (or 6mg/kg if >70kg) **PLUS** IV Gentamicin as per renal function	Guided by culture results	10-14 days
IV Daptomycin 6mg/kg OD **PLUS** IV Gentamicin as per renal function	Guided by culture results	10-14 days
IV Daptomycin 6mg/kg OD	Guided by culture results	7-14 days
IV Teicoplanin 12mg/kg BD for 5 doses **THEN** OD **PLUS** PO Fusidic Acid 500mg TDS	Guided by culture results	6 weeks total (2-4 weeks IV)
IV Daptomycin 6mg/kg OD **PLUS** PO Fusidic Acid 500mg TDS	Guided by culture results	6 weeks total (2-4 weeks IV)

Skin, Soft Tissue, Bone & Joint Infections Cont.	1st Line Antibiotic
Osteomyelitis or Septic Arthritis (in Diabetes or Elderly)	IV Ceftriaxone 1-2g OD If MRSA **ADD** IV Teicoplanin 12mg/kg BD for 5 doses **THEN** OD
Osteomyelitis or Septic Arthritis (Following trauma)	IV Flucloxacillin 1-2g QDS (or 2g 4 hourly if >85kg) **PLUS** IV Metronidazole 500mg TDS
Prosthetic Joint Infection	IV Teicoplanin 12mg/kg BD for 5 doses **THEN** OD **PLUS** PO Rifampicin 300mg BD

Gastrointestinal Infections	1st Line Antibiotic
Clostridium difficile Associated Disease (CDAD)	PO Metronidazole 400mg TDS
Primary Peritonitis or Diverticulitis	IV Co-amoxiclav 1.2g TDS **PLUS** IV Gentamicin as per renal function
Secondary Peritonitis	IV Piptazobactam 4.5g TDS **PLUS** IV Gentamicin as per renal function

2nd line Antibiotic (if 1st line contraindicated)	Oral Treatment (when appropriate)	Duration
IV Meropenem 500mg-1g TDS IF MRSA **ADD** IV Teicoplanin 12mg/kg BD for 5 doses **THEN** OD	Guided by culture results	6 weeks total (2-4 weeks IV)
IV Teicoplanin 12mg/kg BD for 5 doses **THEN** OD **PLUS** IV Metronidazole 500mg TDS	Guided by culture results	6 weeks total (2-4 weeks IV)
IV Daptomycin 6mg/kg OD **PLUS** PO Rifampicin 300mg BD	Guided by culture results	6 weeks total (2-4 weeks IV)

2nd line Antibiotic (if 1st line contraindicated)	Oral Treatment (when appropriate)	Duration
PO Vancomycin 125mg QDS **OR** PO Fidaxomicin 200mg BD	As for 1st and 2nd line	10-14 days
IV Teicoplanin 400mg BD for 3 doses **THEN** OD (or 6mg/kg if >70kg) **PLUS** IV Gentamicin as per renal function **PLUS** IV Metronidazole 500mg TDS	PO Co-amoxiclav 625mg TDS depending on culture results **OR** PO Ciprofloxacin 500mg BD **PLUS** PO Metronidazole 400mg TDS	5-7 days
IV Teicoplanin 400mg BD for 3 doses **THEN** OD (or 6mg/kg if >70kg) **PLUS** IV Gentamicin as per renal function **PLUS** IV Metronidazole 500mg TDS	PO Co-amoxiclav 625mg TDS depending on culture results **OR** PO Ciprofloxacin 500mg BD **PLUS** PO Metronidazole 400mg TDS	5-7 days

Gastrointestinal Infections Cont.	1st Line Antibiotic
Cholecystitis or Cholangitis	IV Amoxicillin 1g TDS **PLUS** IV Gentamicin as per renal function **PLUS** IV Metronidazole 500mg TDS
Necrotising Pancreatitis	IV Piptazobactam 4.5g QDS
Peptic Ulcer Disease	PPI e.g. Lansoprazole 30mg BD **PLUS** Amoxicillin 1g BD **PLUS** Clarithromycin 500mg BD

Other Infections	1st Line Antibiotic
Infective Endocarditis Native Valve (Slow Onset)	IV Amoxicillin 2g 4 hourly **PLUS** IV Gentamicin 1mg/kg BD
Infective Endocarditis Native Valve (Severe Sepsis or Fast Onset)	IV Vancomycin 1g BD (OD if >65 years old) **PLUS** IV Gentamicin 1mg/kg BD
Infective Endocarditis Prosthetic Valve	IV Vancomycin 1g BD (OD if >65 years old) **PLUS** IV Gentamicin 1mg/kg BD **PLUS** PO Rifampicin 300mg BD

2nd line Antibiotic (if 1st line contraindicated)	Oral Treatment (when appropriate)	Duration
IV Teicoplanin 400mg BD for 3 doses **THEN** OD (or 6mg/kg if >70kg) **PLUS** IV Gentamicin as per renal function **PLUS** IV Metronidazole 500mg TDS	PO Co-amoxiclav 625mg TDS depending on culture results **OR** PO Ciprofloxacin 500mg BD **PLUS** PO Metronidazole 400mg TDS	5-7 days
IV Ciprofloxacin 400mg TDS **PLUS** IV Metronidazole 500mg TDS	No oral treatment	2-4 weeks
PPI e.g. Lansoprazole 30mg BD **PLUS** Clarithromycin 500mg BD **PLUS** Metronidazole 400mg BD	As for 1st and 2nd line	7 days

2nd line Antibiotic (if 1st line contraindicated)	Oral Treatment (when appropriate)	Duration
IV Vancomycin 1g BD (OD if >65 years old) **PLUS** IV Gentamicin 1mg/kg BD	No oral treatment	Guided by culture results
IV Daptomycin 6mg/kg OD **PLUS** IV Gentamicin 1mg/kg BD	No oral treatment	Guided by culture results
Microbiology advice required	No oral treatment	Guided by culture results

Emergencies	1st Line Antibiotic
Sepsis	IV Piptazobactam 4.5g QDS **PLUS** IV Gentamicin as per renal function If MRSA **ADD** IV Teicoplanin 400mg BD for 5 doses **THEN** OD (or 6mg/kg if >70kg)
Neutropaenic Sepsis	IV Piptazobactam 4.5g QDS **PLUS** IV Gentamicin as per renal function If MRSA **ADD** IV Teicoplanin 400mg BD for 5 doses **THEN** OD (or 6mg/kg if >70kg)
Neutropaenic Sepsis Previous ESBL or AmpC Producing Bacteria	IV Meropenem 1g TDS **PLUS** IV Gentamicin as per renal function If MRSA **ADD** IV Teicoplanin 400mg BD for 5 doses **THEN** OD (or 6mg/kg if >70kg)
Meningitis	IV Cefotaxime 2g QDS **OR** IV Ceftriaxone 2g BD
Meningitis (if listeria suspected)	IV Cefotaxime 2g QDS **OR** IV Ceftriaxone 2g BD **PLUS** IV Amoxicillin 2g 4 hourly
Meningococcal Sepsis	IV Cefotaxime 2g QDS **OR** IV Ceftriaxone 2g BD
Encephalitis	IV Aciclovir 10mg/kg TDS
Epiglottitis	IV Cefotaxime 2g QDS **OR** IV Ceftriaxone 2g BD
Epidural Abscess	IV Ceftriaxone 1-2g OD If MRSA **ADD** IV Teicoplanin 400mg BD for 5 doses **THEN** OD (or 6mg/kg if >70kg)
Necrotising Fasciitis (in a limb)	IV Benzylpenicillin 1.8g QDS **PLUS** IV Clindamycin 1.2g QDS
Necrotising Fasciitis (in the abdomen)	IV Meropenem 500mg-1g TDS **PLUS** IV Clindamycin 1.2g QDS
Toxic Shock Syndrome (TSS)	IV Clindamycin 600mg-1.2g QDS

2nd line Antibiotic (if 1st line contraindicated)	Duration and Oral Treatment
IV Teicoplanin 400mg BD for 5 doses **THEN** OD (or 6mg/kg if >70kg) **PLUS** IV Gentamicin as per renal function **AND** IV Metronidazole 500mg TDS	Depends on original source of infection No oral treatment
IV Ciprofloxacin 400mg TDS **PLUS** IV Gentamicin as per renal function If MRSA **ADD** IV Teicoplanin 400mg BD for 5 doses **THEN** OD (or 6mg/kg if >70kg)	Depends on original source of infection No oral treatment
IV Ciprofloxacin 400mg TDS **PLUS** IV Amikacin as per renal function If MRSA **ADD** IV Teicoplanin 400mg BD for 5 doses **THEN** OD (or 6mg/kg if >70kg)	Depends on original source of infection No oral treatment
IV Chloramphenicol 25mg/kg QDS	*N. meningitidis* – 5-7 days *S. pneumoniae* – 14 days *H. influenzae* - 10 days No oral treatment
IV Vancomycin 1g BD (OD if >65 years old) **PLUS** IV Meropenem 2g TDS	*L. monocytogenes* - 21 days No oral treatment
IV Chloramphenicol 25mg/kg QDS	7 days No oral treatment
Microbiology advice required	14-21 days No oral treatment
IV Teicoplanin 400mg BD for 5 doses **THEN** OD (or 6mg/kg if >70kg) **PLUS** IV Chloramphenicol 25mg/kg QDS	10-14 days No oral treatment
IV Meropenem 500mg-1g TDS If MRSA **ADD** IV Teicoplanin 400mg BD for 5 doses **THEN** OD (or 6mg/kg if >70kg)	6 weeks total (2-4 weeks IV) Oral treatment guided by culture results
IV Teicoplanin 400mg BD for 5 doses **THEN** OD (or 6mg/kg if >70kg) **PLUS** IV Clindamycin 1.2g QDS	14 days Oral treatment guided by culture results
IV Teicoplanin 400mg BD for 5 doses **THEN** OD (or 6mg/kg if >70kg) **PLUS** IV Clindamycin 1.2g QDS **AND** IV Ciprofloxacin 400mg BD-TDS	14 days Oral treatment guided by culture results
IV Linezolid 600mg BD	Depends on original source of infection No oral treatment

> **Warning**
> Most NHS hospitals have their own paediatric antibiotic guidelines based on national guidelines and local epidemiology. Where possible, use the locally agreed guidelines. The following guidelines are presented to help when there is no access to local guidelines. Doses are taken from the cBNF.

Respiratory Infections	1st Line Antibiotic
Community Acquired Pneumonia (CAP)	PO or IV Co-amoxiclav
Community Acquired Aspiration Pneumonia	IV Co-amoxiclav

Head and Neck Infections	1st Line Antibiotic
Otitis Media	PO Amoxicillin
Otitis Externa	PO Flucloxacillin
Orbital Cellulitis (<6 weeks old)	IV Cefotaxime
Orbital Cellulitis (≥6 weeks old)	IV Ceftriaxone

Urogenital Infections	1st Line Antibiotic
Urinary Tract Infection (UTI) Uncomplicated (>3 months old)	PO Trimethoprim
Pyelonephritis or UTI (<3 months old)	IV Cefotaxime

Paediatric doses are usually based on age, weight or surface area (see section – Antibiotics, Paediatric Antibiotic Doses).

Be very careful when prescribing and always get someone else to check the figures when prescribing doses.

2nd line Antibiotic (if 1st line contraindicated)	Oral Treatment (when appropriate)	Duration
IV Clarithromycin	As for 1st and 2nd line	5-7 days
Microbiology advice required	As for 1st line	5-7 days

2nd line Antibiotic (if 1st line contraindicated)	Oral Treatment (when appropriate)	Duration
PO Clarithromycin	As for 1st and 2nd	5 days
PO Clarithromycin	As for 1st and 2nd	7-10 days
IV Teicoplanin **PLUS** IV Gentamicin	Guided by culture results	7-10 days
IV Teicoplanin **PLUS** IV Gentamicin	Guided by culture results	7-10 days

2nd line Antibiotic (if 1st line contraindicated)	Oral Treatment (when appropriate)	Duration
PO Nitrofurantoin	As for 1st and 2nd line	3 days
IV Gentamicin	PO Cefaclor	7-10 days

Skin, Soft Tissue, Bone and Joint Infections	1st Line Antibiotic
Cellulitis	PO or IV Flucloxacillin
Cellulitis (if MRSA positive)	IV Teicoplanin
Bites	PO or IV Co-amoxiclav
Intravenous Device Associated Infection	IV Teicoplanin
Osteomyelitis or Septic Arthritis	IV Ceftriaxone

Gastrointestinal Infections	1st Line Antibiotic
Primary Peritonitis	IV Co-amoxiclav **PLUS** IV Gentamicin
Secondary Peritonitis	IV Co-amoxiclav **PLUS** IV Gentamicin

2nd line Antibiotic (if 1st line contraindicated)	Oral Treatment (when appropriate)	Duration
IV Teicoplanin	As for 1st line	7-10 days
Microbiology advice required	Guided by culture results	7-10 days
Microbiology advice required	As for 1st line	7 days
Microbiology advice required	Guided by culture results	7-14 days
IV Teicoplanin	Guided by culture results	4 weeks total (3-4 days IV)

2nd line Antibiotic (if 1st line contraindicated)	Oral Treatment (when appropriate)	Duration
IV Teicoplanin **PLUS** IV Gentamicin **PLUS** IV Metronidazole	PO Co-amoxiclav	5-7 days
IV Teicoplanin **PLUS** IV Gentamicin **PLUS** IV Metronidazole	PO Co-amoxiclav	5-7 days

Paediatric Emergencies	1st Line Antibiotic
Sepsis	IV Ceftriaxone **PLUS** IV Gentamicin
Neutropaenic Sepsis	IV Piptazobactam **PLUS** IV Gentamicin
Meningitis (<12 weeks old)	IV Cefotaxime **PLUS** IV Amoxicillin
Meningitis (≥12 weeks old)	IV Ceftriaxone
Meningococcal Sepsis (<6 weeks old)	IV Cefotaxime
Meningococcal Sepsis (≥6 weeks old)	IV Ceftriaxone
Encephalitis	IV Aciclovir
Epiglottitis (<6 weeks old)	IV Cefotaxime
Epiglottitis (≥6 weeks old)	IV Ceftriaxone
Necrotising Fasciitis	IV Benzylpenicillin **PLUS** IV Clindamycin
Toxic Shock Syndrome (TSS)	IV Clindamycin

2nd line Antibiotic (if 1st line contraindicated)	Duration and Oral Treatment
IV Chloramphenicol **PLUS** IV Gentamicin	Depends on original source of infection No oral treatment
Microbiology advice required	Depends on original source of infection No oral treatment
IV Chloramphenicol **PLUS** IV Amoxicillin	*N. meningitidis* – 5-7 days *S. pneumoniae* – 10-14 days *H. influenzae* – 7-10 days *S. agalactiae* – 14-21 days *L. monocytogenes* - 21 days No oral treatment
IV Chloramphenicol	*N. meningitidis* – 5-7 days *S. pneumoniae* – 10-14 days *H. influenzae* – 7-10 days *S. agalactiae* – 14-21 days No oral treatment
IV Chloramphenicol	7 days No oral treatment
IV Chloramphenicol	7 days No oral treatment
Microbiology advice required	14-21 days No oral treatment
Microbiology advice required	10-14 days No oral treatment
Microbiology advice required	10-14 days No oral treatment
IV Teicoplanin **PLUS** IV Clindamycin	14 days oral treatment guided by culture results
Microbiology advice required	Depends on original source of infection No oral treatment

Paediatric Antibiotic Doses

Paediatric doses are usually based on age, weight or surface area.

Antibiotic	1 month to 1 year	1 to 5 years
IV Benzylpenicillin	25mg/kg QDS (double dose in severe infection) (Max 2.4g)	25mg/kg QDS (double dose in severe infection) (Max 2.4g)
IV Flucloxacillin	25mg/kg QDS (double dose in severe infection) (Max 2g)	25mg/kg QDS (double dose in severe infection) (Max 2g)
PO Amoxicillin	62.5mg TDS	125mg TDS
IV Amoxicillin	20-30mg/kg TDS (Max 500mg)	20-30mg/kg TDS (Max 500mg)
IV Amoxicillin (If listeria infection)	50mg/kg 4 hourly (Max 2g)	50mg/kg 4 hourly (Max 2g)
IV Co-amoxiclav	30mg/kg TDS	30mg/kg TDS
IV Piptazobactam	90mg/kg QDS (Max 4.5g)	90mg/kg QDS (Max 4.5g)
PO Cefaclor	62.5mg TDS	125mg TDS
IV Cefotaxime	50mg/kg QDS (Max 2g)	50mg/kg QDS (Max 2g)
IV Ceftriaxone	80mg/kg OD	80mg/kg OD
IV Gentamicin	7mg/kg OD	7mg/kg OD
PO Clindamycin	3-6mg/kg QDS	3-6mg/kg QDS
IV Clindamycin	3.75-6.25mg/kg QDS (Max 1.2g)	3.75-6.25mg/kg QDS (Max 1.2g)
PO Chloramphenicol	25mg/kg QDS	25mg/kg QDS
IV Chloramphenicol	25mg/kg QDS	25mg/kg QDS
IV Teicoplanin	10mg/kg for 3 doses 12 hours apart **THEN** 6mg/kg OD	10mg/kg for 3 doses 12 hours apart **THEN** 6mg/kg OD
PO Trimethoprim	4mg/kg BD (Max 200mg)	4mg/kg BD (Max 200mg)
PO Metronidazole	7.5mg/kg TDS (Max 400mg)	7.5mg/kg TDS (Max 400mg)
IV Metronidazole	7.5mg/kg TDS (Max 500mg)	7.5mg/kg TDS (Max 500mg)

5 to 12 years	12 to 18 years
25mg/kg QDS (double dose in severe infection) (Max 2.4g)	25mg/kg QDS (double dose in severe infection) (Max 2.4g)
25mg/kg QDS (double dose in severe infection) (Max 2g)	25mg/kg QDS (double dose in severe infection) (Max 2g)
250mg TDS	250mg TDS
20-30mg/kg TDS (Max 500mg)	20-30mg/kg TDS (Max 500mg)
50mg/kg 4 hourly (Max 2g)	50mg/kg 4 hourly (Max 2g)
30mg/kg TDS	1.2g TDS
90mg/kg QDS (Max 4.5g)	90mg/kg QDS (Max 4.5g)
250mg TDS	250mg TDS
50mg/kg QDS (Max 2g)	50mg/kg QDS (Max 2g)
<50kg: 80mg/kg OD >50kg: 1-2g OD (BD if severe infection)	<50kg: 80mg/kg OD >50kg: 1-2g OD (BD if severe infection)
7mg/kg OD	7mg/kg OD
3-6mg/kg QDS	150-450mg QDS
3.75-6.25mg/kg QDS (Max 1.2g)	3.75-6.25mg/kg QDS (Max 1.2g)
25mg/kg QDS	25mg/kg QDS
25mg/kg QDS	25mg/kg QDS
10mg/kg for 3 doses 12 hours apart **THEN** 6mg/kg OD	10mg/kg for 3 doses 12 hours apart **THEN** 6mg/kg OD
4mg/kg BD (Max 200mg)	200mg BD
7.5mg/kg TDS (Max 400mg)	400mg TDS
7.5mg/kg TDS (Max 500mg)	7.5mg/kg TDS (Max 500mg)

Paediatric doses are usually based on age, weight or surface area.

Antibiotic	>6 months to 18 years
PO Azithromycin	10mg/kg OD (Max 500mg)

Antibiotic	1 month to 2 years	2 to 10 years	10 to 18 years
PO Flucloxacillin	62.5-125mg QDS	125-250mg QDS	250-500mg QDS

Antibiotic	1 to 3 months	3 months to 12 years	12 to 18 years
PO Nitrofurantoin	No dose available (seek advice)	750 micrograms/kg QDS	50mg QDS
IV Aciclovir	20mg/kg TDS	500mg/m^2 TDS (surface area)	10mg/kg TDS

Antibiotic	1 month to 1 year	1 to 6 years	6 to12 years	12 to 18 years
PO Co-amoxiclav	0.25ml/kg TDS of 125/31 suspension	0.25ml/kg TDS of 125/31 suspension	0.15ml/kg TDS of 250-62 suspension	325mg TDS

Body Surface Area in Children (Boyd Equation)

Body Weight in kg conversion to surface Area in m^2

kg	m^2	kg	m^2	kg	m^2	kg	m^2
1	0.10	9	0.46	24	0.90	40	1.3
1.5	0.13	9.5	0.47	25	0.92	41	1.3
2	0.16	10	0.49	26	0.95	42	1.3
2.5	0.19	11	0.53	27	0.97	43	1.3
3	0.21	12	0.56	28	1.0	44	1.4
3.5	0.24	13	0.59	29	1.0	45	1.4
4	0.26	14	0.62	30	1.1	46	1.4
4.5	0.28	15	0.65	31	1.1	47	1.4
5	0.30	16	0.68	32	1.1	48	1.4
5.5	0.32	17	0.71	33	1.1	49	1.5
6	0.34	18	0.74	34	1.1	50	1.5
6.5	0.36	19	0.77	35	1.2	51	1.5
7	0.38	20	0.79	36	1.2	52	1.5
7.5	0.40	21	0.82	37	1.2	53	1.5
8	0.42	22	0.85	38	1.2	54	1.6
8.5	0.44	23	0.87	39	1.3	55	1.6

Warning
Most NHS hospitals have their own neonatal antibiotic guidelines based on national guidelines and local epidemiology. Where possible use the locally agreed guidelines. Doses are taken from the cBNF.

The following guidelines are presented to help when there is no access to local guidelines. Neonatal doses are usually based on age and weight (see section – Antibiotics, Neonatal Antibiotic Doses.

Be very careful when prescribing and always get someone else to check the figures when prescribing doses.

Gastrointestinal Infections	1st Line Antibiotic	Duration
Suspected Necrotising Enterocolitis (NEC)	IV Benzylpenicillin **PLUS** IV Gentamicin **PLUS** IV Metronidazole	7-10 days depending on persistence of symptoms

Skin and Soft Tissue Infections	1st Line Antibiotic	Duration
Cellulitis	PO or IV Flucloxacillin	5-7 days
Cellulitis (If MRSA positive)	IV Teicoplanin	5-7 days
Intravenous Device Associated Infection	IV Teicoplanin	7-14 days

Neonatal Empirical Antibiotic Guidelines Emergencies

Emergencies	1st Line Antibiotic	Duration
Early Onset Sepsis (≤2 days old)	IV Benzylpenicillin **PLUS** IV Gentamicin	Depends on original source of infection
Late Onset Sepsis (>2 days old)	IV Cefotaxime **PLUS** IV Gentamicin	Depends on original source of infection
Sepsis (in a baby admitted from the community)	IV Cefotaxime **PLUS** IV Amoxicillin	N. meningitidis 5-7 days S. pneumoniae 10-14 days H. influenzae 7-10 days S. agalactiae 14-21 days L. monocytogenes 21 days
Disseminated Herpes Simplex Virus (HSV)	IV Aciclovir	21 days

Antibiotic	<32 Weeks Gestation	>32 Weeks Gestation
IV Gentamicin	4-5mg/kg 36 hourly	4-5mg/kg 24 hourly

Antibiotic	<7 days	7-14 days
IV Benzylpenicillin	25mg/kg BD (double dose in severe infection)	25mg/kg TDS (double dose in severe infection)
PO Flucloxacillin	25mg/kg BD (double dose in severe infection)	25mg/kg TDS (double dose in severe infection)
IV Flucloxacillin	25mg/kg BD (double dose in severe infection)	25mg/kg TDS (double dose in severe infection)
PO Amoxicillin	30mg/kg BD (max 62.5mg)	30mg/kg TDS (max 62.5mg)
IV Amoxicillin	30mg/kg BD	30mg/kg TDS
IV Amoxicillin (if listeria infection)	50mg/kg BD	50mg/kg TDS
PO Co-amoxiclav	0.25ml/kg TDS of 125/31 suspension	0.25ml/kg TDS of 125/31 suspension
IV Co-amoxiclav	30mg/kg BD	30mg/kg TDS
IV Piptazobactam	90mg/kg TDS	90mg/kg TDS
IV Cefotaxime	25mg/kg BD (double dose in severe infection)	25mg/kg TDS (double dose in severe infection)
IV Ceftriaxone	20-50mg/kg OD	20-50mg/kg OD
PO Clindamycin	3-6mg/kg TDS	3-6mg/kg TDS
IV Teicoplanin	16mg/kg single dose **THEN** 8mg/kg OD from 24 hours	16mg/kg single dose **THEN** 8mg/kg OD from 24 hours
PO Trimethoprim	3mg/kg stat **THEN** 1-2mg/kg BD	3mg/kg stat **THEN** 1-2mg/kg BD
PO Metronidazole	15mg/kg loading dose **THEN** 7.5mg/kg BD from 24 hours	15mg/kg loading dose **THEN** 7.5mg/kg BD from 24 hours
IV Metronidazole	15mg/kg loading dose **THEN** 7.5mg/kg BD from 24 hours	15mg/kg loading dose **THEN** 7.5mg/kg BD from 24 hours
IV Aciclovir	20mg/kg TDS	20mg/kg TDS

14-21 days	21-28 days
25mg/kg TDS (double dose in severe infection)	25mg/kg TDS (double dose in severe infection)
25mg/kg TDS (double dose in severe infection)	25mg/kg QDS (double dose in severe infection)
25mg/kg TDS (double dose in severe infection)	25mg/kg QDS (double dose in severe infection)
30mg/kg TDS (max 62.5mg)	30mg/kg TDS (max 62.5mg)
30mg/kg TDS	30mg/kg TDS
50mg/kg TDS	50mg/kg TDS
0.25ml/kg TDS of 125/31 suspension	0.25ml/kg TDS of 125/31 suspension
30mg/kg TDS	30mg/kg TDS
90mg/kg TDS	90mg/kg TDS
25mg/kg TDS (double dose in severe infection)	25mg/kg QDS (double dose in severe infection)
20-50mg/kg OD	20-50mg/kg OD
3-6mg/kg QDS	3-6mg/kg QDS
16mg/kg single dose **THEN** 8mg/kg OD from 24 hours	16mg/kg single dose **THEN** 8mg/kg OD from 24 hours
3mg/kg stat **THEN** 1-2mg/kg BD	3mg/kg stat **THEN** 1-2mg/kg BD
15mg/kg loading dose **THEN** 7.5mg/kg BD from 24 hours	15mg/kg loading dose **THEN** 7.5mg/kg BD from 24 hours
15mg/kg loading dose **THEN** 7.5mg/kg BD from 24 hours	15mg/kg loading dose **THEN** 7.5mg/kg BD from 24 hours
20mg/kg TDS	20mg/kg TDS

Emergencies

How to Recognise the Sick Patient

It is essential that all healthcare staff can recognise when patients are very unwell and worsening. One of the most common reasons for patients dying from sepsis is the failure of healthcare staff to recognise the patient is septic in the first place. **BEWARE** steroids can mask the symptoms and signs of infection as well as suppress the patient's immune system.

Most hospitals in the UK use the National Early Warning Score (NEWS) and a Paediatric Early Warning Score (PEWS) to facilitate recognising the sick patient. These quantify deviations in physiological observations from the normal range and trigger senior review and escalations in medical management of patients.

> **Warning**
> NEWS and PEWS can be affected by medication. Patients on drugs that keep heart rates falsely low (e.g. Beta-blockers) may not display a tachycardia in the face of sepsis and patients who are normally hypertensive may appear normotensive in sepsis. Likewise, patients on Paracetamol may not have a fever. The patient should always be evaluated in terms of their normal baseline physiology wherever possible.

National Early Warning Score (NEWS)

Parameter	3	2	1	0	1	2	3
Respiratory Rate (breaths/min)	≤8		9-11	12-20		21-24	≥25
Oxygen Saturations (%)	≤91	92-93	94-95	≥96			
Any Supplemental Oxygen		Yes		No			
Temperature (°C)	≤35		35.1-36	36.1-38	38.1-39	≥39.1	
Systolic Blood Pressure (mmHg)	≤90	91-100	101-110	111-219			≥220
Pulse (bpm)	≤40		41-50	51-90	91-110	111-130	≥131
Level of Consciousness (AVPU)				A			V, P or U

AVPU =

A =	**A**lert
V =	Only responds to **V**oice
P =	Only responds to **P**ain
U =	**U**nresponsive

Actions from NEWS

Score	Actions
0	No Action
1-4	Qualified nurse to review patient and decide if more frequent monitoring or escalation of clinical care required Minimum 4-6 hourly monitoring of NEWS
5-6 **OR** 3 in single parameter	Qualified nurse to review patient and inform medical team caring for patient Urgent assessment by clinician competent in assessing acutely sick patients Minimum 1 hourly monitoring of NEWS
≥7	Qualified nurse to review patient and immediately inform Specialist Registrar or equivalent caring for patient Emergency assessment by critical care team including clinician competent in advanced airway management skills Consider transfer to a Critical Care Unit e.g. ITU or HDU Continuous monitoring of vital signs

Adapted from: National Early Warning Score UK

Paediatric Early Warning Score (PEWS)

Score **1 point** for each question answered **YES** (total score out of 8 points):
1. Is there a threat to the child's airway e.g. stridor?
2. Does the child require any amount of oxygen to keep SaO_2 >90%?
3. Is the child's respiratory rate outside the normal range for age?
4. Does the child have an abnormal breathing pattern e.g. intercostal or sternal recession, use of accessory muscles?
5. Is the child's heart rate outside of the normal range for age?
6. Is the child's systolic blood pressure outside of the normal range for age?
7. Using AVPU does the child have reduced consciousness i.e. VPU?
8. Is the nurse or doctor concerned about the child's clinical state?

Normal Ranges for Paediatrics

Age (years)	Respiratory Rate (breaths per min)	Heart Rate (bpm)	Systolic Blood Pressure (mmHg)
<1	20-50	90-160	70-90
1-2	15-45	80-150	80-95
3-4	12-40	75-140	80-100
5-11	10-35	60-120	90-110
12-16	10-30	55-100	100-120

Actions from PEWS

Score	Actions
0-1	No action
2	Nurse in charge to review immediately
3	Nurse in charge and Doctor to review immediately
4	Nurse in charge and Doctor to review immediately and inform Consultant
≥5	Nurse in charge and Consultant to review immediately

Adapted from: Cardiff & Vale Paediatric Early Warning Score

Sepsis

Sepsis is defined as life-threatening organ dysfunction caused by a dysregulated host response to infection. Septic shock is sepsis with circulatory, cellular or metabolic dysfunction, and has a high mortality.

Sepsis and septic shock are clinical diagnoses not laboratory diagnoses:
- **Sepsis** - infection with evidence of a systemic response to that infection e.g. hypoxia, oliguria, confusion
- **Septic shock** - sepsis associated with organ dysfunction, hypoperfusion or hypotension

Sepsis and septic shock are medical emergencies and early recognition and treatment improve survival.

Risk Factors for Sepsis
- Age <1 year or >75 years
- Frailty or comorbidities e.g. diabetes, renal failure, liver failure
- Trauma, surgery or other invasive procedure within 6 weeks
- Immunosuppression
- Intravascular device
- Breaches to skin integrity e.g. cuts, burns, blisters
- Current or recent pregnancy (within 6 weeks)

Clinical Features

Potential source of infection OR NEWS ≥4?		
• Pneumonia • Empyema • UTI • Acute abdomen	• Meningitis • Infective endocarditis • CVC infection	• Skin/soft tissue infection • Bone/joint infection • Wound infection • Other

New signs or symptoms of infection? TWO or more of the following:	
• Temperature >38.3°C • Heart Rate >90bpm • WBC <4x10^9/L • Altered mental state	• Temperature <36°C • Respiratory Rate >20 bpm • WBC >12x10^9/L • Blood glucose >7.7mmol/L

Evidence of organ dysfunction remote to the site of infection? ONE of the following or SOFA ≥2 (see opposite):	
• Lactate >2mmol/L • Systolic blood pressure <90mmHg **OR** Mean arterial pressure <65mmHg • Systolic blood pressure >40mmHg below baseline • Creatinine >175mmol/L **OR** urine output 0.5ml/kg/hour for more than 2 hours	• Bilateral pulmonary infiltrates **PLUS** O_2 required to keep O_2 saturations >92% • Bilateral pulmonary infiltrates **PLUS** PaO$_2$/FiO$_2$ ratio <300* • Bilirubin >34 mmol/L • Coagulopathy INR >1.5 **OR** APTT >60 seconds • Platelet count <100x10^9/L

If YES to questions 1 +2 + 3 = criteria for SEPSIS

Note: *PaO$_2$ measured in mmHg (1kPa = 7.5mmHg), FiO$_2$ as % converted into a decimal e.g. 32% = 0.32

Adapted from: Surviving Sepsis Campaign: International Guidelines for Management of Severe Sepsis and Septic Shock www.survivingsepsis.org

Sequential Organ Failure Assessment Score (SOFA)

Parameter	Score				
	0	1	2	3	4
PaO$_2$/FiO$_2$ mmHg	≥400	<400	<300	<200 with respiratory support	<100 with respiratory support
Platelets X 10^9/L	≥150	<150	<100	<50	<20
Bilirubin μmol/L	<20	20-32	33-101	102-204	>204
Cardiovascular status*	MABP ≥70 mmHg	MABP <70 mmHg	Dopamine <5 **OR** Dobutamine any dose	Dopamine 5.1-15 **OR** Epinephrine **OR** Norepinephrine ≤0.1	Dopamine <5 **OR** Epinephrine **OR** Norepinephrine >0.1
Glasgow Coma Scale	15	13-14	10-12	6-9	<6
Creatinine μmol/L or Urine output ml/day	110	110-170	171-299	300-440 <500	>440 <200

Note: *Inotrope doses are in μg/kg/min

Warning
If vasopressors (e.g. Norepinephrine) are required to keep MABP ≥65mmHg **AND** Lactate >2mmol/L despite fluid resuscitation then the patient has **SEPTIC SHOCK**

Hints and Tips
Use the abbreviated qSOFA (quick Sepsis-Related Organ Failure Assessment) to quickly assess sepsis severity, if ≥2 there is an increased risk of death or prolonged ICU stay. Take action!
- Respiratory rate ≥22/min
- Altered mental status
- Systolic blood pressure ≤100mmHg

Causes

Common	• *Staphylococcus aureus* • Group A Beta-haemolytic *Streptococcus* • Enterobacteriaceae e.g. *Escherichia coli, Klebsiella* spp., *Enterobacter* spp., • *Pseudomonas* spp. • *Neisseria meningitidis*

Investigations
- Blood cultures
- Urine for microscopy, culture and sensitivity if able
- Do not unduly delay treatment as mortality increases

Treatment
Antibiotics should be given within 1 hour of the diagnosis of sepsis (see section – Emergencies, Adult Sepsis "Golden-Hour" Management Flowchart)

Adults	
1st line	IV Piptazobactam **PLUS** IV Gentamicin
2nd line (if 1st line contraindicated)	IV Teicoplanin **OR** IV Vancomycin **PLUS** IV Gentamicin **PLUS** IV Metronidazole
If previous ESBL or AmpC positive bacteria	IV Meropenem **PLUS** IV Gentamicin
If MRSA positive	**ADD** IV Teicoplanin **OR** IV Vancomycin

In addition to antibiotics a source of sepsis should be identified and managed as soon as possible e.g. removal of infected CVC, drainage of abscess, repair of perforated abdominal viscus.

For Children (see section – Emergencies, Initial Management of Meningococcal Sepsis in Children)

Children	
1st line	IV Cefotaxime **PLUS** IV Gentamicin
2nd line (if 1st line contraindicated)	IV Chloramphenicol **PLUS** IV Gentamicin

Total Duration
7-10 days
Unless a causative microorganism or focus of infection requires longer treatment e.g. *Staphylococcus aureus* bacteraemia, listeriosis or meningitis (see section – Antibiotics, Adult Empirical Antibiotic Guidelines)

Dosing
See section - Antibiotics, Empirical Antibiotic Guidelines Emergencies.

Warning - Prognosis and Complications
Mortality in sepsis increases if adequate antibiotic treatment is delayed:
- Septic shock - mortality increases by 7% per hour for the first 6 hours that treatment is not adequate
- Sepsis without shock – mortality increases 1-1.5% per hour for the first 6 hours that treatment is not adequate

Adult Sepsis "Golden-Hour" Management Flowchart

First Hour of Surviving Sepsis - "The Golden Hour"

Call for senior support immediately
+/- Critical Care

Give high flow O_2
Aim for SaO_2 >94%
(88-92% if risk of CO_2 retention)

Fluid resuscitate
If hypotensive or lactate >2mmol/L

Target
Systolic blood pressure >90mmHg
MABP ≥65mmHg
Lactate <2mmol/L

Administer
500ml stat **OR** 30ml/kg IV crystalloid to run
over 3 hours

Monitor
Lactate
Urine output

Blood Cultures
Take 2 sets of blood cultures
(at least 1 set peripherally)

DO NOT unnecessarily delay antibiotics

Antibiotics
Give antibiotics within 1hour of diagnosing
sepsis

Warning
Delaying antibiotics in the first 6 hours
increases mortality

Evaluate for focus of infection
Implement source control if possible e.g.
drainage of abscess

Further Treatment
Treat as per the management plan from
seniors or critical care or

Neutropaenic Sepsis and Febrile Neutropaenia

The terms neutropaenic sepsis and febrile neutropaenia are often used synonymously. Neutropaenic sepsis is sepsis in the absence of neutrophils and carries a higher mortality. Febrile neutropaenia is a fever in the absence of neutrophils which may or may not be due to infection. The low neutrophils are due to medical treatment e.g. chemotherapy, bone marrow suppression or haematological malignancy. If a patient has low neutrophils without this being due to a known medical treatment or condition then this is not neutropaenic sepsis but disease.

There are two neutropaenic states in infection:
- **Infection secondary to neutropaenia** (the patient is already neutropaenic due to a medical treatment such as chemotherapy and then develops an infection; this is neutropaenic sepsis)
- **Neutropaenia secondary to infection** (peripheral neutrophil count is low because of infection, this is sepsis and should be treated as sepsis)

> **Warning**
> The causes of infection in sepsis and neutropaenic sepsis are different and therefore the management of these patients is different. Ensure that the correct management plan is followed.

Clinical Features

Neutropaenic sepsis	• Peripheral neutrophil count ≤0.5x10^9/L **PLUS** symptoms or signs of sepsis
Febrile neutropaenia	• Temperature >38°C **PLUS** peripheral neutrophil count ≤0.5x10^9/L

> **Warning**
> Typhlitis (neutropaenic enterocolitis), is a life-threatening infection of the caecum in immunosuppressed patients. Typhlitis should be considered in any patient with a neutrophil count <0.5 x 10^9 per ml **AND** abdominal pain. Treatment includes supportive care, surgical assessment and broad spectrum antibiotics e.g. IV Meropenem **PLUS** IV Metronidazole **PLUS** IV Caspofungin

Causes

Adults and Children	Any microorganism can cause neutropaenic sepsis however the most common and severe bacterial causes are: • *Staphylococcus aureus* • Enterobacteriaceae e.g. *Escherichia coli*, *Klebsiella* spp., *Enterobacter* spp., • *Pseudomonas* spp.

Investigations

- Blood cultures (peripheral and CVC)
- Urine for microscopy, culture and sensitivity if able (**Note:** white blood cell count may be negative due to neutropaenia)
- Urine (for Legionella antigen)
- Sputum for culture and sensitivity
- Stool if diarrhoea
- Swab (if pain or pus at CVC site)
- Chest X-ray (**Note:** chest X-ray may appear normal due to neutropaenia even in severe pneumonia)
- Do not unduly delay treatment as mortality increases

Treatment

Neutropaenic sepsis and febrile neutropaenia are treated with the same antibiotics. Neutropaenic sepsis also requires additional management, as for sepsis (see section – Emergencies, Sepsis).

Antibiotics should be given within 1 hour of the diagnosis.

1st line	IV Piptazobactam **PLUS** IV Gentamicin
If previous ESBL or AmpC positive bacteria	IV Meropenem **PLUS** IV Gentamicin
If suspected pulmonary source	**ADD** IV Clarithromycin 500mg BD
If MRSA positive	**ADD** IV Teicoplanin **OR** IV Vancomycin

2nd line (if 1st line contraindicated)	IV Ciprofloxacin **PLUS** IV Gentamicin
If previous ESBL or AmpC positive bacteria	IV Ciprofloxacin **PLUS** IV Amikacin
If suspected pulmonary source	**ADD** IV Teicoplanin **OR** IV Vancomycin
If MRSA positive	**ADD** IV Teicoplanin **OR** IV Vancomycin

Total Duration

7-10 days
Depends on source of infection, response to treatment and recovery of neutrophil count.

Dosing

See section - Antibiotics, Empirical Antibiotic Guidelines Emergencies.

Neutropaenic Sepsis Antibiotic Flowchart

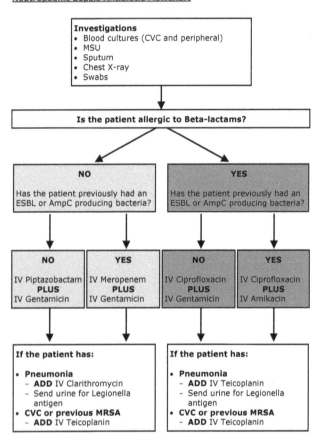

Investigations
- Blood cultures (CVC and peripheral)
- MSU
- Sputum
- Chest X-ray
- Swabs

Is the patient allergic to Beta-lactams?

NO

Has the patient previously had an ESBL or AmpC producing bacteria?

YES

Has the patient previously had an ESBL or AmpC producing bacteria?

NO	**YES**	**NO**	**YES**
IV Piptazobactam **PLUS** IV Gentamicin	IV Meropenem **PLUS** IV Gentamicin	IV Ciprofloxacin **PLUS** IV Gentamicin	IV Ciprofloxacin **PLUS** IV Amikacin

If the patient has:

- **Pneumonia**
  - **ADD** IV Clarithromycin
  - Send urine for Legionella antigen
- **CVC or previous MRSA**
  - **ADD** IV Teicoplanin

If the patient has:

- **Pneumonia**
  - **ADD** IV Teicoplanin
  - Send urine for Legionella antigen
- **CVC or previous MRSA**
  - **ADD** IV Teicoplanin

Warning

Empirical guidelines for neutropaenic sepsis are primarily targeted at treating Gram-negative bacteria because these are what kill neutropaenic patients quickly.

Empirical guidelines provide broad spectrum cover, they **DO NOT** necessarily give the best treatment for specific infections e.g. CVC infections or pneumonia, caused by Gram-positive or non-culturable bacteria. **Once a cause is identified, antibiotics should be targeted** towards that cause rather than continuing empirical treatment.

Toxic Shock Syndrome (TSS)

Toxic shock syndrome (TSS) is fever, rash and shock due to toxins produced by certain strains of bacteria. Toxic shock syndrome has classically been associated with the use of tampons which become colonised with *Staphylococcus aureus* releasing toxins into the blood.

> **Warning**
> Toxic shock syndrome is caused by toxins produced by bacteria. Often the site of infection is not apparent; even small amounts of bacteria can produce a lot of toxins.

Clinical Features

Definite TSS	• Fever >39°C
	• Hypotension (often unresponsive to fluids)
	• Erythroderma (resembling sunburn)
	• Multi-organ failure, **ANY 3** or more:
	  – Renal (acute renal failure)
	  – Gastrointestinal (diarrhoea)
	  – Neurological (encephalopathy)
	  – Cardiac (decreased cardiac output)
	  – Hepatic (liver failure)
	  – Haematogenous (anaemia, thrombocytopaenia)
	• Desquamation 1-2 weeks after illness

Probable TSS	• Lacking one of the above features

Causes

Toxic Shock Syndrome	• Group A Beta-haemolytic *Streptococcus* • *Staphylococcus aureus*

Investigations
If source of infection apparent send pus or tissue for culture and toxin testing.

Treatment
Urgent surgical assessment with a view to surgical resection if source of infection apparent.

1ˢᵗ line	IV Clindamycin
2ⁿᵈ line (if 1ˢᵗ line contraindicated)	IV Linezolid

CONSIDER IV Immunoglobulin 2g/kg **PLUS** a further dose 72 hours after if not improving.

Duration
10-14 days

Dosing
See section - Antibiotics, Empirical Antibiotic Guidelines Emergencies.

Prognosis and Complications
Mortality 2-6% even with treatment.

Meningitis

Meningitis is inflammation of the meninges, the membranes surrounding the brain.

Clinical Features
- Fever
- Headache
- Photophobia
- Neck stiffness
- Pain on extension of the leg (Kernig's sign)
- Decreased conscious level
- Confusion
- Seizures (30% of patients)
- Focal neurological signs (20% of patients)

Causes

Common	• *Neisseria meningitidis* • *Streptococcus pneumoniae* • *Enteroviruses* e.g. *Echovirus* and *Parechovirus* • *Herpes Simplex Virus* (HSV) • *Varicella Zoster Virus* (VZV)
If Elderly or Pregnant	As above plus: • *Listeria monocytogenes*
Neonates	• Group B Beta-haemolytic *Streptococcus* (*Streptococcus agalactiae*) • *Escherichia coli* • *Klebsiella* spp. • *Salmonella* spp. • *Listeria monocytogenes* • *Serratia marcescens* • *Enterovirus* • *Herpes Simplex Virus* (HSV)
If Unvaccinated	• *Mumps Virus* • *Measles Virus* • *Haemophilus influenzae* type b (Hib)

Investigations
- Blood cultures
- Cerebrospinal fluid (CSF) opening pressure, microscopy , culture and sensitivity, glucose, protein and lactate (mark as **URGENT** and inform the microbiology laboratory that the sample has been sent)
    - PCR also routinely available for *N. meningitidis*, *S. pneumoniae*, HSV, VZV and *Enterovirus*
- Peripheral blood glucose to compare to CSF
- EDTA blood for *N. meningitidis* and *S. pneumoniae* PCR
- Bacterial throat swab for *N. meningitidis* culture
- Viral throat swab and stool for *Enterovirus* PCR

Interpretation of CSF

	Bacterial	Viral	TB and Listeria
Opening pressure	>20cm	<20cm	>20cm
WBCs	↑ Neutrophils	↑ Lymphocytes	↑ Lymphocytes
Protein	↑↑	↑ or normal	↑↑↑
Glucose	<50% Blood **OR** <2.2mmol/L	>50% Blood **OR** >2.2mmol/L	<50% Blood **OR** <2.2mmol/L
Lactate	>1.9mmol/L	<1.9mmol/L	>1.9mmol/L

Bacterial Meningitis Score

The Bacterial Meningitis Score (BMS) can be used to predict the likelihood of bacterial meningitis. It is validated in children, and may become validated in adults in the future.

• Does the child have seizures?	
• Is the peripheral neutrophil count ≥10 x 10^9/L?	If **NO** to **ALL** questions then bacterial meningitis is very unlikely, NPV 99.9%
• Are microorganisms seen in the CSF Gram film?	
• Is the CSF neutrophil count ≥1,000x10^6 cells/μl	
• Is the CSF protein ≥0.8g/L	

Treatment (pre-hospital)

If >1 hour delay before hospital admission, signs of septic shock or meningococcal disease (see sections – Emergencies, Sepsis and Meningococcal Sepsis)

1st line	IM or IV Benzylpenicillin stat
2nd line (if 1st line contraindicated)	IM or IV Ceftriaxone stat **OR** IM or IV Cefotaxime stat

Treatment (in hospital within 1 hour of admission)

1st line	IV Cefotaxime **OR** IV Ceftriaxone **PLUS** IV Dexamethasone 6mg QDS*
2nd line (if 1st line contraindicated)	IV Chloramphenicol **PLUS** IV Dexamethasone 6mg QDS*
If listeria suspected	**ADD** IV Amoxicillin
Neonates	IV Benzylpenicillin **PLUS** IV Gentamicin
If travel within 6 months to country with high rates of penicillin resistance in *S. pneumoniae***	**ADD** IV Vancomycin **OR** IV Rifampicin

Note: *IV Dexamethasone should be started just before or with the antibiotics. If antibiotics already started IV Dexamethasone can be started within 12 hours of the first dose. Continue IV Dexamethasone for 4 days in *S. pneumoniae* meningitis, or where *S. pneumoniae* remains the most likely cause; if another cause found stop IV Dexamethasone.

Note: **At the time of writing the main countries include: Canada, China, Croatia, Greece, Italy, Mexico, Pakistan, Poland, Spain, Turkey and USA

> **Warning**
> Meningitis in neonates due to *Serratia marcescens* must be treated with IV Meropenem as it has the enzyme AmpC as well as a relatively high MIC to the aminoglycoside antibiotics.

Total Duration
- *Neisseria meningitidis* – 5-7 days
- *Streptococcus pneumoniae* – 14 days
- *Haemophilus influenzae* type b - 10 days
- Group B Beta-haemolytic *Streptococcus* - 14 days
- *Listeria monocytogenes* - 21 days
- Enterobacteriaceae - 21 days (30% of patients relapse requiring a further 21 days of treatment)

Dosing
See section - Antibiotics, Empirical Antibiotic Guidelines Emergencies.

Prognosis and Complications
Untreated bacterial meningitis has 100% mortality. Even with treatment the mortality from meningitis is 20% (30% with *S. pneumoniae* or *L. monocytogenes*). Long-term sequelae including weakness, sensory loss, seizures and cranial nerve abnormalities occur in 44% *L. monocytogenes*, 30% *S. pneumoniae* and 7% *N. meningitidis*.

Viral meningitis is usually a self-limiting infection, which does not require treatment in patients with normal immune systems.

Complications are more common with bacterial rather than viral meningitis and include:
- Subdural empyema
- Seizures
- Cerebral venous sinus thrombosis

Prevention and Prophylaxis
Many causes of bacterial meningitis can be prevented with the primary course of vaccines, including *S. pneumoniae*, *H. influenzae* type b and *N. meningitidis* types A, B, C, W and Y.

Prophylactic antibiotics are usually given to close contacts, within the previous 7 days, of patients with *N. meningitidis* meningitis; vaccinations are also occasionally given. The decision for this lays with the Consultant in Communicable Disease Control (CCDC) or Public Health Consultant, not the admitting doctors. These antibiotics penetrate into the upper respiratory tract and eliminate carriage from those who might have passed the bacterium onto the patient as well as anyone who might have acquired the bacterium from the patient. Any patient treated for *N. meningitidis* meningitis with Benzylpenicillin alone should be given oropharyngeal decolonisation as for prophylaxis in close contacts below.

1st line	PO Ciprofloxacin • Adults 500mg stat • 5-12 years 250mg stat • <5 years 30mg/kg (max. 125mg) stat
2nd line (if 1st line contraindicated)	PO Rifampicin • >12 years 600mg BD for 2 days • 1-12 years 10mg/kg BD for 2 days • <12 months 5mg/kg BD for 2 days
If pregnant	IM Ceftriaxone 250mg stat

Meningococcal Sepsis

Meningococcal sepsis, which can be rapidly fatal over minutes-to-hours, is caused by the bacterium *Neisseria meningitidis*.

Clinical Features
- Fever
- Hypotension
- Lethargy
- Decreased conscious level
- Confusion
- Prolonged capillary refill time
- Blanching rash **OR** non-blanching petechial rash

> **Warning**
> The non-blanching petechial rash is a sign promoted to aid the diagnosis of meningococcal sepsis; however, due to inflammation when the bacteria initially invade the capillaries supplying the skin, the rash actually starts as a blanching rash. It becomes non-blanching when the bacteria cause blood to leak out of the capillaries causing purpura or have cut off the blood supply to areas of skin causing necrosis. To catch the infection early it is important to consider meningococcal sepsis in patients who are septic with a rapidly spreading rash, even if the rash is blanching.

Causes

UK acquired	• *Neisseria meningitidis* type B • *Neisseria meningitidis* type C
Returned travellers	• *Neisseria meningitidis* type A (Sub-Saharan Africa) • *Neisseria meningitidis* type W135 (Sub-Saharan Africa and Asia – Hajj pilgrimage) • *Neisseria meningitidis* type Y

Investigations
- Blood cultures
- Cerebrospinal fluid (CSF) for microscopy, culture and sensitivity, glucose and protein
  - PCR also routinely available for *Neisseria meningitidis*
- Peripheral blood glucose to compare to CSF
- EDTA blood for *Neisseria meningitidis* PCR
- Throat swab to look for carriage of *Neisseria meningitidis*

Treatment
Antibiotics should be given as soon as possible. In the community, General Practitioners are encouraged to give a dose of IM Benzylpenicillin in patients in whom they suspect meningococcal sepsis as this can be life-saving (see section – Emergencies, Meningitis).

1st line	IV Cefotaxime **OR** IV Ceftriaxone
2nd line (if 1st line contraindicated)	IV Chloramphenicol

Total Duration
5-7 days

Dosing
See section - Antibiotics, Empirical Antibiotic Guidelines Emergencies.

Prognosis and Complications
Untreated meningococcal sepsis has 100% mortality. Up to 57% of patients with meningococcal sepsis experience long term sequelae.

Risk factors for mortality in meningococcal sepsis include:
- Rapidly progressive rash
- Coma
- Hypotension and shock
- Lactate >4mmol/L
- Low peripheral white blood cell count
- Low CRP
- Low platelets
- Coagulopathy
- Absence of meningitis

Prevention and Prophylaxis
- Children are immunised with vaccines for *N. meningitidis* types A, B, C, W and Y as part of their primary immunisation schedule
- Travellers to endemic countries should be offered vaccination against *N. meningitidis* types A, C, W and Y as appropriate to the destination

Prophylactic antibiotics are usually given to close contacts, within the previous 7 days, of patients with meningococcal sepsis; vaccinations are also occasionally given. The decision for this lays with the Consultant in Communicable Disease Control (CCDC) or Public Health Consultant, not the admitting doctors. These antibiotics penetrate into the upper respiratory tract and eliminate carriage from those who might have passed the bacterium onto the patient as well as anyone who might have acquired the bacterium from the patient. Any patient treated for meningococcal sepsis with Benzylpenicillin alone should be given oropharyngeal decolonisation as for prophylaxis in close contacts below.

1st line	PO Ciprofloxacin • Adults 500mg stat • 5-12 years 250mg stat • <5 years 30mg/kg (max. 125mg) stat
2nd line (if 1st line contraindicated)	PO Rifampicin • >12 years 600mg BD for 2 days • 1-12 years 10mg/kg BD for 2 days • <12 months 5mg/kg BD for 2 days
If pregnant	IM Ceftriaxone 250mg stat

Initial Management of Bacterial Meningitis and Meningococcal Sepsis in Adults

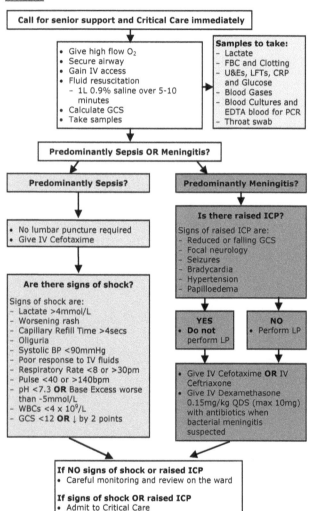

Call for senior support and Critical Care immediately

- Give high flow O$_2$
- Secure airway
- Gain IV access
- Fluid resuscitation
  - 1L 0.9% saline over 5-10 minutes
- Calculate GCS
- Take samples

Samples to take:
- Lactate
- FBC and Clotting
- U&Es, LFTs, CRP and Glucose
- Blood Gases
- Blood Cultures and EDTA blood for PCR
- Throat swab

Predominantly Sepsis OR Meningitis?

Predominantly Sepsis?

- No lumbar puncture required
- Give IV Cefotaxime

Are there signs of shock?

Signs of shock are:
- Lactate >4mmol/L
- Worsening rash
- Capillary Refill Time >4secs
- Oliguria
- Systolic BP <90mmHg
- Poor response to IV fluids
- Respiratory Rate <8 or >30pm
- Pulse <40 or >140bpm
- pH <7.3 **OR** Base Excess worse than -5mmol/L
- WBCs <4 x 10^9/L
- GCS <12 **OR** ↓ by 2 points

Predominantly Meningitis?

Is there raised ICP?

Signs of raised ICP are:
- Reduced or falling GCS
- Focal neurology
- Seizures
- Bradycardia
- Hypertension
- Papilloedema

YES
- **Do not** perform LP

NO
- Perform LP

- Give IV Cefotaxime **OR** IV Ceftriaxone
- Give IV Dexamethasone 0.15mg/kg QDS (max 10mg) with antibiotics when bacterial meningitis suspected

If NO signs of shock or raised ICP
- Careful monitoring and review on the ward

If signs of shock OR raised ICP
- Admit to Critical Care

Note: There are more comprehensive flowcharts available from the Meningitis Research Foundation www.meningitis.org

Initial Management of Bacterial Meningitis in Children

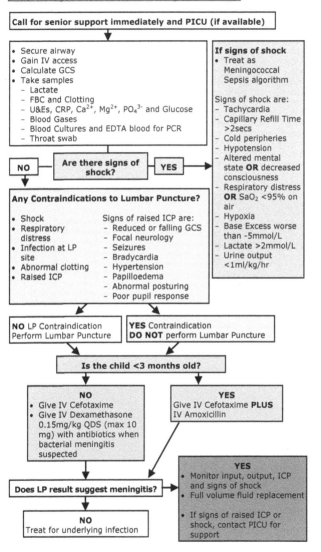

Call for senior support immediately and PICU (if available)

- Secure airway
- Gain IV access
- Calculate GCS
- Take samples
  - Lactate
  - FBC and Clotting
  - U&Es, CRP, Ca^{2+}, Mg^{2+}, PO_4^{3-} and Glucose
  - Blood Gases
  - Blood Cultures and EDTA blood for PCR
  - Throat swab

If signs of shock
- Treat as Meningococcal Sepsis algorithm

Signs of shock are:
- Tachycardia
- Capillary Refill Time >2secs
- Cold peripheries
- Hypotension
- Altered mental state **OR** decreased consciousness
- Respiratory distress **OR** SaO_2 <95% on air
- Hypoxia
- Base Excess worse than -5mmol/L
- Lactate >2mmol/L
- Urine output <1ml/kg/hr

NO | **Are there signs of shock?** | **YES**

Any Contraindications to Lumbar Puncture?

- Shock
- Respiratory distress
- Infection at LP site
- Abnormal clotting
- Raised ICP

Signs of raised ICP are:
- Reduced or falling GCS
- Focal neurology
- Seizures
- Bradycardia
- Hypertension
- Papilloedema
- Abnormal posturing
- Poor pupil response

NO LP Contraindication
Perform Lumbar Puncture

YES Contraindication
DO NOT perform Lumbar Puncture

Is the child <3 months old?

NO
- Give IV Cefotaxime
- Give IV Dexamethasone 0.15mg/kg QDS (max 10 mg) with antibiotics when bacterial meningitis suspected

YES
Give IV Cefotaxime **PLUS** IV Amoxicillin

Does LP result suggest meningitis?

YES
- Monitor input, output, ICP and signs of shock
- Full volume fluid replacement
- If signs of raised ICP or shock, contact PICU for support

NO
Treat for underlying infection

<u>**Initial Management of Meningococcal Sepsis in Children**</u>

Call for senior support immediately and PICU (if available)

- Give high flow O_2 10L/min
- Secure airway
- Insert 2 large IV cannulae **OR** intraosseous access
- Take blood samples
  - FBC and Clotting
  - U&Es, CRP, Ca^{2+}, Mg^{2+}, PO_4^{3-} and Glucose
  - Blood Gases (lactate)
  - Blood Cultures and EDTA blood for PCR
- Estimate weight of child (<10 years old use kg = 2 x [age in years +4])
- Give IV Cefotaxime
- Keep child Nil by Mouth

Are there signs of shock?

Signs of shock are:
- Tachycardia
- Capillary Refill Time >2secs
- Cold peripheries
- Hypotension
- Altered mental state **OR** decreased consciousness
- Respiratory distress **OR** SaO_2 <95% on air
- Hypoxia
- Base Excess worse than -5mmol/L
- Lactate >2mmol/L
- Urine output <1ml/kg/hr

YES
- Give 20ml/kg 0.9% Saline over 5-10 mins

Do signs of shock remain?

YES
- Give another 20ml/kg 0.9% Saline over 5-10 mins

Do signs of shock remain?

YES

→ **NO** →

NO

Is there raised ICP?

Signs of raised ICP are:
- Reduced or falling GCS
- Focal neurology
- Seizures
- Bradycardia
- Hypertension
- Papilloedema
- Abnormal posturing
- Poor pupil response

NO
- Monitor closely for raised ICP or shock
- Perform LP.
- If LP result suggests meningitis, treat as bacterial meningitis algorithm
- Continue antibiotics

YES
- Give Mannitol 0.25g/kg bolus **OR**
- 3% Saline 3ml/kg over 5 minutes

- Call anaesthetist
- Admit to PICU
- Intubate and ventilate

WARNING: Patients with meningococcal sepsis can deteriorate very quickly

Encephalitis

Encephalitis is inflammation of the brain. Encephalitis can be infectious (42%), immune mediated (21%) or of unknown cause (37%). However, up to 90% of infectious encephalitis is caused by just 3 viruses: HSV, VZV and *Enterovirus*.

Clinical Features
- Fever
- Headache
- Neck stiffness
- Decreased conscious level
- Confusion
- Seizures
- Focal neurological signs
- HSV (personality change, hallucinations, aphasia)
- VZV (ophthalmic shingles)
- *Enterovirus* and *Measles Virus* (rash)

Causes

Common	• *Enterovirus* • *Herpes Simplex Virus* (HSV) • *Varicella Zoster Virus* (VZV)
If unvaccinated (rare in the UK)	• *Mumps Virus* • *Measles Virus* • *Mycobacterium tuberculosis*
Rare (usually related to immunodeficiency)	• *Influenza A Virus* and *Influenza B Virus* • *Adenovirus* • *Parechovirus* • *Epstein Barr Virus* • *Cytomegalovirus* • *Human Herpes Virus* 6 and 7 • *JC Virus* • *Lymphocytic Choriomeningitis Virus* • *Human Immunodeficiency Virus* 1 and 2
Non-infectious	• Acute disseminated encephalomyelitis (ADEM) • NMDA (N-methyl-D-aspartate) receptor antibodies • VGKC (voltage-gated potassium channel) antibodies • Vasculitis • Multiple sclerosis (MS) • Paraneoplastic

Investigations
- Cerebrospinal fluid (CSF) for microscopy, culture and sensitivity, glucose and protein
  - PCR for HSV, VZV and *Enterovirus*
- Peripheral blood glucose to compare to CSF
- MRI scan is abnormal in 90% of patients on admission

Recommended Initial Investigations for Encephalitis

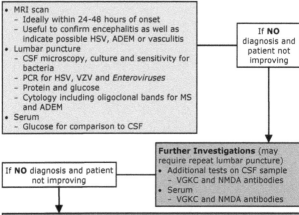

- MRI scan
  - Ideally within 24-48 hours of onset
  - Useful to confirm encephalitis as well as indicate possible HSV, ADEM or vasculitis
- Lumbar puncture
  - CSF microscopy, culture and sensitivity for bacteria
  - PCR for HSV, VZV and *Enteroviruses*
  - Protein and glucose
  - Cytology including oligoclonal bands for MS and ADEM
- Serum
  - Glucose for comparison to CSF

If **NO** diagnosis and patient not improving

Further Investigations (may require repeat lumbar puncture)
- Additional tests on CSF sample
  - VGKC and NMDA antibodies
- Serum
  - VGKC and NMDA antibodies

If **NO** diagnosis and patient not improving

Investigations for rare causes (may require repeat lumbar puncture)
- Additional tests on CSF sample
  - *Mycobacterium tuberculosis* culture (test may be affected by antibiotics) or PCR if sufficient sample
  - PCR for *Influenza Virus, Adenovirus, Parechovirus,* CMV, EBV & HHV6/7
  - PCR for *Measles Virus* and *Mumps Virus* if unvaccinated
- Serum
  - HIV antibodies

Treatment
Do not delay treatment, as delays longer than 6 hours can result in long-term neurological damage.

The only common cause of infectious encephalitis for which there is a specific treatment is HSV.

1ˢᵗ line	IV Aciclovir

Total Duration
14-21 days

> **Warning**
> Do not treat HSV encephalitis with PO Aciclovir or Valaciclovir (an oral pro-drug of Aciclovir); at the time of writing there is no evidence to support their use.
>
> The treatment of encephalitis is IV Aciclovir which, when started quickly, reduces the incidence of permanent brain damage and long-term neurological symptoms.

The British Infection Association recommends repeating the HSV PCR on CSF at 14 days and stopping Aciclovir if the HSV PCR is negative; if positive, continue with weekly LPs until PCR negative. Given that HSV PCR is a Reference Laboratory test for most hospitals the recommendation is difficult to implement because the result can take up to 1 week (taking it up to 21 days treatment).

Hints and Tips
Aciclovir is often started before a diagnosis has been made. Stopping Aciclovir once it has been started can be a difficult decision. The current recommendation is that Aciclovir can be stopped if one the following three criteria are met:

- An alternative diagnosis is made
- HSV PCR on CSF is negative on 2 occasions 24-48 hours apart
  PLUS MRI not characteristic
- HSV PCR on CSF negative >72 hours after symptoms started
  PLUS normal conscious level
  PLUS MRI not characteristic
  PLUS CSF WBCs <5x10^6/L

Adapted from: Management of suspected viral encephalitis in adults, British Infection Association

---

Dosing
See section - Antibiotics, Empirical Antibiotic Guidelines Emergencies.

Prognosis and Complications
Up to 80% of patients have ongoing neurological symptoms, such as headaches and weakness, after HSV encephalitis. These are more common in the elderly and in those in whom treatment with IV Aciclovir is delayed.

Prevention and Prophylaxis
Some causes of encephalitis can be prevented with the normal primary course of vaccines, including *Mumps Virus* and *Measles Virus*.

Epiglottitis

Epiglottitis is life-threatening inflammation and oedema of the epiglottis and surrounding tissue leading to obstruction of the airway.

> **Warning**
> Do not attempt to examine the throat of a patient with suspected epiglottitis as this can precipitate complete obstruction of the airway leading to death; wait until the airway has been secured by an anaesthetist with experience at performing emergency tracheostomy.

Clinical Features
- Stridor
- Fever
- Sore throat
- Drooling
- Toxaemia

Causes

Common	• *Streptococcus pneumoniae* • Beta-haemolytic *Streptococcus* (Groups A, C and G)
If unvaccinated	• *Haemophilus influenzae* type b (Hib)

Investigations
After the airway is secure:
- Blood cultures
- Swab from the epiglottis and surrounding tissue for culture and sensitivity

Treatment

1st line	IV Ceftriaxone **OR** IV Cefotaxime
2nd line (if 1st line contraindicated)	IV Teicoplanin **OR** IV Vancomycin **PLUS** IV Chloramphenicol

Total Duration
10-14 days

Dosing
See section - Antibiotics, Empirical Antibiotic Guidelines Emergencies.

Prognosis and Complications
Delayed diagnosis results in a mortality of 9-18%. However, once the airway is secure the mortality is <1%.

Prevention and Prophylaxis
Epiglottitis due to *Haemophilus influenzae* type b is preventable with the Hib vaccine given to children as part of the primary immunisation schedule.

Spinal Epidural Abscess

Spinal epidural abscess is a collection of pus between the dura mater and the vertebral column which can produce pressure damage to the spinal cord within a few hours.

Clinical Features
- Pain (70-90% of patients) patient usually unable to lie flat
- Fever (60-70% of patients)
- Progressive symptoms from pain and tenderness leading to nerve pain, nerve deficit and sphincter dysfunction, which ultimately leads to paralysis

Causes

Haematogenous	• *Staphylococcus aureus* • *Streptococcus* spp.
Extension from vertebral osteomyelitis	• *Staphylococcus aureus* • *Streptococcus* spp.
If diabetic / elderly	As above plus: • Enterobacteriaceae e.g. *Escherichia coli*, *Klebsiella* spp., *Enterobacter* spp.

Investigations
- Blood cultures
- Pus from abscess for microscopy, culture and sensitivity
- Consider urgent MRI if diagnosis unsure

Treatment
Urgent surgical assessment with a view to surgical decompression to prevent permanent neurological damage

1st line	IV Ceftriaxone **OR** IV Cefotaxime
2nd line (if 1st line contraindicated)	IV Meropenem
If MRSA positive	**ADD** IV Teicoplanin **OR** IV Vancomycin

Total Duration
6 weeks

Dosing
See section - Antibiotics, Empirical Antibiotic Guidelines Emergencies.

Prognosis and Complications
Spinal epidural abscess is a surgical emergency. If neurological signs present for less than 24 hours most patients make a full recovery. However, once neurological damage is sustained it is irreversible.

Necrotising Fasciitis

Necrotising fasciitis is a severe life and limb threatening infection involving superficial and deep fascia as well as other tissues.

> **Warning**
> Necrotising fasciitis is a surgical emergency. Patients should be reviewed by the most senior surgeon available. Do not delay surgery to perform imaging, as even small delays before resecting diseased tissue can cause loss of limb or death.

Clinical Features
- Rapidly progressive infection
- May have a preceding history of sore throat with Group A Beta-haemolytic *Streptococcus* with haematogenous seeding at the site of a minor injury
- Erythema, swelling, heat and pain out of proportion to the other clinical signs leading to discolouration, bullae and eventually gangrene
- Systemic features such as fever, hypotension and tachycardia
- Pus is **NOT** usually a feature with Group A Beta-haemolytic *Streptococcus*; usually only a serosanguinous discharge

Causes

Infection of a limb	• Group A Beta-haemolytic *Streptococcus* • *Clostridium perfringens* (gas gangrene)
Infection of abdomen	• Synergistic gangrene which is caused by mixed anaerobes and Enterobacteriaceae e.g. *Escherichia coli*, *Klebsiella* spp., *Enterobacter* spp.
If diabetic / elderly	• Synergistic gangrene which is caused by mixed anaerobes and Enterobacteriaceae e.g. *Escherichia coli*, *Klebsiella* spp., *Enterobacter* spp.

> **Warning**
> A rapidly progressive soft tissue infection in children, in association with chicken pox, is usually caused by Group A Beta-haemolytic *Streptococcus* and should be treated as necrotising fasciitis.

Investigations
- Blood cultures
- Fluid from tissue for microscopy, culture and sensitivity
- INR often increased with Group A Beta-haemolytic *Streptococcus* (due to production of streptokinase) can be used to monitor progress

Treatment
Urgent surgical assessment for tissue resection which may need to be extensive to reveal healthy tissue.

If there is any doubt as to whether the tissue is viable, it should be removed. Surgeons should have a low threshold for taking patients back to theatre if they are not improving.

If a Limb is affected

1st line	IV Benzylpenicillin **PLUS** IV Clindamycin
2nd line (if 1st line contraindicated)	IV Teicoplanin **PLUS** IV Clindamycin

If the Abdomen is affected or if Diabetic/Elderly

1st line	IV Meropenem **PLUS** IV Clindamycin
2nd line (if 1st line contraindicated)	IV Teicoplanin **PLUS** IV Ciprofloxacin **PLUS** IV Clindamycin

For Group A Beta-haemolytic *Streptococcus* and *Clostridium perfringens* consider IV Immunoglobulin 2g/kg **PLUS** a further dose 72 hours after if not improving.

Duration
10-14 days

Dosing
See section - Antibiotics, Empirical Antibiotic Guidelines Emergencies.

Prognosis and Complications
Necrotising fasciitis has a high mortality rate (up to 70%) if not managed aggressively enough with surgical intervention; amputation can be a life-saving intervention.

Malaria

Malaria is a parasitic infection seen in travellers returning to the UK from abroad (see section – Clinical Scenarios, Fever in a Returned Traveller). A diagnosis of malaria should be considered in any febrile or unwell patient who has been in a malaria-endemic area. All patients with suspected malaria should be admitted to hospital and evaluated immediately. Malaria is a potentially severe and life-threatening infection.

Clinical Features
- Fever
- Headache
- Muscle pains
- Nausea and vomiting
- Dry cough
- Occasionally – sore throat, shortness of breath, gastrointestinal disturbance

---

Warning
Features of severe malaria include:
- >2% parasitaemia
- Decreased consciousness **OR** seizures
- Renal failure (oliguria <0.4ml/kg/hr **OR** creatinine >265μmol/L)
- Acidosis (pH <7.3)
- Hypoglycaemia (blood glucose <2.2mmol/L)
- Pulmonary oedema **OR** Acute Respiratory Distress Syndrome (ARDS)
- Haemoglobin <80g/L
- Disseminated Intravascular Coagulation
- Shock (blood pressure <90/60 mmHg)
- Haemoglobinuria

Malaria in pregnancy is more likely to be severe as parasites concentrate in the placenta making diagnosis and treatment difficult. There is a high rate of still births and premature labour as well as high maternal mortality and morbidity.

If the patient has evidence of severe malaria (or is pregnant) discuss with an Infectious Diseases Physician and transfer to a Critical Care Unit for monitoring and supportive care including:
- Oxygen
- 4 Hourly observations, fluid balance, blood glucose
- Continuous ECG
- Daily FBC, U&Es, LFTs and % parasitaemia
- IV antibiotics to cover for possible Gram-negative sepsis e.g. Ceftriaxone, Piptazobactam, Meropenem or combination therapy including Gentamicin

---

Causes

Falciparum	• Plasmodium falciparum
Non-falciparum	• Plasmodium vivax • Plasmodium malariae • Plasmodium ovale • Plasmodium knowlesi (rare - only found in some forested areas of South East Asia)

Incubation Period

6 days – 1 month (rarely up to 6 months)	• *Plasmodium falciparum* • *Plasmodium knowlesi* • *Plasmodium malariae*
6 days - >6 months	• *Plasmodium vivax* • *Plasmodium ovale*

Investigations

Antimalarial prophylaxis should be stopped until malaria excluded otherwise malaria tests can be falsely negative. Remember to restart antimalarial prophylaxis if diagnosis of malaria excluded.

- Malaria detection
  - Combination of rapid diagnostic test **PLUS** thick and thin films
  - If positive, obtain estimate of percentage red blood cells infected with parasites (parasitaemia) from laboratory
  - If original test negative then repeat tests at approximately 24 and 48 hours before excluding a diagnosis of malaria
- Consider investigations to rule out additional travel related infections (see section – Clinical Scenarios, Fever in a Returned Traveller)
- FBC, U&Es, LFTs and blood glucose
- If patient unwell – blood gas, lactate, clotting and ECG
- If pregnancy a possibility do a pregnancy test as malaria in pregnancy has a high rate of severe disease as well as miscarriages and stillbirths

> **Warning**
> Rapid diagnostic tests are very good for diagnosing falciparum malaria but they are less good for non-falciparum malaria. A negative rapid diagnostic test **does not** rule out a diagnosis of malaria. All malaria tests should include thick and thin films, as well as any rapid diagnostic test, as these give an indication of severity.

Treatment

ALL patients with malaria in the UK should be admitted to hospital for at least 24 hours and be discussed with an Infectious Diseases Consultant.

Treatment for Falciparum Malaria or Unknown Malaria Species

Mild/Moderate (adults)	
1st Line	PO Riamet® (Co-artem or Artemether-lumefantrine) 4 tablets stat **THEN** 4 tablets at 8, 24, 36, 48 and 60 hours **OR** PO Eurartesim® (Dihydroartemisinin-piperaquine*) 4 tablets/day for 3 days
2nd Line (if 1st Line Contraindicated or Unavailable)	PO Quinine 600mg TDS for 7 days **PLUS** PO Doxycycline 200mg OD for 7 days **OR** PO Clindamycin 450mg TDS for 7 days **OR** PO Malarone® (Atovaquone-Proguanil) 4 tablets/day for 3 days

Note: *Eurartesim (Dihydroartemisinin-piperaquine*) is an unlicensed treatment in UK, complicated dosing regimen based on body weight – seek specialist advice

Severe or Patient Nil By Mouth (adults)	
1st Line	IV Artesunate 2.4mg/kg stat **THEN** at 12 and 24 hours **THEN** OD
2nd Line (if 1st Line Contraindicated or Unavailable)	IV Quinine loading dose 20mg/kg (max 1.4g) **THEN** 10mg/kg TDS (max 700mg) for 2 days **THEN** 10mg/kg BD (max 700mg) **PLUS** PO Doxycycline 200mg OD for 7 days **OR** PO Clindamycin 450mg TDS for 7 days If Nil By Mouth, **ADD** orals as soon as able

Note: Convert IV Quinine or IV Artesunate to oral therapy (as per Mild/Moderate) as soon as the patient is no longer Nil By Mouth or classed as severe

Mild/Moderate (children)	
1st Line	PO Riamet® (Co-artem or Artemether-lumefantrine) **OR** PO Eurartesim® (Dihydroartemisinin-piperaquine*)
2nd Line (if 1st Line Contraindicated or Unavailable)	PO Quinine 10mg/kg (max 600mg) TDS for 7 days **PLUS** PO Clindamycin 7-13mg/kg (max 450mg) TDS for 7 days **OR** PO Malarone® (Atovaquone-Proguanil)

Note: *Eurartesim (Dihydroartemisinin-piperaquine*) is an unlicensed treatment in UK, complicated dosing regimen based on body weight – seek specialist advice

Severe or Patient Nil By Mouth (children)	
1st Line	IV Artesunate* 2.4mg/kg stat **THEN** at 12 and 24 hours **THEN** OD (if <20kg use 3mg/kg)
2nd Line (if 1st Line Contraindicated or Unavailable)	IV Quinine loading dose 20mg/kg (max 1.4g) **THEN** 10mg/kg (max 700mg)TDS for 2 days **THEN** 10mg/kg (max 700mg) BD **PLUS** PO Clindamycin 7-13mg/kg (max 450mg) TDS for 7 days If Nil By Mouth, **ADD** orals as soon as able

Note: *Artesunate in children is an unlicensed treatment in UK
Note: Convert IV Quinine or IV Artesunate to oral therapy (as per Mild/Moderate) as soon as the patient is no longer Nil By Mouth or classed as severe

Treatment for Non-Falciparum Malaria

Adults	
Control of parasitaemia	PO Chloroquine 600mg **THEN** 300mg at 6, 24 and 48 hours after initial dose
Eradication of parasites from hepatocytes	P. ovale – PO Primaquine* 15mg OD 14 days P. vivax – PO Primaquine* 30mg OD 14 days

Children	
Control of parasitaemia	PO Chloroquine 10mg/kg **THEN** 5mg/kg at 6, 24 and 48 hours after initial dose
Eradication of parasites from hepatocytes	P. ovale – PO Primaquine* 0.25mg/kg OD 14 days P. vivax – PO Primaquine* 0.5mg/kg OD 14 days

Note: *Primaquine is contraindicated in pregnancy and G6PD deficiency. Screen for G6PD (glucose-6-phosphate dehydrogenase) deficiency before giving Primaquine
Note: If Chloroquine unavailable, treat as Falciparum malaria **PLUS** Primaquine to eradicate parasites from hepatocytes as above

Warning
Haemolysis occurs in 10-15% of patients treated with IV Artesunate, therefore haemoglobin should be checked 14 days after treatment and any anaemia treated according to local guidelines.

Prognosis and Complications
If diagnosed and treated the mortality is 1%. However, in severe malaria the mortality, even with treatment, is up to 10%.

Prevention and Prophylaxis
Travellers should take malaria prophylaxis appropriate to their destination and avoid mosquito bites by using insect repellents, mosquito nets, long sleeved shirts and long trousers when mosquitoes are active and feeding.

Glossary

Acid-fast	Staining red using the Ziehl-Neelsen method, used to identify bacteria with mycolic acid in their cell wall
Aerobic	Grows in the presence of oxygen
Alpha-haemolytic *Streptococcus* spp.	Previously known as Viridans *Streptococcus* spp.
Anaerobic	Grows in the absence of oxygen
Bacillus	Shaped like a rod
Bacteraemia	Presence of bacteria in blood
Bactericidal	Kills bacteria
Bacteriostatic	Stops bacteria growing without killing them
Biofilm	Collection of microorganisms sticking to a surface
Blanching	Redness which disappears with pressure
Blood-borne Virus	Virus which can be transmitted between people via blood
Bullae	Large fluid-filled blister >5mm diameter
Clone	Genetically indistinguishable bacterium
Coccus	Shaped like a sphere
Communicability	Ability to be transmitted between people
Critical Care Unit	A department looking after a mixture of High Dependency and Intensive Care patients
Culture	Microorganisms grown under laboratory conditions
Decontamination	Free from any microorganism or substance that may harm health
Donor	A person who is the source of a body fluid in a needlestick injury
Empirical Antibiotics	Antibiotics that treat the most common causes of infection before the actual cause is known
Endemic	Present in the population all the time
Epidemic	An outbreak of an infectious disease that exceeds the normal background rate of that disease within a population
Erythema	Redness of the skin
Facultative Anaerobe	Grows in the presence or absence of oxygen
Flora	Bacteria living in a specific place
Fomite	An inanimate object capable of transferring microorganisms
Fungaemia	Presence of fungi in blood
Genotype	Classification of viruses based on their genetic material
Gram-negative	Staining red with Gram's method, cell membrane outside of a thin cell wall
Gram-positive	Staining purple with Gram's method, thick cell wall with no cell membrane
In vitro	In the laboratory, literally means "in glass"
Incident form	Method of recording adverse events in healthcare settings in order to monitor trends and implement corrective changes
Incubation period	Time from when exposed to a microorganism until the development of symptoms of infection
Lysing	Killing a cell by breaking the cellular membrane
Macules	Area of red skin <5mm diameter

Microaerophilic	Grows in the presence of oxygen at lower concentrations than in air
Mode of transmission	The process by which a microorganism transfers between people
Morbidity	Ill health
Mortality	Death
Necrosectomy	Surgical removal of dead tissue e.g. necrotic pancreas
Nephrotoxigenic	Bacteria produces toxins that damage the kidney
Nocté	At night / take at night
Non-blanching	Redness which does not disappear with pressure
Nucleic Acid	The main constituents of human genes
Opportunist	A microorganism causing infection which does not normally cause an infection
Out-of-hours	The time period of medical care when staffing levels are reduced, usually from 5pm-9am and at weekends
Pandemic	An outbreak of an infectious disease across a large geographical area, e.g. multiple continents
Papules	Raised area of skin <5mm diameter
Pathogen	A microorganism causing disease
Petechiae	Haemorrhage <3mm diameter
Piptazobactam	A Beta-lactam-Beta-lactamase inhibitor combination of Piperacillin + Tazobactam
Predisposing	Criteria that come before the acquisition of a disease
Prosthetic	An artificial device or material which replaces part of the human body
Purpura	Haemorrhage >3mm diameter
Purulent	The presence of white blood cells forming pus
Pyuria	The presence of white blood cells in urine
Recipient	A person who receives the body fluid in a needlestick injury
Seasonal	Occurring at a particular time of year
Sensitivity	A test's ability to identify positive results
Slough	Dead tissue overlying healthy tissue
Specificity	A test's ability to identify negative results
Spore	An asexual form of a microorganism, which is able to survive for prolonged periods in unfavourable conditions
Sterile	Free from any living microorganisms
Toxin	A poisonous substance produced in a microorganism
Transposon	A mobile genetic element
Turnaround time	The time taken from a laboratory receiving a sample to when the laboratory releases the result of any tests performed on that sample
Vacutainer	A glass tube containing a vacuum used to collect blood samples from patients
Vesicle	Small fluid-filled blister <5mm diameter
Vesico-ureteric Reflux	Abnormal movement of urine from the bladder into the ureters
Virulence	The ability of a microorganism to cause disease
Wild-type	The naturally occurring form of a microorganism
Zoonotic	Derived from animals

A simple method to systematically read chest X-rays:

A	Airways and lung fields
B	Bones
C	Cardiac outline and blood vessels
D	Diaphragm, air under the diaphragm, effusions etc.
E	Everything else. CVCs, pacemakers, stents and heart valves, sternal wires and surgical staples, ET tubes, NG tubes, ECG lines, piercings

Appendix 2 Bristol Stool Chart

Diarrhoea is stool loose enough to take the shape of the container (types 5-7 on the Bristol Stool Chart below:

Bristol Stool Chart

Type 1	Separate hard lumps, like nuts (hard to pass)
Type 2	Sausage-shaped but lumpy
Type 3	Like a sausage but with cracks on the surface
Type 4	Like a sausage or snake, smooth and soft
Type 5	Soft blobs with clear-cut edges
Type 6	Fluffy pieces with ragged edges, a mushy stool
Type 7	Watery, no solid pieces. **Entirely Liquid**

Old name	New name
Haemophilus aphrophilus	*Aggregatibacter aphrophilus*
Haemophilus paraphrophilus	*Aggregatibacter paraphrophilus*
Streptococcus milleri group	*Streptococcus anginosus* group
Propionibacterium spp.	*Cutibacterium* spp.
Clostridium difficile	*Clostridioides difficile*
Chlamydia pneumoniae	*Chlamydophila pneumoniae*
Chlamydia psittaci	*Chlamydophila psittaci*
Pneumocystis carinii	*Pneumocystis jirovecii*
Klebsiella ornithinolytica	*Raoultella ornithinolytica*
Enterobacter aerogenes	*Klebsiella aerogenes*
Streptococcus bovis biotype 1	*Streptococcus gallolyticus*
Streptococcus bovis biotype 2	*Streptococcus equinus* *Streptococcus infantarius* *Streptococcus pasteurianus* *Streptococcus lutetiensis*
Staphylococcus intermedius	*Staphylococcus pseudintermedius* *Staphylococcus delphini* *Staphylococcus intermedius*

New name	Old name
Aggregatibacter aphrophilus	*Haemophilus aphrophilus*
Aggregatibacter paraphrophilus	*Haemophilus paraphrophilus*
Streptococcus anginosus group	*Streptococcus* milleri group
Cutibacterium spp.	*Propionibacterium* spp.
Clostridioides difficile	*Clostridium difficile*
Chlamydophila pneumoniae	*Chlamydia pneumoniae*
Chlamydophila psittaci	*Chlamydia psittaci*
Pneumocystis jirovecii	*Pneumocystis carinii*
Raoultella ornithinolytica	*Klebsiella ornithinolytica*
Klebsiella aerogenes	*Enterobacter aerogenes*
Streptococcus gallolyticus	*Streptococcus bovis* biotype 1
Streptococcus equinus *Streptococcus infantarius* *Streptococcus pasteurianus* *Streptococcus lutetiensis*	*Streptococcus bovis* biotype 2
Staphylococcus pseudintermedius *Staphylococcus delphini* *Staphylococcus intermedius*	*Staphylococcus intermedius*

Zoonoses are infections where the infecting microorganism has been transmitted from an animal to a human. There are many different types of zoonoses but some of the more common or serious are shown in the table below:

Type of microorganism	Name	Infection	Animal
Bacteria	*Salmonella enteritidis*	Salmonella gastroenteritis	Poultry e.g. chickens, ducks, geese
	Salmonella bongori	Salmonella gastroenteritis	Reptiles
	Campylobacter spp.	Campylobacter gastroenteritis	Poultry e.g. chickens, ducks, geese
	Pasteurella multocida	CAP Septic arthritis Osteomyelitis Sepsis	Cats Dogs Komodo dragons
	Capnocytophaga canimorsus	Sepsis	Dogs
	Streptobacillus moniliformis	Rat bite fever	Rodents
	Bartonella henselae	Cat scratch fever	Cats
	Staphylococcus pseudintermedius	Skin, bone, joint or IV device infection	Dogs
Viruses	*Rabies Virus*	Rabies	Mammals Bats
	Ebola Virus	Ebola	Primates Bats
	SARS Coronavirus	Severe acute respiratory syndrome	Masked palm civets Horseshoe bats
	MERS Coronavirus	Middle-East respiratory syndrome	Camels
Fungi	*Histoplasma capsulatum*	Histoplasmosis	Bats
	Microsporidium canis	Dermatophytosis (fungal skin infection, ringworm)	Dogs
Parasites	*Toxocara cati*	Toxocariasis	Cats
	Toxocara canis	Toxocariasis	Dogs
	Toxoplasma gondii	Toxoplasmosis	Cats
	Giardia lamblia	Giardiasis (gastrointestinal infection)	Ruminants e.g. cows, sheep, goats
	Taenia saginata	Tapeworm	Cows

Index

A

Numbers & Notes

Sources of Information, Guidelines and Further Reading

- EUCAST Disk Diffusion Method for Antimicrobial Susceptibility Testing Version 6.0 January 2017
- British National Formulary (BNF) www.bnf.org
- British National Formulary for Children (cBNF)
- Mandell, Douglas, and Bennett's Principles and Practice of Infectious Diseases, 8th edition. Saunders, 2014
- The Renal Drug Handbook, 5th edition. Ashley C, Dunleavy A. CRC Press, 2018
- Control of Communicable Diseases Manual, 20th edition. Heymann D. American Public Health Association, 2014
- Immunisation Against Infectious Disease, Salisbury D, Ramsay M. Department of Health, 2006
- The Flesh and Bones of Medical Microbiology. Guyot A, Schelenz S, Myint S, Mosby, 2010

There is no single library where all national guidelines are kept. Guidelines are often set by professional associations and experts in their clinical fields. The following are those considered important for microbiology purposes. The website www.microbiologynutsandbolts.co.uk will be up-dated with new guidelines as they become available.

Infection Control Guidelines
- *Clostridium difficile* infection objectives for NHS organisations in 2014/2015 and guidance on sanction implementation. NHS England 2014
- Updated guidance on the management and treatment of *Clostridium difficile* infection. Public Health England 2013
- Updated guidance on the diagnosis and reporting of *Clostridium difficile*. Department of Health UK 2012
- Acute trust toolkit for the early detection, management and control of carbapenemase-producing Enterobacteriaceae. Public Health England 2013
- UK guideline for the use of Post-Exposure Prophylaxis for HIV following sexual exposure (2011). British Association for Sexual Health and HIV (BASHH), International Journal of STD & AIDS 2011; 22: 695-708
- HIV Post-Exposure Prophylaxis: Guidance from the UK Chief Medical Officers' Expert Advisory Group on AIDS. Department of Health 2008
- Management of Hazard Group 4 viral haemorrhagic fevers and similar human infectious diseases of high consequence. Advisory Committee on Dangerous Pathogens, Department of Health UK. 2015

Antibiotic Guidelines
- Antibiotic duration and timing of the switch from intravenous to oral route for bacterial infections in children: systematic review and guidelines. McMullan B, Andresen D, Blyth C, *et al*. The Lancet Infectious Diseases 2016; 16: e139-152

Clinical Scenarios & Emergencies Guidelines
- Guidelines for the management of community acquired pneumonia in adults: update 2009. British Thoracic Society, Thorax, Oct 2009, Vol. 64; Supplement III
- Pneumonia in adults: diagnosis and management, clinical guideline 191. National Institute for Health and Care Excellence 2014
- Guidelines for the management of hospital-acquired pneumonia in the UK: report of the Working Party on Hospital-Acquired Pneumonia of the British Society for Antimicrobial Chemotherapy. Journal of Antimicrobial Chemotherapy 2008; 62: 5-34
- Clinical diagnosis and management of tuberculosis, and measures for its prevention and control: clinical guideline 117. National Institute for Health and Care Excellence 2011
- UK National Guideline for the Management of Pelvic Inflammatory Disease 2001. British Association for Sexual Health and HIV (BASHH)
- UK national guideline for the management of gonorrhoea in adults, 2011. British Association for Sexual Health and HIV (BASHH), International Journal of STD & AIDS 2011; 22: 541-547

- 2006 UK National Guideline for the Management of Genital Tract Infection with *Chlamydia trachomatis*. British Association for Sexual Health and HIV (BASHH)
- UK national guidelines on the management of syphilis 2015. International Journal of STD & AIDS 2015; 27: 421-446
- Diagnosis and Management of Prosthetic Joint Infection: Clinical Practice Guidelines by the Infectious Diseases Society of America, Osmon D, Berbari E, Berendt A *et al*. Clinical Infectious Diseases 2013; 56: 1-25
- 2012 Infectious Diseases Society of America Clinical Practice Guideline for the Diagnosis and Treatment of Diabetic Foot Infections. Lipsky B, Berendt A, Cornia P *et al*. Clinical Infectious Diseases 2012; 54: 132-173
- Guidelines for the diagnosis and antibiotic treatment of endocarditis in adults: a report of the Working Party of the British Society for Antimicrobial Chemotherapy. Gould F, Denning D, Elliott T, *et al*. Journal of Antimicrobial Chemotherapy 2012; 67: 269-289
- Fever in returned travellers presenting in the United Kingdom: Recommendations for investigation and initial management. Johnston V, Stockley J, Dockrell D, *et al*. Journal of Infection 2009; 59: 1-18
- UK malaria treatment guidelines. Lalloo D, Shingadia D, Bell D, *et al*. Journal of Infection 2016; 72: 635-649
- Surviving Sepsis Campaign: International guidelines for the management of severe sepsis and septic shock: 2016. Rhodes A, Evans L, Alhazzani W, *et al*. Critical Care Medicine 2017; 45 (3): 486-552
- Antibiotics for early-onset neonatal infection: clinical guideline 149. National Institute for Health and Care Excellence 2012
- Sexually transmitted infections in primary care 2nd edition. Royal College of General Practitioners (RCGP), British Association for Sexual Health and HIV (BASHH), 2013
- British HIV Association and British Infection Association guidelines for the treatment of opportunistic infection in HIV-seropositive individuals 2011. British HIV Association (BHIVA)
- National Early Warning Score (NEWS) Standardising the assessment of acute-illness severity in the NHS, Royal College of Physicians 2012
- The UK joint specialist society's guideline on the diagnosis and management of acute meningitis and meningococcal sepsis in immunocompetent adults. McGill F, Heyderman R, Michael B, *et al*. Journal of Infection 2016; 72: 405-438
- Lyme disease, NICE guideline 95. National Institute for Health and Care Excellence 11th April 2018
- American College of Gastroenterology Guideline: Management of Acute Pancreatitis. Tenner S, Baillie J, DeWitt J, *et al*. Am J Gastro July 2013

Useful websites

- Infectious Diseases Society of America, www.idsociety.org
- British Society for Antimicrobial Chemotherapy, www.bsac.org.uk
- The Hospital Infection Society, www.his.org.uk
- British Infection Association www.britishinfection.org
- Learn Infection (British Infection Association) www.learninfection.org.uk
- Surviving Sepsis Campaign www.survivingsepsis.org
- Meningitis Research Foundation www.meningitis.org
- National Institute for Health and Care Excellence www.nice.org.uk

Commonly Used 1st Line Antibiotics

The list below is not exhaustive and may be used when there is no access to local guidelines. See sections – Antibiotics, Adult Empirical Antibiotic Guidelines for 2nd line antibiotics and Paediatrics Guidelines for children.

Infections	1st Line Antibiotic
Community Acquired Pneumonia (CAP) (CURB-65 score 0-2)	PO Amoxicillin 500mg-1g TDS **PLUS** PO Clarithromycin 500mg BD (If Nil By Mouth use IV)
Community Acquired Pneumonia (CAP) (CURB-65 score 3-5)	IV Co-amoxiclav 1.2g TDS **PLUS** IV Clarithromycin 500mg BD If MRSA **ADD** IV Teicoplanin 400mg BD for 3 doses **THEN** OD (or 6mg/kg if >70kg)
Hospital Acquired Pneumonia (HAP) Onset 2-4 days after admission	IV Co-amoxiclav 1.2g TDS If MRSA **ADD** IV Teicoplanin 400mg BD for 3 doses **THEN** OD (or 6mg/kg if >70kg)
Hospital Acquired Pneumonia (HAP) Onset ≥4 days after admission	IV Piptazobactam 4.5g TDS If MRSA **ADD** IV Teicoplanin 400mg BD for 3 doses **THEN** OD (or 6mg/kg if >70kg)
Infective Exacerbation of	PO Amoxicillin 500mg TDS
Pyelonephritis	IV Co-amoxiclav 1.2g TDS **PLUS** IV Gentamicin as per renal function
Cellulitis	IV Flucloxacillin 1-2g QDS
Cellulitis (if MRSA positive)	IV Teicoplanin 400mg BD for 3 doses **THEN** OD (or 6mg/kg if >70kg)
Osteomyelitis or Septic Arthritis	IV Flucloxacillin 1-2g QDS **PLUS** PO Fusidic Acid 500mg TDS
Osteomyelitis* or Septic Arthritis* (*if MRSA positive)	IV Teicoplanin 12mg/kg BD for 3 doses **THEN** OD **PLUS** PO Fusidic Acid 500mg TDS
Clostridium difficile Associated Disease	PO Metronidazole 400mg TDS
Emergencies	
Sepsis	IV Piptazobactam 4.5g QDS **PLUS** IV Gentamicin as per renal function If MRSA **ADD** IV Teicoplanin 400mg BD for 5 doses **THEN** OD (or 6mg/kg if >70kg)
Meningitis	IV Cefotaxime 2g QDS **OR** IV Ceftriaxone 2g BD
Meningitis (if Listeria suspected)	IV Cefotaxime 2g QDS **OR** IV Ceftriaxone 2g BD **PLUS** IV Amoxicillin 2g 4 hourly

First Hour of Surviving Sepsis – "The Golden Hour"

Call for senior support immediately
+/- Critical Care

Give high flow O$_2$
Aim for SaO$_2$ >94%
(88-92% if risk of CO$_2$ retention)

Fluid resuscitate
If hypotensive or lactate >2mmol/L

Target
Systolic blood pressure >90mmHg
MABP ≥65mmHg
Lactate <2mmol/L

Administer
500ml stat **OR** 30ml/kg IV crystalloid to run
over 3 hours

Monitor
Lactate
Urine output

Blood Cultures
Take 2 sets of blood cultures
(at least 1 set peripherally)

DO NOT unnecessarily delay antibiotics

Antibiotics
Give antibiotics within 1hour of diagnosing
sepsis

Warning
Delaying antibiotics in the first 6 hours
increases mortality

Evaluate for focus of infection
Implement source control if possible e.g.
drainage of abscess

Further Treatment
Treat as per the management plan from
seniors or critical care or

Useful Telephone Numbers

FY1/HO/Intern	
FY2/SHO/Resident	
Registrar/StR/Fellow	
Consultant	
Outreach Team	
Critical Care/ITU	
Microbiology Lab	
Biochemistry Lab	
Haematology Lab	
Transfusion	
Radiology	
Pharmacy	

Please feel free to alert me to items you feel this book misses and that are needed via www.microbiologynutsandbolts.co.uk. They will be considered for future editions.